POLYMER APPLICATIONS IN MEDICINE

Revolutionizing Treatment and Therapeutics

POLYMER APPLICATIONS IN MEDICINE

Revolutionizing Treatment and Therapeutics

Mohd. Imran Ahamed

Faheem Ahmad

Ishaat M. Khan

Editors

APPLE ACADEMIC PRESS

First edition published 2026

Apple Academic Press Inc.
1265 Goldenrod Circle, NE,
Palm Bay, FL 32905 USA

760 Laurentian Drive, Unit 19,
Burlington, ON L7N 0A4, Canada

CRC Press
2385 NW Executive Center Drive,
Suite 320, Boca Raton FL 33431

4 Park Square, Milton Park,
Abingdon, Oxon, OX14 4RN, UK

Library and Archives Canada Cataloguing in Publication

CIP data on file with Canada Library and Archives

Library of Congress Cataloging-in-Publication Data

CIP data on file with US Library of Congress

ISBN: 978-1-77964-086-4 (hbk)
ISBN: 978-1-77964-087-1 (ebk)
DOI: 10.1201/9781779640871

About the Editors

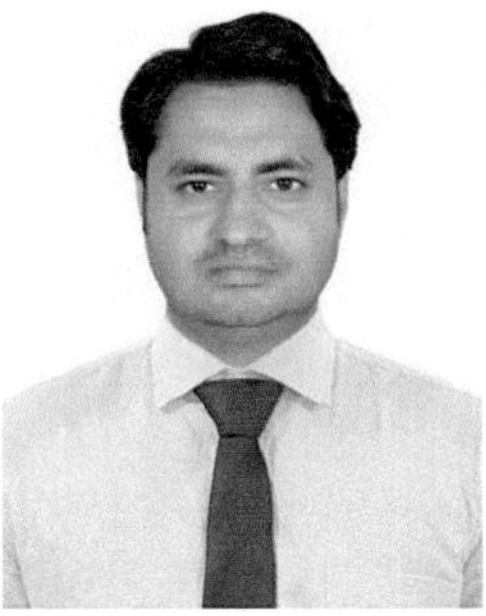

Mohd. Imran Ahamed, PhD
Department of Chemistry, Faculty of Science, Aligarh Muslim University, Aligarh, Uttar Pradesh, India

Mohd. Imran Ahamed, PhD, is a distinguished Research Associate at the Department of Chemistry, Aligarh Muslim University, India, specializing in materials science and sustainable chemistry. He obtained his doctoral degree in 2019, focusing on the synthesis and characterization of inorganic–organic composites as heavy metal–selective cation-exchangers. Dr. Ahamed's expertise is evident from his impressive h-index of 20 and a citation score of 1600. He has published over fifteen research articles in international journals and contributed seventeen book chapters to renowned publishers. With a passion for disseminating knowledge, he has also edited over forty books. Dr. Ahamed's dedication to academia is further demonstrated through his affiliations with editorial boards of prestigious academic journals, establishing him as a distinguished and influential figure in chemistry.

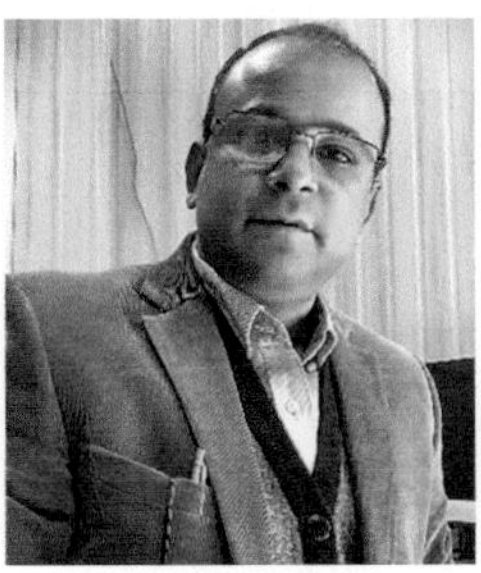

Faheem Ahmad, PhD
Department of Botany, Faculty of Life Sciences, Aligarh Muslim University, Aligarh, Uttar Pradesh, India

Faheem Ahmad, PhD, is a Senior Assistant Professor at the Department of Botany, Aligarh Muslim University, India. He obtained his doctoral degree in 2009. He also worked as a Postdoctoral Research Associate at Ehime University, Japan. Before that, he was a Postdoctoral Fellow at North-West University, Mafikeng Campus (South Africa), and at National Sun Yat-Sen University, Kaohsiung (Taiwan).

At present, Dr. Ahmad is involved in both teaching and research. He has published more than 50 peer-reviewed research papers.

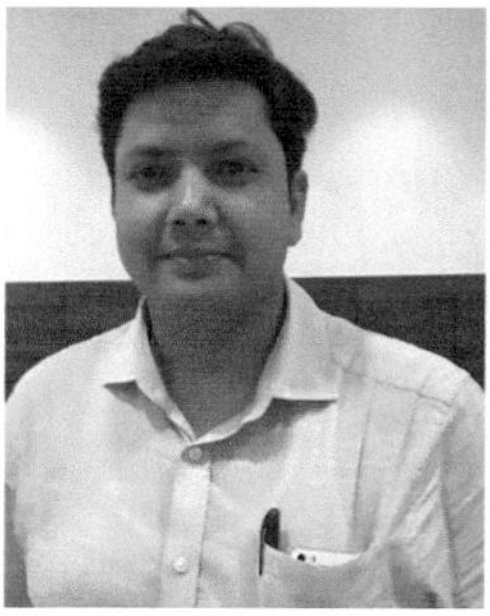

Ishaat M. Khan, PhD
Department of Chemistry, Faculty of Science, Aligarh Muslim University, Aligarh, Uttar Pradesh, India

Ishaat M. Khan, PhD, is an Associate Professor at the Department of Chemistry, Aligarh Muslim University, India. With a strong academic background, he completed his bachelor's degree (with honors) and master's degree in physical chemistry from the same institution. In 2009, Dr. Khan earned his PhD, specializing in designing, spectral investigations, and crystallographic studies of novel CT complexes. Alongside his research, he passionately imparts knowledge as a dedicated teacher of physical chemistry to undergraduate and postgraduate students at Aligarh Muslim University. Dr. Khan's expertise in his field and his commitment to education have established him as a respected figure in the realm of chemistry.

Contents

Contributors

Nisat Alam
Department of Biochemistry, School of Chemical and Life Sciences, Jamia Hamdard, New Delhi, India

Arshi Amin
Department of Chemistry, Noida International University, Greater Noida, Uttar Pradesh, India

Aparajita Banerjee
Department of Zoology, Changu Kana Arts, Commerce and Science College, New Panvel, Raigad, Maharashtra, India

Aditya Dam
Department of Applied Chemistry, Delhi Technological University, New Delhi, Delhi, India

Sonalee Das
Central Institute of Petrochemicals Engineering & Technology (CIPET)-IPT Lucknow, Amausi Indl. Area, Lucknow

S. Brindha Devi
Division of Physics, School of Advanced Sciences, Vellore Institute of Technology (VIT), Chennai, Tamil Nadu, India

Md. Wamique Hossain
School of Biotechnology, Jawaharlal Nehru University, New Delhi, India

Iram
Department of Chemistry, DSB Campus, Kumaun University, Nainital, Uttarakhand, India

Maidul Islam
Department of Chemistry, Faculty of Science, Aligarh Muslim University, Aligarh, Uttar Pradesh, India

Mohammad S. Javed
Department of Chemistry, DSB Campus, Kumaun University, Nainital, Uttarakhand, India

M. S. Kamali
Department of Biotechnology, Kalaignarkarunanidhi Institute of Technology (KIT), Coimbatore, Tamil Nadu, India

Arif Khan
Department of Chemistry, School of Chemical and Life Sciences (SCLS), Jamia Hamdard, New Delhi, India

Ishaat M. Khan
Department of Chemistry, Faculty of Science, Aligarh Muslim University, Aligarh, Uttar Pradesh, India

Mohd. Arham Khan
Interdisciplinary Nanotechnology Centre, Faculty of Engineering and Technology, Aligarh Muslim University, Aligarh, Uttar Pradesh, India

Mohd. Farhan Khan
Department of Science, Gagan College of Management and Technology, Aligarh, Uttar Pradesh, India

Rafi Ullah Khan
Institute of Polymer and Textile Engineering, University of the Punjab, Lahore, Pakistan

K. Kowsuki
Division of Physics, School of Advanced Sciences, Vellore Institute of Technology (VIT), Chennai, Tamil Nadu, India

Christian Lunetta
NeMO Lab, ASST Niguarda Cà Granda Hospital, Milan, Italy; NEuroMuscular Omnicenter (NEMO), Fondazione Serena Onlus, Milan, Italy

Hasina Najnin
Department of Biochemistry, School of Chemical and Life Sciences, Jamia Hamdard, New Delhi, India

R. Navamathavan
Division of Physics, School of Advanced Sciences, Vellore Institute of Technology (VIT), Chennai, Tamil Nadu, India

R. Nirmala
Department of Biotechnology, Hindustan College of Arts and Science, affiliated to University of Madras, Padur, Chennai, Tamil Nadu, India

Raffaele Pugliese
NeMO Lab, ASST Niguarda Cà Granda Hospital, Milan, Italy

M. Ramesh
Department of Mechanical Engineering, Mahendra Engineering College, Mallasamudram, Namakkal, Tamil Nadu, India

Stefano Regondi
NeMO Lab, ASST Niguarda Cà Granda Hospital, Milan, Italy; NEuroMuscular Omnicenter (NEMO), Fondazione Serena Onlus, Milan, Italy

Aneela Sabir
Institute of Polymer and Textile Engineering, University of the Punjab, Lahore, Pakistan

K. Sakthishobana
Department of Biotechnology, Bannari Amman Institute of Technology, Sathyamangalam, Tamil Nadu, India

Riccardo Sala
NeMO Lab, ASST Niguarda Cà Granda Hospital, Milan, Italy

Shabnam
School of Biotechnology, Jawaharlal Nehru University, New Delhi, India

Muhammad Shafiq
Institute of Polymer and Textile Engineering, University of the Punjab, Lahore, Pakistan

Sonam Shakya
Department of Chemistry, Faculty of Science, Aligarh Muslim University, Aligarh, Uttar Pradesh, India

Habiba Sultana
Department of Chemistry, Vidyasagar University, Midnapore, West Bengal, India

Maria Wasim
Institute of Polymer and Textile Engineering, University of the Punjab, Lahore, Pakistan

Rana Zaidi
Department of Biochemistry, School of Chemical and Life Sciences, Jamia Hamdard, New Delhi, India

Abbreviations

AM	additive manufacturing
ART	Artenisimin
BNC	bio-nanocomposite
CA	camphoric acid
CID	chronic inflammatory disease
CT	chemotherapy
DDS	drug delivery system
EPR	enhanced permeability and retention
FDM	fused deposition modeling
HA	hyaluronic acid
HAS	human serum albumin
ICG	indocianine green
MDR	multidrug resistance
MRI	magnetic resonance imaging
MSN	mesoporous silica nanoparticle
NCD	non-communicable disease
PAH	polyanhydride
PC	polymer conjugate
PCL	polycaprolactone
PDC	polymer-drug conjugate
PEG	polyethylene glycol
PES	polyethersulfone
PGA	poly glycolic acid
PHB	poly hydroxybutyrate
PLA	polylactic acid
PLGA	poly lactic-co-glycolic acid
PMC	polymer matrix composite
PMMA	polymethylmethacrylate
PPE	personal protective equipment
PTT	particularly photothermal therapy
PUR	polyester/ether urethane
PVA	polyvinyl alcohol
ROS	reactive oxygen species
SLA	stereolithography
SLS	selective laser sintering
SP	supramolecular polymer

TME	tumor microenvironment
TNF	tumor necrosis factor
WHO	World Health Organization

Preface

The field of medicine has witnessed remarkable advancements in recent years, driven by the application of polymers in various aspects of health-care. Polymers, with their diverse properties and versatile nature, have revolutionized the development of novel therapies, drug delivery systems, diagnostic tools, and medical devices. This volume, *Polymer Applications in Medicine: Revolutionizing Treatment and Therapeutics,* explores the profound impact of polymers in the medical field and delves into the multidisciplinary aspects of their utilization.

This book encompasses a wide range of topics, each shedding light on different areas where polymers have made significant contributions. The chapters cover diverse subjects, including the role of polymers in inflammatory disease therapy, 3D-printed polymers for medical applications, biodegradable polymers in drug delivery, supramolecular polymers in drug delivery and biomedical applications, polymers and their nanocomposites in cancer therapy, polymer-based nanocomposites in clinical diagnosis, polymers in tissue engineering, and the role of polymers in combating the COVID-19 pandemic. Each chapter provides a comprehensive overview of the topic, highlighting recent advancements, challenges, and future prospects.

The chapters on polymers in inflammatory disease therapy discuss the tailored formulations of polymers and their ability to address the complex nature of inflamed tissues. The utilization of 3D-printed polymers in medicine showcases the potential of this emerging technology in manufacturing patient-specific medical devices, tissue engineering scaffolds, and drug delivery systems. The exploration of biodegradable polymers used in drug delivery elucidates the compatibility and degradable nature of these materials, along with their clinical applicability. Supramolecular polymers and their applications in drug delivery and tissue engineering offer new possibilities for controlled release systems and complex tissue regeneration. The chapters on polymers and their nanocomposites in cancer therapy emphasize the challenges in drug delivery and the potential of polymer-based systems to overcome these obstacles. Polymer-based nano-composites in clinical diagnosis provide insights into the fabrication and application of polymer nanocomposites for diagnostic purposes. The use of polymers in tissue engineering elucidates the role of these materials in creating functional biological structures for various medical applications. Finally, the chapter on polymer chemistry in relation to the COVID-19 pandemic demonstrates how polymers and additive manufacturing technologies have played a crucial role in addressing the shortage of medical supplies during this global crisis.

Each chapter of this book is written by experts in their respective fields, presenting a wealth of knowledge and cutting-edge research. The book aims to serve as a valuable resource for researchers, scientists, clinicians, and students interested in the applications of polymers in medicine. It provides a comprehensive overview of the advancements, challenges, and potential future directions in this rapidly evolving field.

We hope that this book serves as a valuable resource for researchers, students, and professionals seeking a deeper understanding of the diverse and significant role of polymers in medicine. It is our sincere belief that the knowledge shared in this book will inspire further research, innovation, and advancements in this exciting field.

—Editors

CHAPTER 1

Polymers in Inflammatory Diseases

IRAM,[1] ARIF KHAN,[2,*] and MOHAMMAD S. JAVED[1]

[1]*Department of Chemistry, DSB Campus, Kumaun University, Nainital, Uttarakhand, India*

[2]*Department of Chemistry, School of Chemical and Life Sciences (SCLS), Jamia Hamdard, New Delhi, India*

*Corresponding author

ABSTRACT

Various types of polymers with tailored formulations, such as desirable molecular weight, crosslinking degree, blends, and bioactive surface functionalization, agree with an extensive range of biological applications. Wide research in recent years has led to the advancement of diverse inflammatory disease therapies. Polymers and nano-polymers exhibit the ability to carry out inflammatory activities, supported by multiple clinical trials with cost-effectiveness. Pathologically inflamed tissues are characterized by lower pH (~6.4), 10–1000 times higher reactive oxygen species (ROS), matrix remodeling enzymes, and the evolution of inflammation-sensitive polymers based on skin surface inflammation. A more advanced property of polymers is biodegradation, which is increasing in number of fields, from suture materials, and they may disappear after they have fulfilled their function and defined triggers with controlled drug release.

Polymer Applications in Medicine: Revolutionizing Treatment and Therapeutics.
Mohd. Imran Ahamed, Faheem Ahmad, and Ishaat M. Khan (Eds.)

DOI: 10.1201/9781779640871-1

1.1 INTRODUCTION

1.1.1 WHAT IS POLYMER?

In the current scenario, there's an exaggerated consumption and accumulation of polymer-derived urban waste that has drawn the attention of many fields, particularly that of organized social groups. By means of mobilization and empowerment, the environment has become more confined towards the use and removal of polymeric materials [1]. Polymeric materials are commonly used in a number of fields, such as auto electronics, stationery, civil engineering, pharmaceuticals, therapeutics, self-healing materials, and so forth [2]. To improve the therapeutic potential of drugs and low molecular weight proteins, the development of polymeric therapies has become an exciting area of research [3]. Polymers have attracted the attention of therapeutic delivery researchers all over the world. The 20th century saw recent strides in polymer synthesis. Nowadays, polymers are widely used in the drug industry; they are used to treat several diseases caused by inflammation [4]. In the past two decades, polymer drug delivery systems (DDS) have made great strides. It is defined as the technology that enables a pharmacotherapy component to be introduced into the body. Biodegradable and bio-reducible polymers are excellent choices for a variety of new DDS [5]. They show an immense contribution to the drug delivery system. It has been observed that these polymers improve medication pharmacokinetics and reduce side effects [6]. Biodegradable polymers have many applications in medicine and pharmacy due to their ability to reduce inflammatory reactions, be nontoxic, and be degraded by enzymes in the body [7]. Various strategies are used to advance biomedical applications of polymer drugs, including chemically attaching drugs to polymer scaffolds, generating polymers directly from polymerizable drugs, and using polymers to bind and remove toxic compounds. Polymeric drugs in this category are in or near clinical application [8]. Newly discovered polymers are constantly being developed for new medicinal applications. At the same time, new and modified polymeric chemicals that provide unique drug degradation and delivery are being recognized and analyzed [6]. Future research prospects for practical applications require development in this field.

1.1.2 CLASSIFICATION OF POLYMER

In addition, there are several polymers with different behaviors that can be found naturally or synthetically, and as indicated in the chart (Figure

1.1), they can be categorized in a variety of ways. Polymers are grouped according to their structure. They may have a carbon chain backbone or a heterocyclic backbone. Another basis of classification is based on origin; they can be natural polymers or synthetic polymers. They are also called biodegradable polymers.

1.1.2.1 BIODEGRADABLE POLYMER

Recently, the use of biodegradable polymers has increased. Biodegradable polymers are becoming increasingly essential in a wide range of applications, including medical implants, DDS, as well as disposable packaging and consumer plastics [9]. Biodegradation is the chemical breakdown of a material in a physiological environment by enzymes or hydrolysis. It is classified into two types based on the source: synthetic polymers and natural polymers [10].

1. **Natural Polymers:** These are those produced by organic systems such as microbes, plants, and animals. Plant-derived polymers are used in pharmaceutical formulations to make solid monolithic matrix systems, implants, films, beads, microparticles, nanoparticles, and viscous liquid formulations. They are used in the biomedical field due to their intrinsic properties such as biodegradability, biocompatibility, and non-toxicity. Examples include collagen, keratin, albumin, chitosan, dextrin, polysaccharides, poly(glycolic acid), poly(lactic acid), hyaluronic acid, and so forth [5, 11, 12].

2. **Synthetic Polymers:** These are chemical substances that are manufactured in large quantities and are made up of a number of molecules that are joined together by covalent bonds. For patients who are allergic to natural polymers, synthetic polymers are the best substitutes. Synthetic polymers are less immunogenic than natural polymers and do not cause chronic immunogenic inflammation, such as polyester, polyanhydrides, polyamides, polyglycolic acid, polylactic acid (PLA), polyvinyl alcohol (PVA), polycaprolactone (PCL), and polylactic-co-glycolic acid (PLGA) [11, 13].

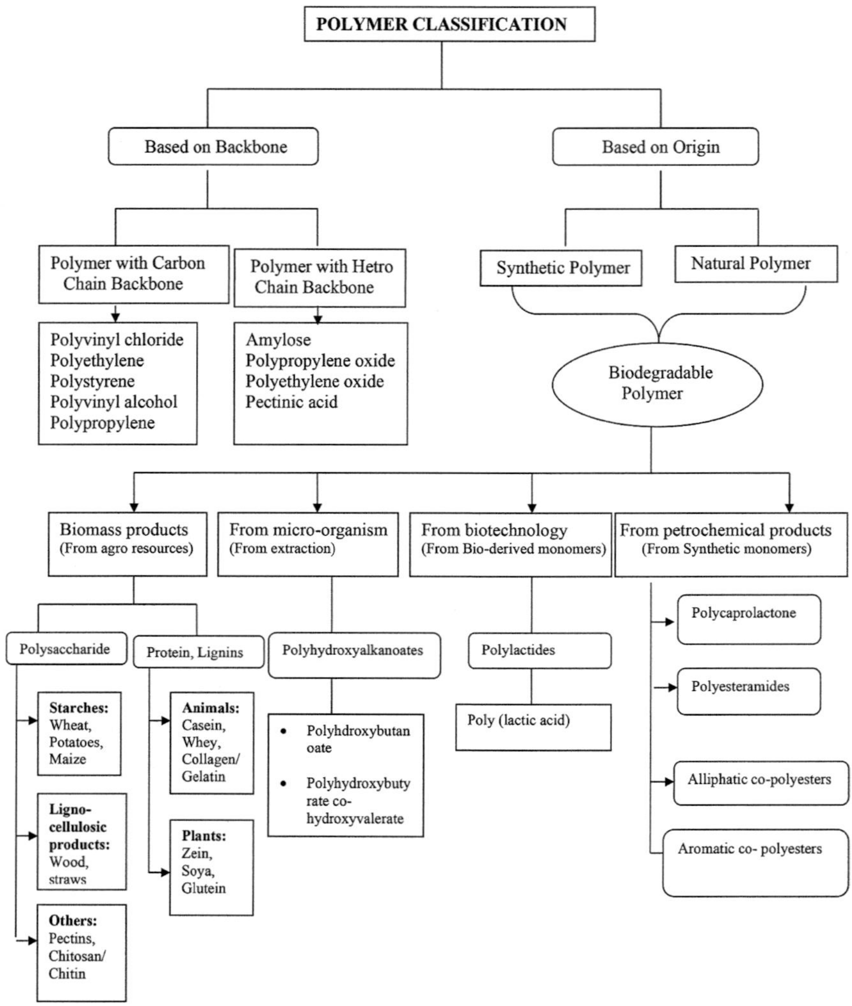

FIGURE 1.1 Classification of polymers.

1.2 INFLAMMATORY DISEASES

World Health Organization (WHO) reports that more than 235 million people suffer from chronic, acute, and other inflammatory diseases worldwide. Inflammation is an innate immune response to unfavorable stimuli such as noxious stimuli, damaged cells, irritants, and microorganisms. It is a biological mechanism that not only eliminates the cause of tissue damage but also helps in healing the damaged tissue [14]. It is a requisite defensive measure in all life forms. Chronic inflammation, on the other hand, can result in severe pathological processes and eventually lead to various chronic inflammatory diseases (CIDs), such as rheumatoid arthritis, multiple sclerosis, or certain types of cancer [4]. Chronic inflammation caused by long-term stress, such as infection, physiological stress, and malnutrition, activates immune cells to reorganize tissues and plays a critical role in the treatment of inflammatory disorders [15]. Inflammation begins as soon as pathogens and damaged tissue are recognized by innate immune cells that activate signaling pathways that produce pro-inflammatory effectors such as cytokines, chemokines, and proteinoids [16]. COVID-19 infection, which has been linked to a significant cytokine storm and uncontrolled systemic inflammation, resulting in acute respiratory distress in some cases, is an example of such a severe reaction [17].

1.2.1 TYPES OF INFLAMMATION

Inflammation is a complicated physiological process characterized by five distinct symptoms: pain, redness, swelling, heat, and functional loss. Inflammatory processes are usually characterized as either acute or chronic inflammation (Figure 1.2).

1. **Acute Inflammation:** It occurs rapidly at the site of the body's direct injury and lasts for a short period of time, usually 2–5 days. There are typical causes of acute inflammation, such as pathogens, allergens, toxins, burns, and frostbite. It generally occurs after a skin injury or wound, a sprained ankle, or a sore throat caused by bacterial infection. During acute inflammation, the blood vessels in the affected area dilate, blood flow increases, and white blood cells cover the injured area to promote healing [18].

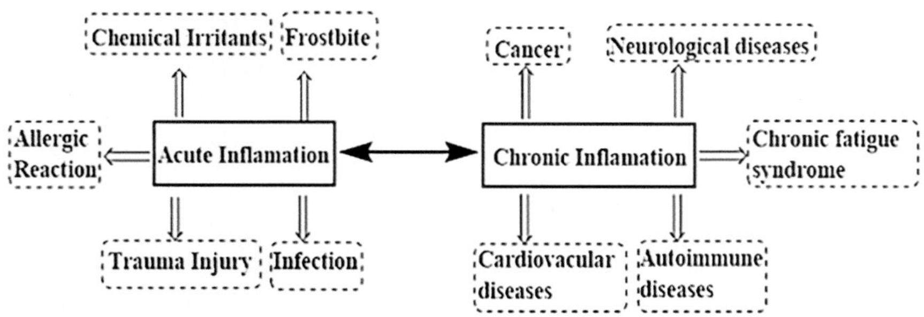

FIGURE 1.2 Classification of inflammation.

2. **Chronic Inflammation:** It is a long-term response; it is usually a mild, persistent form of inflammation that can last for months or even years. It represents a progressive inflammatory response that can eventually lead to irreversible changes, such as fibrosis, due to extensive local synthesis of collagen, connective tissue matrix proteins, and so forth [19].

1.2.2 CAUSES OF INFLAMMATION

The main cause of inflammation is pure mechanical pressure, which includes blunt trauma, foreign bodies, vibrations, and low-intensity chronic pressure. The primary mechanism by which pressure causes inflammation is most likely tissue hypoxia [20]. The most common causes of inflammation are pathogens such as viruses, bacteria, or fungi, as well as chemicals or radiation that affect the lungs or body.

1.3 POLYMER CONJUGATES

Polymer conjugates (PCs), also called polymeric prodrugs, are high molecular weight (HMW) conjugates, which typically contain several molecules of low molecular weight drugs or combinations thereof linked to a polymeric backbone and are designed to optimize pharmacokinetics (Figure 1.3) [4]. Polymer-Drug Conjugates (PDCs) show clinical and commercial success in drug delivery [21]. Polymer conjugation is used to overcome the constraints of previously found low-molecular-weight medicines with promising therapeutic potential in a variety of major human diseases [22].

1.3.1 INFLAMMATORY TREATMENT VIA POLYMER–DRUG CONJUGATES

Conjugation is a concept that has been widely applied in the context of inflammation and other related diseases. It is used as PDCs in inflammation due to the pathophysiological resemblance between inflamed tissue and cancer [23]. Clinical benefit has been exemplified with PCs holding conventional cancer therapy agents. Cancer therapy involves the inhibition of specific kinases, apoptotic pathways, and angiogenesis. Polymer–drug conjugates have fascinating and prospective uses in the treatment of diabetes, hypertension, infections, digestive tract illnesses, and inflammation, as well as new potential applications in regenerative medicine. To develop effective therapies that can enable patients to recover or at least significantly improve patient quality, an understanding of the molecular basis associated with age-related diseases, combination therapies, PC design, and multidisciplinary research must be considered [4, 22, 24]. In recent years, their application has been greatly expanded because polymer drug conjugates are growing exponentially as macromolecular pro-drugs that have discovered anticancer and anti-inflammatory agents. Providing new anti-cancer agents, combination therapies, treatments for non-cancer diseases, and new polymer structures are exciting and promising areas. Some of these new approaches are expected to reach clinical evaluation in the next decade [25].

1.4 POLYMERIC NANOPARTICLES

Polymers can be easily customized and synthesized, making them versatile building blocks for NP design. Their physicochemical properties can be easily altered, which enables the development of self-assembled and individualized therapeutic NPs via controlled release [26]. Polymer nanoparticles (NPs) have received a great deal of attention in recent years due to their small size, ranging from 1 to 1000 nm. They can be encapsulated in polymer cores or filled with active substances adsorbed on the surface. They are gaining popularity because of their biocompatibility, biodegradability, and versatility, and offer a wide range of materials that can have the properties required for specific applications [27]. The term "nanoparticle" includes both nano-capsules and nanospheres in different morphologies. Nano-capsules consist of an oily core in which the drug is normally dissolved and are surrounded by a polymer shell that controls the release profile of the drug from the core. Nanospheres are based on a continuous polymer network that allows the active drug to be retained internally or adsorbed on the surface (Figure 1.3) [28]. They have shown great potential in targeted drug delivery to treat a number of diseases. There are numerous reports of 'smart' nanoparticles that respond rapidly and selectively to various specific pathogenic stimuli; however, there is a shortage of nanoparticles capable of specifically targeting inflammation [29]. The use of NPs in the treatment of autoimmune and inflammatory diseases provides innovative solutions to improve the effectiveness of current immunosuppressive therapies and overcome the side effects associated with such therapies. Some experimental examples show that NP-based drug delivery is more effective in treating autoimmune and inflammatory diseases compared to current therapies [30]. Non-steroidal anti-inflammatory drugs (NSAIDs) such as diclofenac, celecoxib, ibuprofen, aspirin, and many other substances are used to prevent and treat cancer to control the inflammatory component of the disease [31]. Nanomedicine-based polymers, an area concerned with the use of polymer NPs, polymeric micelles, polyplexes, polymer-lipid hybrid systems, and PDCs to improve therapeutic efficacy in cancer, have been widely explored. In both preclinical and clinical research stages, polymer-based nano-carriers show excellent therapeutic effects [32].

1.4.1 ADVANTAGES OF POLYMERIC NANOPARTICLES

- They are more efficient and effective than conventional oral and intravenous delivery methods.
- They deliver higher concentrations of drugs to the desired location.
- The choice of polymers and their ability to alter drug release from polymer nanoparticles make them ideal candidates for cancer treatment, vaccine delivery, contraceptives, and targeted antibiotic delivery.
- Polymeric nanoparticles can easily be integrated into other drug delivery processes.
- Nanomedicines have been found to increase the solubility and toxicity of low-soluble pharmaceuticals by dissolving them in their hydrophobic or hydrophilic compartments [28, 33].

1.4.2 LIMITATION OF POLYMERIC NANOPARTICLES

Despite their advantages and enormous potential, several disadvantages can be found in their use due to their extensively distributed agglomerate state with limited morphology, chemical composition, size, and electro-magnetic properties, including oral bioavailability, circulatory instability, and inadequate distribution [34]. Nanoparticle size, polydispersity, and charges depend on measurement technique and hydration state. There is a heterogeneous population of nanoparticles within a particular sample. Nanoparticle assembly and degradation is a dynamic process that changes during storage, blood circulation, and tissue and cell distribution. Changing one of the properties of nanoparticles (such as size) affects the other properties. Premature release of bound fluorophore: stability of links used to mark nanoparticles in blood and tissues. Impure fluorophore results in monitoring two populations (free and conjugated dyes) [35]. A polymeric nanoparticle as a universal nanocarrier has a wide range of therapeutic biomedical applications. Easy control of shape, charge, size, structure, geometry, and composition ensures future development and success.

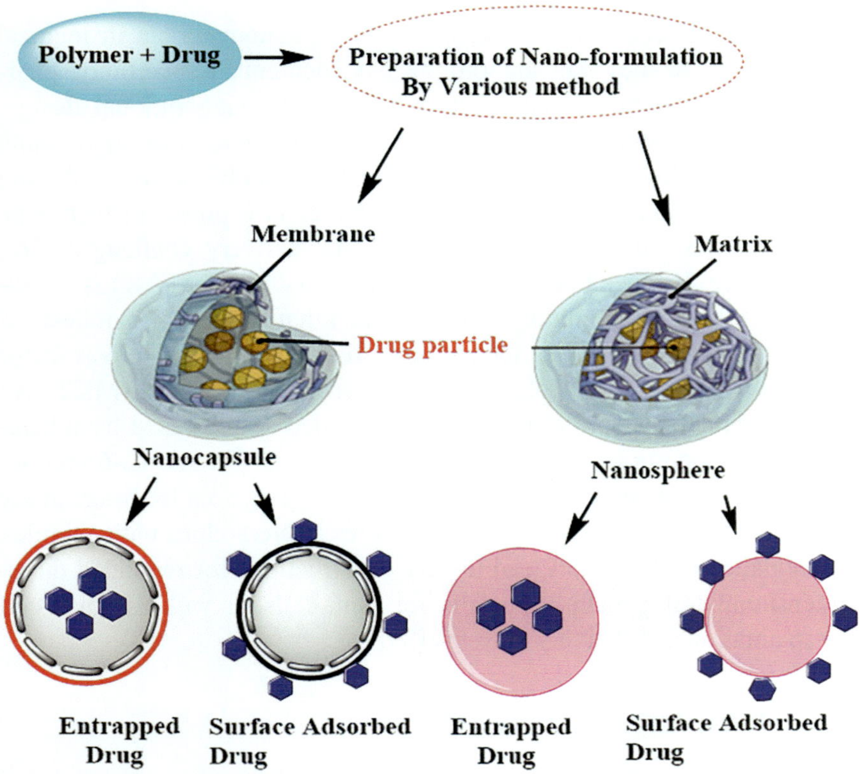

FIGURE 1.3 Various types of polymer-based nanoparticles with drugs.

1.5 CONTRIBUTION OF POLYMERIC NANOMEDICINES IN INFLAMMATORY DISEASES

The inflammatory responses of molecular and cellular activities have opened up new avenues for treating inflammation, particularly through the creation of well-designed nano-therapies. Nanoparticle formulations that modulate the expression of anti-inflammatory chemicals and target inflammatory sensors or macrophages via phagocytosis have a lot of potential for treating inflammatory disorders [17]. Significant interest in the development of nano-anti-inflammatory drugs that are more effective in overcoming the side effects commonly found in conventional therapies has led to the development of nano-anti-inflammatory drugs.

1.5.1 ANTI-INFLAMMATORY PEPTIDES NANOMEDICINES

Peptides are effective in the management of nanomaterials in medical science because they can incorporate physiochemical specificity, pharmacotherapy functions, and crystal structures through rational design. Even though peptides, with the exception of antibodies, are tiny enough to fit in a shallow binding pocket or are hydrophobic without altering affinity, combining peptides and nanoparticles is a powerful technique for overcoming many standard medications' delivery challenges [36]. For example, KAFAKLAARLYRKALARQLGVAA (KAFAK) is a cell-penetrating anti-inflammatory peptide (CPP) that blocks the synthesis of pro-inflammatory cytokines such as IL-1, IL-6, and tumor necrosis factor (TNF) α by means of a protein kinase activated by mitogens (MK2). An anti-inflammatory peptide (KAFAK) was loaded and released from heat-sensitive nanoparticles and was shown to inhibit TNFα and IL-6 production levels in monocytes [37, 38]. Another intriguing area for future study is the use of bioactive peptide nanostructures in hierarchies with complex functionalities. This could lead to new constructions for regulated three-dimensional cell growth, especially for stem cells, as well as novel cell transplantation and delivery systems [39].

1.5.2 BIOMIMETIC NANOPARTICLES

Recently, biomimetic nanoparticles for the clinical field have seen a lot of intriguing advancements. Inflammation is a defense mechanism to injury and infection in which immune cells, blood vessels, and cellular immunity are involved, and it is intimately connected to many pathogens. As a result, they can be used to mimic immune cells, which can help with molecular imaging and targeted medication management to sensitive areas [40]. Biomimetic nanoparticles are designed to mimic the behavior of cells or exosomes. They are an emerging new type of nanostructure that intends to overcome current nanomedicine issues by emulating the biomimicry of native cells [41]. The anti-inflammation and targeted antiviral effects of a biomimetic nanocarrier-based drug delivery system seem favorable, suggesting that it could have a broad therapeutic benefit in the treatment of COVID-19 [42]. These biomimetic nanoparticles, as a new type of nano therapy, acquire specialized bioactivities from the source cells such as red blood cells, immune cells, cancerous cells, and platelets. These avoid immune rejection, prolong circulation, and even target the pathological area due to the endocytotic tendency of cellular membrane polypeptides. Biomimetic cell membrane nanoparticles for therapeutics, with a special emphasis on their application in the treatment of infections and cancer. We anticipate a broader range of applications of biomimetic approaches to cell membranes due to the very diverse functions of cell membranes in nature [43].

1.5.3 ANTI-INFLAMMATORY MEDIATORS IN NANO-ENCAPSULATION

Anti-inflammatory mediators are a promising new therapy option for inflammatory disorders. Nano-encapsulation can be described as the entrapment, confinement, or covering of biologically active compounds on nanoscale carriers. Advances in microscale to nanoscale encapsulation have been inspired by those with more precise site targeting, as seen in the treatment of cancer with chemotherapeutic drugs [44]. They have better entrapment efficiency in drug delivery due to increased solubility of bioactive molecules in the core, low polymer content compared to other nanomolecular systems like nanoparticles, protection of the drug's polymer shell from degradation factors, and reduced tissue irritation caused by the polymer shell [45]. The anti-inflammatory and antioxidant activity of Cur and Nano responsible for inhibiting the inflammatory skin response induced by croton oil (CO) nanocur inhibited the inflammatory response at eight times lower dose than Cur, suggesting that nanoencapsulation of curcuminoids is important to protect against their biodegradation after oral administration, increasing their bioavailability [46]. Nano-encapsulated diclofenac has a stronger anti-inflammatory effect than the free form of diclofenac. Encapsulation of diclofenac can assist in improving the drug's efficacy and decrease the dosage to minimize the drug's side effects. Inflammatory mediators such as prostaglandins, histamine, serotonin, and bradykinin are inhibited, resulting in an anti-inflammatory effect [47].

1.6 APPLICATIONS

In this era, biomedical applications of biodegradable polymers have improved their biocompatibility, biodegradability, flexibility, and very few unintended consequences. These polymers can be used to make skin, cartilage scaffolds, blood vessels, and drug delivery nano-systems, and they can also cause inflammatory responses in cells. Other biodegradable polymeric nanoparticles improve bioavailability and stability [48]. Smart polymers were developed very quickly in medical devices (cell/drug/protein carriers), 3D printing, and cell therapy for precision medicine. Smart polymers have performed as shape memory performance, bioprinting, minimally invasive surgery, injectability, and precision medicine, with tailorable mechanical strength and precise shapes [49]. Polymer encapsulation of Ru, Pt, and Ag metal complexes has been used in biological and medicinal applications [50]. N-(2-hydroxypropyl) methacrylamide conjugates of camptothecin, doxorubicin, paclitaxel, and platinum complexes have been enhancing the therapeutic index of clinical recognition [3, 50]. Polymer with protein conjugates, drug with PCs, and supramolecular drug-delivery systems of polymer have raised stability and pharmacokinetic properties. Polyethylene glycol components (PEGylation) form of adenosine deaminase. Polyanionic polymers inhibit virus attachment, polycationic complexes with DNAs or RNAs (polyplexes), and dendritic core-shell architectures for the encapsulation of drugs [3]. The cancer-targeted DDS and cell therapy platforms for inflammation-related diseases have been revealed by ROS potential in the biomedical field [51, 52].

1.7 CONCLUSION

In the conclusion, based on the recent literature, synthetic and hybrid polymers are used for multiple medical applications as distinguishing features of inflammatory diseases. Polymeric systems have extraordinary potential for the treatment of most inflammation-related disorders. Biomedical polymer coatings and pharmaceutical nano-carriers enhance the bioavailability of inflammatory drugs due to their hydrophobicity for cardiovascular diseases, obesity, cancer, and neurodegenerative diseases. Here, we focus on advances in polymer and nano-polymer design that improve efficacy in general drug delivery applications in inflammation therapies.

KEYWORDS

- **bioavailability**
- **biodegradable polymeric nanoparticles**
- **inflammation**
- **inflammation-related diseases**
- **multidisciplinary**
- **nanoencapsulation**
- **pharmaceutical nano-carriers**
- **polymer**

REFERENCES

1. Corrêa, H. L., & Corrêa, D. G. (2020). Polymer applications for medical care in the COVID-19 pandemic crisis: Will we still speak ill of these materials. *Frontiers in Materials*, *7*, 1–6.
2. Zhu, M., Liu, J., Gan, L., & Long, M. (2020). Research progress in bio-based self-healing materials. *European Polymer Journal*, *129*, 0014–3057.
3. Haag, R., & Kratz, F. (2006). Polymer therapeutics: Concepts and applications. *Angewandte Chemie–International Edition*, *45*, 1198–1215.
4. Koziolová, E., Venclíková, K., & Etrych, T. (2018). Polymer-drug conjugates in inflammation treatment. *Physiological Research*, *67*, 281–292.
5. Sharma, P., Negi, P., & Mahindroo, N. (2018). Recent advances in polymeric drug delivery carrier systems. In *Advances in Polymers for Biomedical Applications*, *20*, 369–388.

6. Prajapati, S. K., Jain, A., Jain, A., & Jain, S. (2019). Biodegradable polymers and constructs: A novel approach in drug delivery. *European Polymer Journal, 120*, 109–191.
7. Asghari, F., Samiei, M., Adibkia, K., Akbarzadeh, A., & Davaran, S. (2017). Biodegradable and biocompatible polymers for tissue engineering application: A review. *Artificial Cells, Nanomedicine and Biotechnology*, *45*, 185–192.
8. Kiick, K. L. (2007). Materials science: Polymer therapeutics. *Science*, *317*, 1182.
9. Patwary, M. A. S., Surid, S. M., & Gafur, M. A. (2020). Properties and applications of biodegradable polymers. *Journal of Research Updates in Polymer Science*, *9*, 32–41.
10. Sowjanya, M., Debnath, S., Lavanya, P., Thejovathi, R., & Babu, M. N. (2017). Polymers used in the designing of controlled drug delivery system. *Research Journal of Pharmacy and Technology*, *10*, 903–912.
11. Sanjay, P. D., & Vasantrao, P. P. (2016). Polymers used in pharmaceuticals: A brief review Pawar. *International Journal of Pharma and Chemical Research*, *2*, 233–238.
12. Criado-Gonzalez, M., Mijangos, C., & Hernández, R. (2021). Polyelectrolyte multilayer films based on natural polymers: From fundamentals to bio-applications. *Polymers*, *13*, 1–30.
13. Kalirajan, C., Dukle, A., Nathanael, A. J., Oh, T. H., & Manivasagam, G. (2021). A critical review on polymeric biomaterials for biomedical applications. *Polymers*, *13*, 1–27.
14. Baek, J. S., Yeo, E. W., Lee, Y. H., Tan, N. S., & Loo, S. C. J. (2017). Controlled-release nanoencapsulating microcapsules to combat inflammatory diseases. *Drug Design, Development and Therapy*, *11*, 1707–1717.
15. Fukuda, D., & Sata, M. (2021). Frontiers of inflammatory disease research: Inflammation in cardiovascular–cerebral diseases. *Inflammation and Regeneration*, *41*, 0–1.
16. Chen, Y. C., Gad, S. F., Chobisa, D., Li, Y., & Yeo, Y. (2021). Local drug delivery systems for inflammatory diseases: Status quo, challenges, and opportunities. *Journal of Controlled Release*, *330*, 438–460.
17. Brusini, R., Varna, M., & Couvreur, P. (2020). Advanced nanomedicines for the treatment of inflammatory diseases. *Advanced Drug Delivery Reviews*, *157*, 161–178.
18. Fernandes, E. F. A., & Özcelik, D. (2021). Imaging biomarkers for monitoring the inflammatory redox landscape in the brain. *Antioxidants*, *10*, 528–547.
19. Zetoune, F. S., Serhan, C. N., & Ward, P. A. (2014). Inflammatory disorder. In *Reference Module in Biomedical Sciences* Issue July. Elsevier Inc. https://www.elsevier.com (accessed on 4th July 2025).
20. Stankov, V. S. (2012). Definition of inflammation causes of inflammation and possible anti-inflammatory strategies. *The Open Inflammation Journal*, *5*, 1–9.
21. Lautenschläger, C., Schmidt, C., Fischer, D., & Stallmach, A. (2014). Drug delivery strategies in the therapy of inflammatory bowel disease. *Advanced Drug Delivery Reviews*, *71*, 58–76.
22. Sanchis, J., Canal, F., Lucas, R., & Vicent, M. J. (2010). Polymer-drug conjugates for novel molecular targets. *Nanomedicine*, *5*, 915–935.
23. Natfji, A. A., Osborn, H. M. I., & Greco, F. (2017). Feasibility of polymer-drug conjugates for non-cancer applications. *Current Opinion in Colloid and Interface Science*, *31*, 51–66.

24. Rojo, L., Fernandez-Gutierrez, M., Deb, S., Stevens, M. M., & San Roman, J. (2015). Designing dapsone polymer conjugates for controlled drug delivery. *Acta Biomaterialia*, *27*, 32–41.
25. Greco, F., & Vicent, M. J. (2008). Polymer-drug conjugates: Current status and future trends. *Frontiers in Bioscience*, *13*, 2744–2756.
26. Kamaly, N., Fredman, G., Subramanian, M., Gadde, S., Pesic, A., Cheung, L., Fayad, Z. A., Langer, R., Tabas, I., & Farokhzad, O. C. (2013). Development and *in vivo* efficacy of targeted polymeric inflammation-resolving nanoparticles. *National Academy of Sciences*, *110*, 6506–6511.
27. Zielinska, A., Carreiró, F., Oliveira, A. M., Neves, A., Pires, B., Nagasamy Venkatesh, D., Durazzo, A., Lucarini, M., Eder, P., Silva, A. M., Santini, A., & Souto, E. B. (2020). Polymeric nanoparticles: Production, characterization, toxicology and ecotoxicology. *Molecules*, *25*, 3731–3751.
28. Begines, B., Ortiz, T., Pérez-Aranda, M., Martínez, G., Merinero, M., Argüelles-Arias, F., & Alcudia, A. (2020). Polymeric nanoparticles for drug delivery: Recent developments and future prospects. *Nanomaterials*, *10*, 1–41.
29. Mahmoud, E. A., Sankaranarayanan, J., Morachis, J. M., Kim, G., & Almutairi, A. (2011). Inflammation responsive logic gate nanoparticles for the delivery of proteins. *Bioconjugate Chemistry*, *22*, 1416–1421.
30. Prosperi, D., Colombo, M., Zanoni, I., & Granucci, F. (2018). Drug nanocarriers to treat autoimmunity and chronic inflammatory diseases. *HHS Public Access*, *34*, 61–67.
31. Lee, A., Di Mascolo, D., Francardi, M., Piccardi, F., Bandiera, T., & Decuzzi, P. (2016). Spherical polymeric nano constructs for combined chemotherapeutic and anti-inflammatory therapies. *Nanomedicine: Nanotechnology, Biology, and Medicine*, *12*, 2139–2147.
32. Prabhu, R. H., Patravale, V. B., & Joshi, M. D. (2015). Polymeric nanoparticles for targeted treatment in oncology: Current insights. *International Journal of Nanomedicine*, *10*, 1001–1018.
33. Nagavarma, B. V. N., Yadav, H. K. S., Ayaz, A., Vasudha, L. S., & Shivakumar, H. G. (2012). Different techniques for preparation of polymeric nanoparticles–A review. *Asian Journal of Pharmaceutical and Clinical Research*, *5*, 16–23.
34. Lee, S., Stubelius, A., Hamelmann, N., Tran, V., & Almutairi, A. (2018). Inflammation-responsive drug-conjugated dextran nanoparticles enhance anti-inflammatory drug efficacy. *ACS Applied Materials and Interfaces*, *10*, 40378–40387.
35. Elsabahy, M., & Wooley, K. L. (2012). Design of polymeric nanoparticles for biomedical delivery applications. *Chemical Society Reviews*, *41*, 2521–3012.
36. Chung, E. J. (2016). Targeting and therapeutic peptides in nanomedicine for atherosclerosis. *Experimental Biology and Medicine*, *241*, 891–898.
37. He, Z., Zang, H., Zhu, L., Huang, K., Yi, T., Zhang, S., & Cheng, S. (2019). An anti-inflammatory peptide and brain-derived neurotrophic factor-modified hyaluronan-methylcellulose hydrogel promotes nerve regeneration in rats with spinal cord injury. *International Journal of Nanomedicine*, *14*, 721–732.
38. Poh, S., Lin, J. B., & Panitch, A. (2017). Release of anti-inflammatory peptides from thermosensitive nanoparticles with degradable cross-links suppresses pro-inflammatory cytokine production. *HHS Public Access*, *176*, 139–148.

39. Webber, M. J., Kessler, J. A., & Stupp, S. I. (2010). Emerging peptide nanomedicine to regenerate tissues and organs. *Journal of Internal Medicine*, *267*, 71–88.
40. Jin, K., Luo, Z., Zhang, B., & Pang, Z. (2018). Biomimetic nanoparticles for inflammation targeting. *Acta Pharmaceutica Sinica B*, *8*, 23–33.
41. Zinger, A., Sushnitha, M., Naoi, T., Baudo, G., De Rosa, E., Chang, J., Tasciotti, E., & Taraballi, F. (2021). Enhancing inflammation targeting using tunable leukocyte-based biomimetic nanoparticles. *ACS Nano*, *15*, 6326–6339.
42. Tan, Q., He, L., Meng, X., Wang, W., Pan, H., Yin, W., Zhu, T., Huang, X., & Shan, H. (2021). Macrophage biomimetic nanocarriers for anti-inflammation and targeted antiviral treatment in COVID-19. *Journal of Nanobiotechnology*, *19*, 1–16.
43. Wang, H., Liu, Y., He, R., Xu, D., Zang, J., Weeranoppanant, N., Dong, H., & Li, Y. (2021). Cell membrane biomimetic nanoparticles for inflammation and cancer targeting in drug delivery. *Biomaterials Science*, *8*, 552–568.
44. Ngwuluka, C. N., Abu-Thabit, N. Y., Uwaezuoke, J. O., Erebor, O. O., Ilomuanya, M. O., Mohamed, R. R., Soliman, M. A., Abu Elella, M. H., & Ebrahim, A. A. A. (2021). Natural polymers in micro- and nanoencapsulation for therapeutic and diagnostic applications: Part I: Lipids and fabrication techniques. In *Nano- and Microencapsulation–Techniques and Applications*.
45. Bayraktar, O., Erdogan, I., Köse, M. D., & Kalmaz, G. (2017). Nanocarriers for plant-derived natural compounds. In *Nanostructures for Antimicrobial Therapy* (pp. 395–412).
46. Lima, E. P., Gonçalves, O. H., Ames, F. Q., Castro-Hoshino, L. V., Leimann, F. V., Cuman, R. K. N., Comar, J. F., & Bersani-Amado, C. A. (2021). Anti-inflammatory and antioxidant activity of nano encapsulated curcuminoids extracted from *Curcuma longa* L. in a model of cutaneous inflammation. *Inflammation*, *44*, 604–616.
47. Zuraini, A., Zakariai, Z. A., Kadir, A. A., Chiong, H. S., & Fauzee, M. S. O. (2013). Enhanced anti-inflammatory effects of nano encapsulated diclofenac. *European Journal of Inflammation*, *11*, 855–861.
48. Caballero-George, C., & Marin, B. (2013). Critical evaluation of biodegradable polymers used in nanodrugs. *International Journal of Nanomedicine*, *8*, 3071.
49. Huang, H. J., Tsai, Y. L., Lin, S. H., & Hsu, S. H. (2019). Smart polymers for cell therapy and precision medicine. *Journal of Biomedical Science*, *26*, 1–11.
50. Espinosa-Cano, E., Aguilar, M. R., Portilla, Y., Barber, D. F., & Román, J. S. (2020). Anti-inflammatory polymeric nanoparticles based on ketoprofen and dexamethasone. *Pharmaceutics*, *12*, 1–18.
51. Xu, Q., He, C., Xiao, C., & Chen, X. (2016). Reactive oxygen species (ROS) responsive polymers for biomedical applications. *Macromolecular Bioscience*, *16*, 635–646.
52. Pridgen, E. M., Alexis, F., & Farokhzad, O. C. (2015). Polymeric nanoparticle drug delivery technologies for oral delivery applications. *Expert Opinion on Drug Delivery*, *12*, 1459–1473.

CHAPTER 2

3D Printed Polymers for Medical Applications: Recent Achievements and Challenges

RAFFAELE PUGLIESE,[1,*] RICCARDO SALA,[1] STEFANO REGONDI,[1,2] and CHRISTIAN LUNETTA1,[2]

[1]*NeMO Lab, ASST Niguarda Cà Granda Hospital, Milan, Italy*

[2]*NEuroMuscular Omnicenter (NEMO), Fondazione Serena Onlus, Milan, Italy*

*Corresponding author

ABSTRACT

Polymer 3D printing is an emerging technology that is revolutionizing the field of medicine because it allows for specific production for each patient with high resolution at the microstructure level. Research in this field has led to the development of reinforcing and biocompatible polymeric materials, achieved by modifying printing process parameters. With cheaper production than traditional techniques, 3D printing is gaining ground as a versatile manufacturing technology for healthcare, tissue engineering, regenerative medicine, rehabilitation, drug delivery systems, medical apparatus, and instruments. In this chapter, the current additive manufacturing (AM) technologies, printable polymer-based materials, and their applications in the medical field will be discussed. Finally, the challenges, barriers, and regulatory controversies of polymer printing in medicine will be addressed.

Polymer Applications in Medicine: Revolutionizing Treatment and Therapeutics.
Mohd. Imran Ahamed, Faheem Ahmad, and Ishaat M. Khan (Eds.)

DOI: 10.1201/9781779640871-2

2.1 INTRODUCTION

Additive Manufacturing (AM), also called 3D printing, was first introduced by Charles Hull in 1984 [1, 2] to cope with the needs of modeling and rapid prototyping (Figure 2.1).

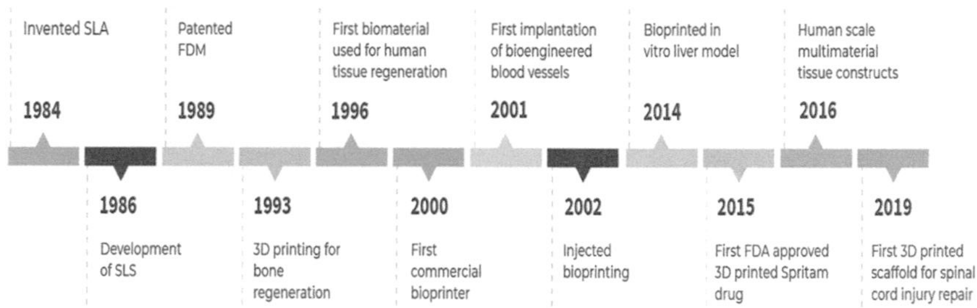

FIGURE 2.1 3D printing milestones since the invention of 3D printing by Charles Hull in 1984.

The AM allows the production of 3D structures with high shape complexity from polymers, metals, composites, and ceramics without the need for molds or machining typical of conventional manufacturing processes [3]. Furthermore, AM is able to 3D print customized and inexpensive objects. This is particularly valuable in medicine, where patient-specific products are required [4]. In fact, Wohlers Associates reported that about 50% of AM in 2021 is associated with custom devices [5]. However, it is only in recent years that 3D printing has been adopted in different industries, from research and development to prototypes and products, as reported by Jabil [6] in their yearly survey submitted to the key players of the AM community (Figure 2.2A). As evidence of these developments, the scientific impact of 3D printing has also increased dramatically (Figure 2.2B).

Medical applications for 3D printing are expanding at an accelerating pace and are expected to revolutionize health care [7, 8]. In particular, 3D printed polymers have shown many advantages in various medical areas, including craniofacial implants [9–11], dental molds [12, 13], orthoses [14–16], medical devices [17], surgical models [18–20], scaffolds for regenerative medicine [21, 22], organoids [23], and tissue models for drug discovery [24].

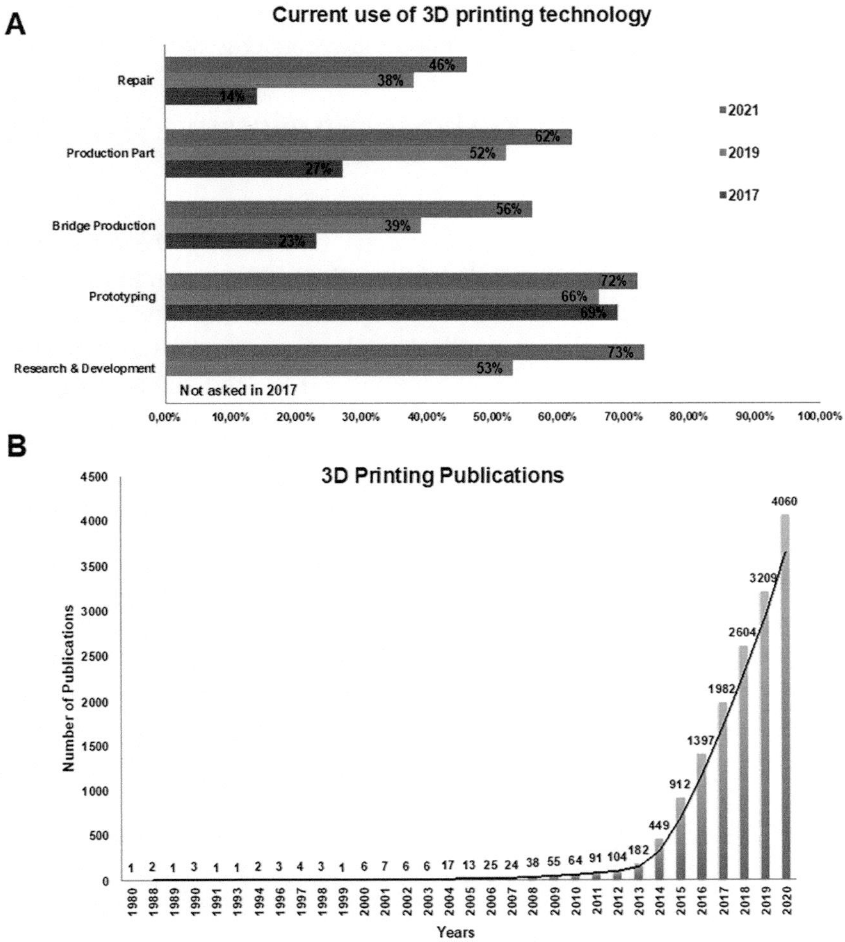

FIGURE 2.2 A) Percentage of current use of 3D printing technology in various industries field as reported by Jabil in the yearly survey. B) Timeline of publications dealing with the topic of 3D printing and additive manufacturing retrieved by querying PubMed.

All this is possible because polymer-based materials have: (1) adequate biomechanics for printability, (2) tunable compressive and shear loads, (3) are nontoxic, and (4) have a tunable degradation rate [25]. In this chapter, we summarize the currently available AM techniques and 3D printable polymer-based materials, analyzing their printability features. Furthermore, some medical applications, including tissue scaffolds, dental implants, drug delivery, and surgical models, are summarized. Finally, regulatory standpoints, patent, and copyright concerns will be discussed.

2.2 CURRENT AM TECHNOLOGIES AND PRINTABLE MATERIALS

2.2.1 PRINTING PROCESSES

All AM technologies offer pros and cons, and usually, the type of 3D printer chosen for a specific application—whether industrial or medical—depends on the feedstock materials to be used. The most commonly used 3D printing technologies in medical applications are: fused deposition modeling (FDM), selective laser sintering (SLS), and stereolithography (SLA). Below is a brief discussion of each of these technologies.

2.2.1.1 FUSED DEPOSITION MODELING (FDM)

Extrusion-Based 3D Printing (Figure 2.3A), also referred to as Fused Deposition Modeling (FDM) or Fused Filament Fabrication (FFF), is the most extensively used 3D printing technique [4]. A polymeric filament (commonly PLA, ABS, PET, and PC) is fed into the printer, where it is melted until reaching a semi-liquid state and extruded through a nozzle [26]. The printhead moves on a platform, and the extruded filament (i.e., 1.5 or 1.75 mm diameter) is deposited on the printer platform, creating a layer-by-layer object [27]. The nozzle follows a defined path obtained from a CAD model in order to build up a 3D object; subsequent layers of material are then deposited upon, thus bonding to the underlying layers [28]. The platform moves down each time a layer is completely deposited until the final shape is obtained. In order to use different kinds of polymers, the printhead temperature can be adjusted in each printer. The printing accuracy can be controlled by changing printing parameters, such as layer thickness, printing orientation, raster, and voids [26]. Typically, FDM is suitable for only pure thermoplastics; however, nowadays, reinforced feedstocks are also commercially available (i.e., polyamides reinforced with carbon fibers). The main advantages of this technology are the low cost, good strength, and multi-material capability, due to the possibility of employing multiple printheads, whereas the main drawbacks are the anisotropy, voids, interlayer distortions, and weak mechanical properties [29].

2.2.1.2 SELECTIVE LASER SINTERING (SLS)

SLS (Figure 2.3B) is widely used in the industrial field since it is able to print different materials (such as polymers, ceramics, and metals) into complex structures [27]. The main components of the SLS technology are (1) the building platform, (2) the material powder (ranging from 10 to 100 μm), and (3) the laser beam to provide the required energy for particle bonding. For this latter, a CO_2 laser is often employed in order to raise the particles' temperature to above their melting temperature. The laser moves in a two-dimensional plane, following a peculiar path predetermined by a software program. The laser scans the powder bed, melting a localized zone to create a customized product [8], and when one layer is completed, the build platform moves down, enabling the deposition of a new one via a roller to be heated up and solidified. The untreated portion of the bed remains unmachined and provides support during the process for subsequent layers [30]. Due to the adoption of the laser, the process does not require any solvent and fabricates objects with optimal resolution. The quality characteristics are influenced by the process conditions, such as laser power and scan speed. Despite these features, SLS printers are slow and require a large amount of material; for this reason, they are mostly used within manufacturing industries.

2.2.1.3 STEREOLITHOGRAPHY (SLA)

SLA is a technique based on the hardening of layers of resin under liquid shape by photo-polymerization using UV light [4] (Figure 2.3C). The SLA method is considered the progenitor of AM, as it was developed and marketed in the mid-1980s by Charles Hull. Since then, different configurations of SLA machines exist depending on the position of the laser and the movement of the building platform. If the laser is located on the top of the printer, the building platform moves down when each layer is completed, while if the laser is placed on the bottom, the platform moves upward. The laser moves using scanning mirrors, making the resin photocured on the platform or on the previous layer in order to obtain the final shape. The movement of the building platform allows the previous layer to be covered by a thin quantity of uncured resin to be processed. The mechanism continues until the final shape is obtained. The advantages of this process are the high resolution (25 μm) and lower stress concentration in the object [27]. The main drawbacks of this technology are the sensitivity to the exposure of UV light and the possibility of having trapped uncured resin inside the final shape.

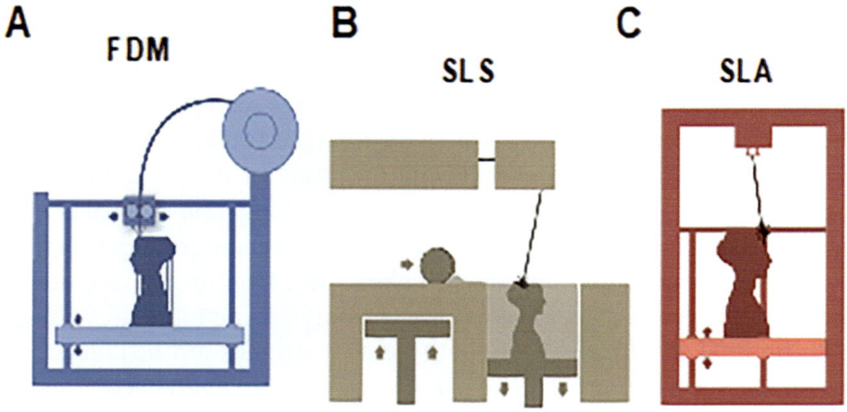

FIGURE 2.3 Simplified representation of 3D printing techniques: A) fused deposition modeling (FDM), B) selective laser sintering (SLS), and C) stereolithography (SLA).

2.2.2 3D PRINTABLE POLYMERS

Polymers are the widely used AM materials as they can be manufactured in different form (such as filaments, powder, and solutions). As reported in the section 2.2.1. printing processes, each of these techniques requires peculiar printing parameters. Polymers for FDM must have (1) a specific diameter of 1.75 mm or 3 mm (for thermoplastic polyurethanes), (2) a fast solid-to-melt transition, (3) a ration of elastic modulus and viscosity below $5{\times}10^5$ s^{-1}[30]. Instead, polymer beads for SLS must have a diameter ranging from 10 to 100 μm to allow particle flow during printing, with a melt temperature achievable by the laser (usually ≤200°C). Finally, for SLA, polymers must be stable and possibly photo-cross-linkable. Based on these design parameters, here we describe some commonly used 3D printed polymers for medical applications (Table 2.1).

TABLE 2.1 Properties of 3D Printed Polymers

Polymers Name	Melting Point	Mechanical Properties
PLA	175°C	Young's modulus: 230 MPa Tensile Strength: 26 MPa
PCL	60°C	Young's modulus: 216 MPa Tensile Strength: 37 MPa
ABS	105°C	Young's modulus: 30 MPa Tensile Strength: 29 MPa
PP	165°C	Young's modulus: 1.6 GPa Tensile Strength: 40 MPa
PEEK	350°C	Young's modulus: 3.6 GPa Tensile Strength: 100 MPa

Polylactic acid (PLA) is the most used polymer in FDM and can be easily extruded at 190°C (melting temperature of 175°C). The 3D printed PLA constructs exhibit compressive moduli between 20 and 500 MPa, which is useful for orthopedics. However, the hydrophobicity of PLA results in poor cell adhesion, as well as potential bacterial adhesion [31]. Thus, 3D printed PLA-based constructs can be functionalized with biomolecules (i.e., collagen, peptides, minocycline, and hydroxyapatite, to name a few) to overcome these issues. Another concern with PLA is its long-term biocompatibility due to the release of lactic acid byproducts during degradation [32].

Polycaprolactone (PCL) is another polymer at the forefront of the FDM technique, thanks to its superior mechanical features (tensile strength 37 MPa, elongation at break 746%) and its low melting temperature of 60°C. Furthermore, PCL is highly used as a scaffold for tissue regeneration or wound healing, as it has a long degradation time (≈3 years) [33]. PCL is also a good choice for manufacturing prosthetic devices via FDM, SLS, and DIW, as it forms entangled networks of fibers at the nanoscale level, leading to a final construct with tunable porosity and mechanical properties [34].

Acrylonitrile butadiene styrene (ABS) is a thermoplastic copolymer derived from styrene [35], with a melting temperature of 105°C and the ability to withstand temperatures up to 80°C, making it useful for both FDM and SLA technologies. Furthermore, due to its toughness, ABS is widely used in cartilage and nucleus pulposus engineering. Polypropylene (PP) is a crystalline thermoplastic polymer with a melting point of 165°C, a stiffness of 1.2 GPa, and a tensile strain at break of ~40 MPa [36]. PP is a lightweight polymer, which is why it is widely used in orthopedics [37].

Lastly, the evolution of 3D printing technologies has allowed the development of high-performance polymers (namely Poly-Ether-Ether-Ketone – PEEK) with mechanics similar to those of metals (i.e., Young's modulus of 3.6 GPa and tensile strength of 100 MPa) [38]. For this reason, PEEK is widely used for bone tissue engineering and craniofacial implants [39, 40].

2.2.3 MEDICAL APPLICATIONS

2.2.3.1 DENTAL IMPLANTS

It has been estimated that worldwide there are about 276 million patients suffering from tooth loss [41], and 3D-printed polymers may provide a valuable opportunity to fabricate economical and precise dental implants compared to conventional dental stone [42]. For instance, PLA and PEEK are adopted for dental implant fabrication and for oral cavity implantation due to their (1) high mechanical properties, (2) resistance against impact, and (3) good biocompatibility [30]. However, the water absorption of such polymer-based materials can lead to the formation of bacterial biofilms on the surface of dental prostheses. To overcome this issue, as reported by Du-Hyeong Lee and co-workers, chlorhexidine-loaded polydimethylsiloxane (PDMS)-based coating can be applied to the surface of polymer microstructures, thus improving antibacterial activity [43]. In addition, some results demonstrate that SLS and polyjet printing processes could provide accuracy close to that of conventionally manufactured dental implants. Moreover, the possibility of using CAD software enables customization of the implant for the patient, thus providing a helpful tool for dentists, which allows for reduced fabrication time, selection of the required depth and width of teeth, accurate sizing for implants, and higher quality at lower costs.

2.2.3.2 TISSUE SCAFFOLDS

In the last two decades, polymers and biopolymers have been widely used in tissue engineering and regenerative medicine, since they provide ideal synthetic and bio-resorbable extracellular matrix (ECM) microenvironments for tissues and organs [7, 44]. Thanks to 3D printing, polymers have gained increasing interest in tissue engineering applications, as 3D printing design processes and strategies play a key role in customizing scaffold structures and producing optimized designs. Indeed, by using 3D printing techniques, it is now possible to consider scaffold features across scales (from micro- to macro-scale), thus precisely tuning the scaffold's topology for cell migration, infiltration, and nutrient transport. In doing so, a computer-aided system for tissue scaffolds (namely CASTS) has been developed for creating tunable porous 3D scaffold models for bone, cartilage, skin, vasculature, neurons, and skeletal muscle [45–47]. Using such CASTS-designed tissue-engineered scaffolds, materials were fabricated with PCL, PLLA, PVA, PLGA, PEEK, PEEK/HA, PVA/HA, and PCL/HA by both SLS and FDM processes.

2.2.3.3 SAFETY EQUIPMENT

The COVID-19 pandemic has recently highlighted the key benefits of rapid prototyping of safety equipment because of the inadequate supply in certain regions, where the demand exceeds conventional production. The first safety equipment produced by 3D printing was the PP particle filters and masks [48]. Then, some studies were conducted on respirators and helmets integrating breathing filters built with TPU, ABS, and PLA filaments. Furthermore, Jacopo Profili et al. explored different 3D printed design concepts focused on personal protective equipment (PPE) such as facemasks and air-purifying respirator (PAPR) hoods, and hospital respiratory support equipment like venturi valves, ventilator splitters, adjustable flow control valves, and non-invasive respiratory systems (NIV) [49].

Already existing devices were readapted in order to be functional in hospitals, such as snorkeling masks, rearranged with different kinds of 3D printed valves to allow the air coming inside and the exhaust air to leave the device. Different configurations of valves were created, most of them built via the FDM method, utilizing PLA or PETG as building materials [49]. It is important to note that, in order to make such devices functional, it is necessary to set the proper design parameters and pay particular attention to the removal of support and debris that can be inhaled by the patient. After that, each device needs to be sterilized before use in order to compensate for the uncontrolled manipulations during printing and assembling.

2.2.3.4 SURGICAL PLANNING

3D printing is also having a significant impact on medical education and surgical planning, as 3D anatomical models can be printed by perfectly reproducing the microscopic anatomical structures of tissues and organs, thus having a positive impact in terms of time required, efficiency, accuracy, and success of the surgery. Further, 3D printed anatomical models can be used for training new surgeons. Patient-specific 3D printed organ models have been used in various medical fields including cardiac surgery and neurology [50–55]. For instance, ABS has been adopted in cardiology to fabricate patient-specific hearts in order to improve the implantation procedure [51]. In addition, PLA filaments have been used to manufacture 3D-printed aneurysm models for studying the patient-specific hydrodynamics system [53].

2.2.3.5 DRUG DELIVERY

3D printed drug development is another exciting topic in medicine, as it would allow for patient-specific drug needs with customizable dosage forms and/or release profiles [56]. Drug delivery is also possible on the skin by using a 3D printed micro-needle array. This delivery approach generally remains painless and promotes efficient drug transportation. In fact, the micro-needles are manufactured with a tip width ranging from 65 to 84 μm, a pitch of 700 μm, and a height of 400 μm [57].

2.3 ADVANTAGES OF 3D PRINTING IN MEDICINE

The greatest advantage of 3D printers in medical applications is the freedom to produce custom-made medical products, implants, and orthoses, which is unparalleled compared to traditional technology. This leads to new therapeutic, surgical, and rehabilitative solutions available for different branches of medicine, providing great value for both patients and physicians, as it can improve patient recovery time and reduce hospitalization, as well as having a positive impact in terms of time required, efficiency, accuracy, and success of the surgery [28]. Moreover, 3D printing has the ability to produce items quickly (products can be made within several hours) and cheaply. This is particularly advantageous for medical applications that have to produce highly complex products that require frequent changes. In addition, 3D printing technology is attractive compared to traditional methods of producing prostheses, orthoses, and implants, since the latter require milling, forging, and long delivery times, while 3D printing ignores these constraints, thanks to the 3D scanning technologies and CAD, which allow the immediate modification or customization of the part to be printed according to the requests and needs of the individual patient, reducing implementation times and costs.

Finally, an unprecedented opportunity provided by 3D printing is the nature of the STL files that can be shared among researchers, physicians, engineers, materials scientists, and orthopedists all over the world, thus reducing the costly waste of time associated with trial and error in reproducing the parameters described in scientific papers. The STL files can be downloaded from an open-source database, allowing for the exact replica of a model or medical device. For instance, the National Institutes of Health (NIH) has set up the 3D Print Exchange (3dprint.nih.gov) to guarantee the open-source sharing of 3D printing files for medical and anatomical models, aids, laboratory equipment, and models of proteins and viruses [58].

2.4 CHALLENGES, BARRIERS, AND CONTROVERSIES

AM applications have been subject to patent, industrial design, copyright, and trademark law [59]. However, there is still not much experience regarding how these laws can be applied not only by individuals but also within hospitals and research centers. In addition, approval from regulators is another critical barrier that may hinder the use of 3D printing in medicine. Some 3D-printed medical devices have received the 510(k) approval from the FDA, demonstrating that such devices are safe and effective and can be placed on the market [60]. New challenges arise here as 3D printing aims to provide patient-specific devices, so it will be necessary to demonstrate whether regulatory standards on production quality also apply to these custom devices. On the other hand, manufacturing regulations and state legal requirements could hinder the dispensing of 3D-printed medications. In this case, 3D printers will need to be legally defined as biomedical equipment [60].

2.5 CONCLUDING REMARKS

3D printing has caught on as a leading technology for fabricating parts to be used in medicine, dentistry, orthopedics, surgery, tissue engineering, and drug-delivery applications. From our point of view, we have only scratched the surface of the countless potential that 3D printing for medical applications has. Despite many important achievements in this field, we are confident that there are still numerous untapped applications that have yet to emerge, but if exploited correctly, they can positively affect millions of lives and provide a higher quality of healthcare. On the other hand, we are aware that there are still several challenges, both related to the regulatory process and to the development of polymers with tunable mechanical and biological features for the advancement of this technology.

KEYWORDS

- **3D printing**
- **additive manufacturing**
- **fused deposition modeling**
- **fused filament fabrication**
- **polymers**
- **rapid prototyping**
- **selective laser sintering**
- **stereolithography**

REFERENCES

1. Hull, C. W. (2015). The birth of 3D printing. *Research-Technology Management, 58.*
2. Hull, C., Feygin, M., Baron, Y., Sanders, R., Sachs, E., Lightman, A., & Wohlers, T. (1995). Rapid prototyping: Current technology and future potential. *Rapid Prototyping Journal, 1*, 11–19.
3. Ligon, S. C., Liska, R., Stampfl, J., Gurr, M., & Mulhaupt, R. (2017). Polymers for 3D printing and customized additive manufacturing. *Chemical Reviews, 117*, 10212–10290.
4. Vaz, V. M., & Kumar, L. (2021). 3D printing as a promising tool in personalized medicine. *AAPS PharmSciTech, 22*, 49.

5. Wohlers Report. (2021). 3D printing and additive manufacturing: Global state of the industry. https://www.wohlersassociates.com (accessed on 4th July 2025).
6. Jabil. (2021). 3D printing technology trends: A survey of additive manufacturing decision-makers, *3*, 1–38. https://www.jabil.com (accessed on 4th July 2025).
7. Pugliese, R., Beltrami, B., Regondi, S., & Lunetta, C. (2021). Polymeric biomaterials for 3D printing in medicine: An overview. *Annals of 3D Printed Medicine*, *2*, 100011.
8. Fan, D., Li, Y., Wang, X., Zhu, T., Wang, Q., Cai, H., Li, W., Tian, Y., & Liu, Z. (2020). Progressive 3D printing technology and its application in medical materials. *Frontiers in Pharmacology*, *11*, 122.
9. Sutradhar, A., Park, J., Carrau, D., Nguyen, T. H., Miller, M. J., & Paulino, G. H. (2016). Designing patient-specific 3D printed craniofacial implants using a novel topology optimization method. *Medical & Biological Engineering & Computing*, *54*, 1123–1135.
10. Chamo, D., Msallem, B., Sharma, N., Aghlmandi, S., Kunz, C., & Thieringer, F. M. (2020). Accuracy assessment of molded, patient-specific polymethylmethacrylate craniofacial implants compared to their 3D printed originals. *Journal of Clinical Medicine*, *9*.
11. Tamimi, F., Torres, J., Gbureck, U., Lopez-Cabarcos, E., Bassett, D. C., Alkhraisat, M. H., & Barralet, J. E. (2009). Craniofacial vertical bone augmentation: A comparison between 3D printed monolithic monetite blocks and autologous onlay grafts in the rabbit. *Biomaterials*, *30*, 6318–6326.
12. Yang, Y., Li, H., Xu, Y., Dong, Y., Shan, W., & Shen, J. (2019). Fabrication and evaluation of dental fillers using customized molds via 3D printing technology. *International Journal of Pharmaceutics*, *562*, 66–75.
13. Kaye, R., Goldstein, T., Zeltsman, D., Grande, D. A., & Smith, L. P. (2016). Three-dimensional printing: A review on the utility within medicine and otolaryngology. *International Journal of Pediatric Otorhinolaryngology*, *89*, 145–148.
14. Vujaklija, I., & Farina, D. (2018). 3D printed upper limb prosthetics. *Expert Review of Medical Devices*, *15*, 505–512.
15. Ribeiro, D., Cimino, S. R., Mayo, A. L., Ratto, M., & Hitzig, S. L. (2021). 3D printing and amputation: A scoping review. *Disability and Rehabilitation: Assistive Technology*, *16*, 221–240.
16. Cuellar, J. S., Smit, G., Zadpoor, A. A., & Breedveld, P. (2018). Ten guidelines for the design of non-assembly mechanisms: The case of 3D-printed prosthetic hands. *Proceedings of the Institution of Mechanical Engineers, Part H: Journal of Engineering in Medicine*, *232*, 962–971.
17. Salmi, M. (2021). Additive manufacturing processes in medical applications. *Materials (Basel)*, *14*.
18. Werz, S. M., Zeichner, S. J., Berg, B. I., Zeilhofer, H. F., & Thieringer, F. (2018). 3D printed surgical simulation models as educational tool by maxillofacial surgeons. *European Journal of Dental Education*, *22*, 500–505.
19. Sun, Z. (2020). Clinical applications of patient-specific 3D printed models in cardiovascular disease: Current status and future directions. *Biomolecules*, *10*.
20. Martin-Noguerol, T., Paulano-Godino, F., Riascos, R. F., Calabia-Del-Campo, J., Marquez-Rivas, J., & Luna, A. (2019). Hybrid computed tomography and magnetic

resonance imaging 3D printed models for neurosurgery planning. *Annals of Translational Medicine*, *7*, 684.
21. Do, A. V., Khorsand, B., Geary, S. M., & Salem, A. K. (2015). 3D printing of scaffolds for tissue regeneration applications. *Advanced Healthcare Materials*, *4*, 1742–1762.
22. Laird, N. Z., Acri, T. M., Chakka, J. L., Quarterman, J. C., Malkawi, W. I., Elangovan, S., & Salem, A. K. (2021). Applications of nanotechnology in 3D printed tissue engineering scaffolds. *European Journal of Pharmaceutics and Biopharmaceutics*, *161*, 15–28.
23. Pennarossa, G., Arcuri, S., De Iorio, T., Gandolfi, F., & Brevini, T. A. L. (2021). Current advances in 3D tissue and organ reconstruction. *International Journal of Molecular Sciences*, *22*.
24. Peng, W., Datta, P., Ayan, B., Ozbolat, V., Sosnoski, D., & Ozbolat, I. T. (2017). 3D bioprinting for drug discovery and development in pharmaceutics. *Acta Biomaterial*, *57*, 26–46.
25. Trenfield, S. J., Awad, A., Goyanes, A., Gaisford, S., & Basit, A. W. (2018). 3D printing pharmaceuticals: Drug development to frontline care. *Trends in Pharmacological Sciences*, *39*, 440–451.
26. Wang, X., Jiang, M., Zhou, Z., Gou, J., & Hui, D. (2017). 3D printing of polymer matrix composites: A review and prospective. *Composites Part B: Engineering, 110.*
27. Guvendiren, M., Molde, J., Soares, R. M., & Kohn, J. (2016). Designing biomaterials for 3D printing. *ACS Biomaterials Science & Engineering*, *2*, 1679–1693.
28. Ventola, C. L. (2014). Medical applications for 3D printing: Current and projected uses. *Pharmacy and Therapeutics*, *39*, 704–711.
29. Ngo, T. D., Kashani, A., Imbalzano, G., Nguyen, K. T. Q., & Hui, D. (2018). Additive manufacturing (3D printing): A review of materials, methods, applications and challenges. *Composites Part B: Engineering*, *145*, 172–196.
30. Arefin, A. M. E., Khatri, N. R., Kulkarni, N., & Egan, P. F. (2021). Polymer 3D printing review: Materials, process, and design strategies for medical applications. *Polymers (Basel)*, *13*.
31. Ramot, Y., Haim-Zada, M., Domb, A. J., & Nyska, A. (2016). Biocompatibility and safety of PLA and its copolymers. *Advanced Drug Delivery Reviews*, *107*, 153–162.
32. da Silva, D., Kaduri, M., Poley, M., Adir, O., Krinsky, N., Shainsky-Roitman, J., & Schroeder, A. (2018). Biocompatibility, biodegradation and excretion of polylactic acid (PLA) in medical implants and theragnostic systems. *Chemical Engineering Journal*, *340*, 9–14.
33. Serrano, M. C., Pagani, R., Vallet-Regí, M., Peña, J., Ramila, A., Izquierdo, I., & Portolés, M. T. (2004). *In vitro* biocompatibility assessment of poly(ε-caprolactone) films using L929 mouse fibroblasts. *Biomaterials*, *25*, 5603–5611.
34. Williams, J. M., Adewunmi, A., Schek, R. M., Flanagan, C. L., Krebsbach, P. H., Feinberg, S. E., Hollister, S. J., & Das, S. (2005). Bone tissue engineering using polycaprolactone scaffolds fabricated via selective laser sintering. *Biomaterials*, *26*, 4817–4827.
35. Casavola, C., Cazzato, A., Moramarco, V., & Renna, G. (2019). Mechanical behaviour of ABS-fused filament fabrication compounds under impact tensile loadings. *Materials (Basel)*, *12*.

36. Wang, L., Sanders, J. E., Gardner, D. J., & Han, Y. (2018). Effect of fused deposition modeling process parameters on the mechanical properties of a filled polypropylene. *Progress in Additive Manufacturing*, *4*.
37. Lin, H., Shi, L., & Wang, D. (2015). A rapid and intelligent designing technique for patient-specific and 3D-printed orthopedic cast. *3D Printing in Medicine*, *2*, 4.
38. Deng, X., Zeng, Z., Peng, B., Yan, S., & Ke, W. (2018). Mechanical properties optimization of poly-ether-ether-ketone via fused deposition modeling. *Materials (Basel)*, *11*.
39. Gu, X., Sun, X., Sun, Y., Wang, J., Liu, Y., Yu, K., Wang, Y., & Zhou, Y. (2020). Bioinspired modifications of PEEK implants for bone tissue engineering. *Frontiers in Bioengineering and Biotechnology*, *8*, 631616.
40. Kang, J., Zhang, J., Zheng, J., Wang, L., Li, D., & Liu, S. (2021). 3D-printed PEEK implant for mandibular defects repair–A new method. *Journal of the Mechanical Behavior of Biomedical Materials*, *116*, 104335.
41. Kessler, A., Hickel, R., & Reymus, M. (2020). 3D printing in dentistry—State of the art. *Operative Dentistry*, *45*.
42. Vasamsetty, P., Tejaswini, P., Kukkala, D., Singamshetty, M., & Gajula, S. (2020). 3D printing in dentistry–Exploring the new horizons. *Materials Today: Proceedings*, *26*.
43. Mai, H. N., Hyun, D. C., Park, J. H., Kim, D. Y., Lee, S. M., & Lee, D. H. (2020). Antibacterial drug-release polydimethylsiloxane coating for 3D-printing dental polymer: Surface alterations and antimicrobial effects. *Pharmaceuticals (Basel)*, *13*.
44. Sharma, D., Saha, S., & Satapathy, B. K. (2021). Recent advances in polymer scaffolds for biomedical applications. *Journal of Biomaterials Science, Polymer Edition*, 1–49.
45. Cheah, C. M., Chua, C. K., Leong, K. F., & Chua, S. W. (2003). Development of a tissue engineering scaffold structure library for rapid prototyping. Part 1: Investigation and classification. *The International Journal of Advanced Manufacturing Technology*, *21*.
46. Cheah, C. M., Chua, C. K., Leong, K. F., & Chua, S. W. (2003). Development of a tissue engineering scaffold structure library for rapid prototyping. Part 2: Parametric library and assembly program. *The International Journal of Advanced Manufacturing Technology*, *21*, 302–331.
47. Cheah, C. M., Chua, C. K., Leong, K. F., Cheong, C. H., & Naing, M. W. (2004). Automatic algorithm for generating complex polyhedral scaffold structures for tissue engineering. *Tissue Engineering*, *10*.
48. Swennen, G. R. J., Pottel, L., & Haers, P. E. (2020). Custom-made 3D-printed face masks in case of pandemic crisis situations with a lack of commercially available FFP2/3 masks. *International Journal of Oral and Maxillofacial Surgery*, *49*, 673–677.
49. Profili, R. J., Dubois, É., Groenhuis, V., & Hof, L. (2021). Use of 3D printed connectors to redesign full face snorkeling masks in the COVID-19 era: A preliminary technical case-study. *Annals of 3D Printed Medicine*, *3*, 100023.
50. Rubio-Perez, I., & Diaz Lantada, A. (2020). Surgical planning of sacral nerve stimulation procedure in presence of sacral anomalies by using personalized polymeric prototypes obtained with additive manufacturing techniques. *Polymers (Basel)*, *12*.

51. Vukicevic, M., Mosadegh, B., Min, J. K., & Little, S. H. (2017). Cardiac 3D printing and its future directions. *JACC: Cardiovascular Imaging*, *10*, 171–184.
52. Farooqi, K. M., Lengua, C. G., Weinberg, A. D., Nielsen, J. C., & Sanz, J. (2016). Blood pool segmentation results in superior virtual cardiac models than myocardial segmentation for 3D printing. *Pediatric Cardiology*, *37*, 1028–1036.
53. Anderson, J. R., Thompson, W. L., Alkattan, A. K., Diaz, O., Klucznik, R., Zhang, Y. J., Britz, G. W., Grossman, R. G., & Karmonik, C. (2016). Three-dimensional printing of anatomically accurate, patient-specific intracranial aneurysm models. *Journal of Neurointerventional Surgery*, *8*, 517–520.
54. Wake, N., Chandarana, H., Huang, W. C., Taneja, S. S., & Rosenkrantz, A. B. (2016). Application of anatomically accurate, patient-specific 3D printed models from MRI data in urological oncology. *Clinical Radiology*, *71*, 610–614.
55. Bernhard, J. C., Isotani, S., Matsugasumi, T., Duddalwar, V., Hung, A. J., Suer, E., Baco, E., Satkunasivam, R., Djaladat, H., Metcalfe, C., Hu, B., Wong, K., Park, D., Nguyen, M., Hwang, D., Bazargani, S. T., de Castro Abreu, A. L., Aron, M., Ukimura, O., & Gill, I. S. (2016). Personalized 3D printed model of kidney and tumor anatomy: A useful tool for patient education. *World Journal of Urology*, *34*, 337–345.
56. Palo, M., Hollander, J., Suominen, J., Yliruusi, J., & Sandler, N. (2017). 3D printed drug delivery devices: Perspectives and technical challenges. *Expert Review of Medical Devices*, *14*, 685–696.
57. Economidou, S. N., Lamprou, D. A., & Douroumis, D. (2018). 3D printing applications for transdermal drug delivery. *International Journal of Pharmaceutics*, *544*, 415–424.
58. 3D Print Exchange. National Institutes of Health. (2014). http://3dprint.nih.gov (accessed on 4th July 2025).
59. Hoy, M. B. (2013). 3D printing: Making things at the library. *Medical Reference Services Quarterly*, *32*, 94–99.
60. Di Prima, M., Coburn, J., Hwang, D., Kelly, J., Khairuzzaman, A., & Ricles, L. (2016). Additively manufactured medical products–The FDA perspective. *3D Printing in Medicine*, *2*.

CHAPTER 3

Biodegradable Polymers Used in Drug Delivery

MARIA WASIM,* ANEELA SABIR, MUHAMMAD SHAFIQ, and RAFI ULLAH KHAN

Institute of Polymer and Textile Engineering, University of the Punjab, Lahore, Pakistan

*Corresponding author

ABSTRACT

Utilization of biodegradable polymers, mainly in the medical field, has been extensive owing to their compatible and degradable nature. The classification of biodegradable polymers consists of natural and synthetic polymers. Meanwhile, both synthetic and natural polymers are employed for drug delivery, and a few of them have been successfully developed for clinical applicability. This chapter mainly focuses on biodegradable polymers and their prime characteristics that are primarily responsible for their applicability in drug delivery applications. Furthermore, advanced methods for nano- or micro-based synthesis enable the advancement of a wide range of biodegradable polymers, primarily in the drug delivery field.

3.1 INTRODUCTION

The expansion of a variety of biodegradable polymers for applications in drug delivery has been substantial, but hurdles persist for scientists who anticipate the production of effective drug release systems while escaping the toxicological and pharmacological influences from the

Polymer Applications in Medicine: Revolutionizing Treatment and Therapeutics.
Mohd. Imran Ahamed, Faheem Ahmad, and Ishaat M. Khan (Eds.)

DOI: 10.1201/9781779640871-3

polymeric matrix. This has ensured plentiful synthetic substitutes for polymeric biomaterials with *in vivo* bioactivity. Hitherto, with progressive hybrid technology, pharmaceutical researchers are now reconnoitering genetically modified polymeric materials. A key therapeutic attribute of biologically degradable polymeric materials to be used in advanced drug release is the schematic degradation phenomenon into monomeric forms or oligomers. Drug carriers composed of biodegradable materials are designed to deliver drugs and then usually degrade via hydrolysis or other means for clearance. However, the applicability of biologically degradable polymeric materials for drug release systems is not widely employed, partially due to the fear of systemic retention and the inability to eradicate the polymer from the body, commonly designated as macromolecular syndrome [1–5]. Within the cellular context, the residence period of the polymer has been a subject of concern regarding biocompatibility and potential long-term toxic influence; accordingly, biocompatibility remains a major issue of concern for sustained drug delivery. Consequently, there are various drug delivery applications for which polymers that are biocompatible and biodegradable in nature are included, based on the fundamental principle of controlled drug delivery via controlled polymeric degradation phenomena. This chapter will focus on the major synthetic and recombinant systems of biodegradable polymers, with comprehensive design, synthesis, degradation, and existing standing in the literature.

3.2 BIODEGRADABLE POLYMERS

They are termed as polymers that have the ability to break down within a restricted time period in the body system and are fabricated to provide temporary support. In the year 2001, the predicted consumption of 68 million kg/year of biodegradable polymers was reported in the field of tissue engineering and biomedical devices [6]. They can either exist in nature or be synthesized. The preference for synthetic polymers over natural ones offers numerous benefits. Primarily, synthetic biodegradable polymers can be fabricated through procedures that can yield the same results with the same formulation every time. They can have infinite availability and can offer a wide range of flexibility over physiochemical and mechanical characteristics that can be altered based on their application.

The most commonly employed synthetic biodegradable polymers belong to the polyester family, which may include Poly Glycolic Acid (PGA) and Poly Lactic Acid (PLA) and their copolymers, like PGLA [7]. The most commonly employed cell and drug delivery systems (DDS) have been manufactured using biodegradable polymers.

3.2.1 GENERAL POLYMER CHARACTERISTICS

Such polymers that can degrade could undergo hydrolysis *in vivo* and are normally categorized on the basis of the source from which they are obtained: synthetic or natural. Generally employed polymers are α-hydroxy acids, natural sugars (chitosan), poly(anhydride), and many other types. The synthetic-based polymers are more preferred in tissue engineering or drug release systems, as the variation is less likely to differ in various batches in contrast to degradable polymers obtained from nature [8]. Polymers can also be made degradable via the incorporation of alterable anhydride, ester, and amide linkages that are vulnerable to degradation phenomena through hydrolytic or enzymatic cleavage reactions. These can be used to make polymers that can degrade. In order to study the breakdown of chemical bonds (scission) of polymeric chains, drug release from biodegradable polymers can be controlled by:

- Breakdown of polymeric bonds present onto the surface or within bulk of polymeric matrix.
- Surface erosion of polymer.
- Dissipation of corporally entwined drug.

Though the delivery of drugs is basically the synchronized amalgamation of all three factors [9]. To overall design the biodegradable polymer, monomer chemistry plays a vital role, as polymer breakdown to monomeric units and its biocompatibility and toxicity can affect the body system. The number of monomeric units can be described by the degree of polymerization, which is normally $>$ 100 for high molecular weight polymers [10]. Several parameters like glass transition temperature (Tg), crystallinity, solubility, and molecular weight can alter the rate of drug release, and a thorough understanding of these factors can affect the polymeric matrix characteristics, which is vital to progress biodegradation and release phenomena.

3.2.2 CRYSTALLINITY OF POLYMER

Polymers are composed of partially aligned polymeric chains in their structure that can be attributed to polymer crystallinity, influencing the physico-chemical properties of the polymer. It basically designates the degree of crystallinity within the polymer matrix in connection to amorphous areas. It is one of the significant concepts in drug delivery, as only the amorphous areas have permeability and are hence accessible to molecules of water [11]. Several factors that are dependent on this property are swelling phenomena, mechanical strength, hydrolytic activity, and the rate of biodegradation. When polymer chains have a stereoregular nature (regular monomeric repetition), linear polymeric chains are arranged into a crystallite structure [12]. Polymers can never reach 100% crystallinity, so they always have a semi-crystalline nature. Crystallinity can be detected via the X-ray diffraction (XRD) process, a vital feature as it may alter the rate of release of drugs from polymers. It can be heavily influenced by the orientation and size of polymeric chains. Slow drug release is studied in the case of high crystallinity of low molecular weight polymers. On the other hand, at high molecular weight, crystallinity has very low influence on drug release as porosity is higher [10].

3.2.3 GLASS TRANSITION TEMPERATURE

The class of polymer and operating temperature determine whether the amorphous area acts like a rubbery material or a glassy material. This factor is mostly dependent on the glass transition temperature (Tg), which can be characterized via differential scanning calorimetry (DSC) [10]. Below the range of Tg, the polymer exists in a glass-like state (has restricted mobility and a lower rate of diffusion). While above the Tg, the polymer behaves like rubber, promoting the mass transfer rate of molecules of water and drugs through the polymer matrix [13]. For the successful fabrication of biodegradable polymers for drug release systems, an equilibrium should be present between the amorphous and crystalline states, as these factors contribute to a direct influence on the mechanical strength and the rate at which the drug is released. Due to these circumstances, polymeric nanoparticles can also be prepared from copolymers composed of both hydrophilic and hydrophobic parts, making physical characteristics like the rate of drug release more foreseeable [14]. The glass transition temperature of polymers like PLGA declines with the increment of the content of lactide monomer and molecular weight; numerous studies have suggested the influence of glass transition temperature on the rate of drug release [15–17].

3.2.4 HYDROPHILIC AND HYDROPHOBIC CHARACTER

The fundamental notion for the design of biodegradable polymers for drug release systems is solubility. It is governed by the chemical structure, its nature, and the degree of crystallinity present in the polymer matrix. The hydrophobic character of polymers usually rises with molecular weight and branching of the backbone structure, resulting in water-soluble polymers [18]. When hydrophobic polymers are employed for drug release systems, they are governed by surface erosion phenomena. While the equilibrium between hydrophilic and hydrophobic parts in the polymer matrix results in degradation occurring from within the bulk of the polymer [19].

In the case of micro or macroscale polymeric drug release systems, the degree of hydrophilic character in the polymer matrix is vital. Even though the physical features at the nanoscale, such as a high surface-to-volume ratio, reduce the stability of polymer colloids in the aqueous phase, a variety of hydrophobic polymers can still be applied [20]. Moreover, the mixing of hydrophilic and hydrophobic polymers can enhance pore generation, ultimately increasing degradation phenomena and its rate along with the discharge of drugs. The constitution of the polymer is also vital for its solubility phenomena. For instance, an increment in the glycolic acid part in the case of PLGA causes an increase in hydrophilic character, thus resulting in a higher rate of degradation [21]. The solubility of the monomer is consequently a critical feature for the drug release rate from the polymer system [22].

3.2.5 MOLECULAR WEIGHT OF POLYMER

Most of the physical characteristics, such as solubility, crystallinity, Tg, viscosity, mechanical strength, and rate of degradation, are connected to the molecular weight of the polymer. The low molecular weight causes a faster rate of degradation [12]. The drug release rate from biodegradable polymers is interconnected with their mechanical strength. A higher molecular weight of polymers yields a low modulus of elasticity while producing a non-deformable matrix that hinders the numerical figure of the formation of pore-creating channels. In contrast, a lower molecular weight of polymers yields a high modulus of elasticity, thus generating a deformable matrix and creating expandable pores as a consequence of osmotic pressure [23].

3.3 NATURALLY OCCURRING BIODEGRADABLE POLYMERS

Most of the biodegradable polymers that are present in nature are widely employed in the drug delivery field, owing to their abundance in nature and biocompatibility. They mostly include protein-based polymers that may consist of gelatin, collagen, albumin, and polysaccharides (alginate, hyaluronic acid, chitosan, carrageenan, agarose, dextran, and cyclodextrins) [24]. Specifically, nature-based polysaccharides have been extensively employed for tissue engineering and the design of bio scaffolds, along with the fabrication of nanoparticles for drug release. Even though they have high biodegradability, the restriction of natural polymers is the batch-to-batch inconsistency and broader range of molecular weight distributions, thus making them less favorable than synthetic ones, as the latter have high reproducibility and flexibility. The most commonly employed polysaccharide polymers are hyaluronic acid (HA) and chitosan.

3.3.1 CHITOSAN

Chitosan is considered one of the fundamental polysaccharides with a broad range of applicability, mainly acquired naturally from the exoskeletons of crustaceans (Figure 3.1) [25]. The deacetylation of chitin yields the random recurring entities of D-glucosamine and N-acetyl glucosamine. The degree of deacetylation is associated with the degradation and crystallinity of chitosan [26]. Owing to its crystalline nature, chitosan does not solubilize in water but does so in dilute acidic solutions before use. One of the applications is in the development of oral drug release systems [27, 28]. It is further broken down via lysozyme. The remaining chitosan with a low degree of acetylation can persist *in vivo* for multiple months [29]. The breakdown of chitosan may also be augmented by disordering substantial linkages of H-bonding through the addition of large side chains. The most noteworthy application of chitosan is in healing and wound dressing due to its antibacterial and anti-inflammatory properties [30], gene delivery (as it consists of a positive charge) [31], delivery of oral drugs [32], and pulmonary drug release because of its muco-adhesive characteristics [33]. The versatility with which the side chains can be altered and deacetylated, along with its ability to blend with several polymers, makes chitosan a flexible bioactive polymer [34].

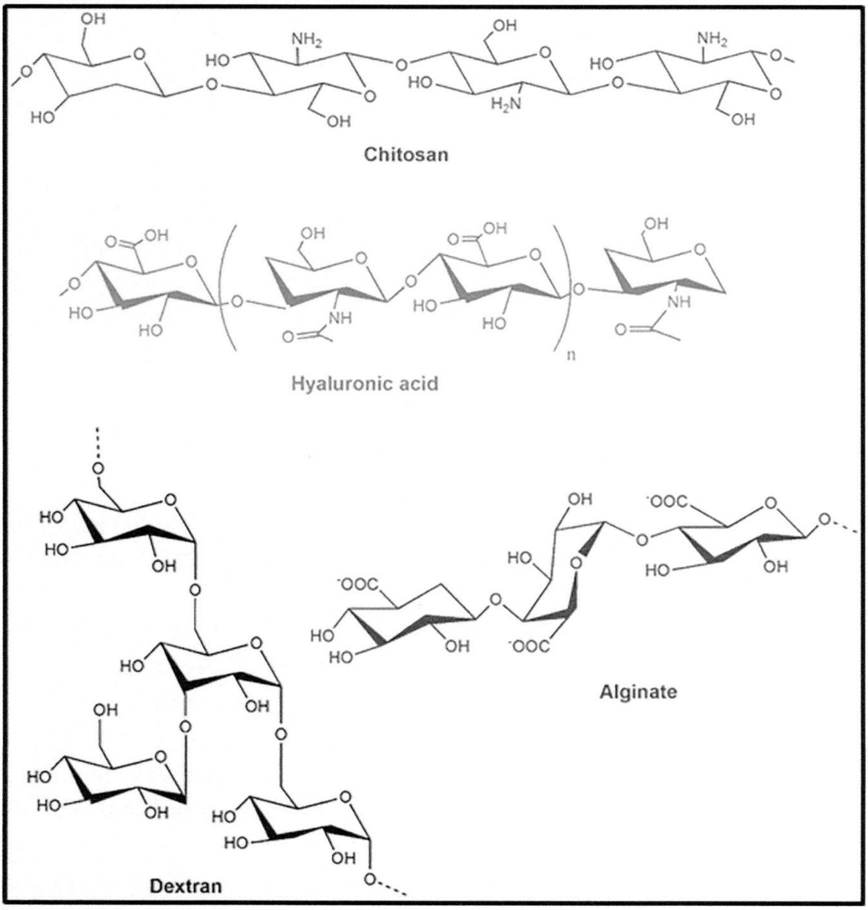

FIGURE 3.1 Chemical structures of various biodegradable polymers.

3.3.2 HYALURONIC ACID-BASED POLYMERS

HA is the linear polysaccharide polymer that exists naturally, consisting of D-glucuronic acid and N-acetyl-D-glucosamine disaccharide (Figure 3.1) [35]. The reason for HA to be considered to have a wide range of applications is its biocompatibility, biodegradability, non-toxic nature, and non-immunogenicity. Moreover, it is employed for tissue engineering, drug release systems, and surgical applications [36]. For the last few decades, HA has been used for the development of a variety of drugs or biologic conjugates and hydrogels for drug release systems. Bioconjugation of HA to therapeutics enhances drug solubility, pharmacokinetics, and clearance from the body system [37]. The value of the acid dissociation constant (pKa) for carboxyl groups lies in the range of three to four, creating a negative charge on the polymer at pH 7 [38]. Consequently, HA has high hydrophilicity because of its capability to absorb water and can enlarge 1000 times its original volume, leading to the formation of a loose hydrated network [38]. These characteristics of HA enable it to be a striking material for hydrogel preparation employed for drug release systems. Moreover, due to its intrinsic targeting capability, it can selectively intermingle with the CD44 receptor, also called hyaluronan receptors, for endocytosis. It is mainly employed for cancer treatment by selectively targeting cancer cells [39].

3.3.3 HYDROXYPROPYL-METHYLCELLULOSE

Hydroxypropyl-methylcellulose (HPMC) has gained worldwide attention for drug release via the oral pathway owing to its hydrophilic nature. Due to this property, it can retain water, thus having remarkable swelling capability and surface characteristics [40]. The swelling nature of HPMC can greatly affect the drug release phenomena. As HPMC interacts with the fluids of the body, chains of the polymer tend to relax; consequently, volume extension may lead to the diffusion of the drug into the fluid media. Moreover, it has been studied that HPMC has the ability to adhere to surfaces/substrates via the adsorption process of drugs or biomolecules [41]. Particularly, the cellulose ether that has methoxy or hydroxypropyl functional groups can simply adhere to the hydrophobic surfaces of drugs. In several drugs having solid dispersions, HPMC has been used to adjust drug release.

3.3.4 ALGINATES

Alginates are types of polysaccharides that are acquired naturally from seaweeds. Structurally, they are composed of a linear arrangement of α-L-guluronic acid and β-D-mannuronic acid chains via (1–4) covalent links (Figure 3.1). Owing to their anionic nature, they have the capability to form microparticles or microcapsules when multivalent, especially divalent cations such as Ca^{2+}, are added [41]. Several properties of alginate microcapsules, like muco-adhesiveness and biocompatibility, ensure their applicability in the field of biomedicine [33]. They have also been utilized for the advancement of controlled drug release systems, primarily for protein release or small molecules [42]. Additionally, they are used for the advancement of scaffolds, mostly for organ or tissue regeneration [43]. Even though alginates are not considered immunogenic by nature, they are acquired naturally, thus contaminations of proteins are common. Advanced studies have depicted that the immunogenic nature of alginates can be reduced by eradicating the residual protein [44].

3.3.5 DEXTRAN

They are branched polysaccharides that are composed of α-D-glucopyranosyl straight chain units and branches at α-1,3 linkages (Figure 3.1). Their remarkable hydrophilic character and appropriate degradation methods enable a wide range of uses for this polymer. It has been extensively studied as a core material for the development of controlled and sustained drug or biomolecule release systems [45].

3.3.6 GELATIN

Gelatin is a protein by nature, mostly present as a constituent of connective tissues, bone, and skin. It can be acquired by the denaturation of collagen in a controlled way. Because of its water solubility, biocompatibility, biodegradability, and non-toxicity, it has a variety of uses in the pharmaceutical and medical fields [33]. Furthermore, the variety of functional groups present in the gelatin structure can expedite the formation of chemical derivatives [34]. For the controlled or sustained release of hydrophobic-based drugs, macromolecules such as proteins and gelatin have shown tremendous success [46]. These methods have some limitations that may include poor mechanical strength. Conversely, the integration of cross-linkers such as glutaraldehyde facilitates improved stability and shape in gelatin-involved designs. The extent of cross-linking can influence the erosion and swelling phenomena of gelatin-based media during discharge inside the media. It can promote various release profiles of encapsulated drugs [47].

3.4 SYNTHETIC BIODEGRADABLE POLYMERS

3.4.1 POLYESTER AND POLYETHER-BASED POLYMERS

Synthetic polymers, mostly polyester, are widely used for the delivery of drugs, proteins, or any bio-based molecules. As time progresses, PGA, poly lactic acid (PLA), and their copolymerization product PLGA (Figure 3.2 a) have developed along with other distinguished polymers for the advancement of different carrier systems. Various forms of PLGA can be acquired depending on the relevant concentration of lactic and glycolic acid employed during the polymerization step. PLGA can be available in crystalline or amorphous forms, and it is totally dependent on the structure of the block and the molar concentration of the copolymer. One of the foremost characteristics of PLGA is the Tg, which exists in the range of 40–60°C. It degrades in the presence of water via the cleavage of ester links by the hydrolysis process, so the polymers that have their ends capped take a longer duration for half-life degradation [48]. Microspheres of PLGA may release antigens for various days to weeks or months via continuous or unsteady/pulsatile kinetics [49]. As studied, pulsatile release of antigens is designed by influencing the polymer properties that may mimic mandatory booster dosages in most non-live vaccines [50]. Moreover, PLGA microspheres can promote the stimulation of immune responses as they are recognized and consumed by dendritic cells and macrophages [51].

Polyethylene oxide (PEO) or Polyethylene glycol (PEG) are polyether-based polymer, named based on their molar mass. PEG consists of oligomers and polymers that have MW < 20,000 g/mol, on the other hand PEO holds polymers > 20,000 g/mol. PEG exist in three diverse conformations which are:

- Branched PEG that is composed of small number of PEG chains (around 3–10) that are adhered to central chain.
- Star shaped PEG consist of higher number of PEG chains (around 10–100) adhered to central structure.
- Comb shaped structure of PEG composed of various PEG chains connected against the polymeric support [52].

Figure 3.2 b represent the star polymer structure (hydroxyl- terminated 6 arm PEO).

Block copolymerization of PEG and PLA is termed as the poly (lactic acid) PEG (PELA) offer stability of protein along with the enhanced drug or protein loading efficacy. PEG constituent of PELA provides the biocompatibility. PELA block copolymer has developed as a suitable contender for the advancement of controlled discharge system due to their biocompatibility and biodegradability [53].

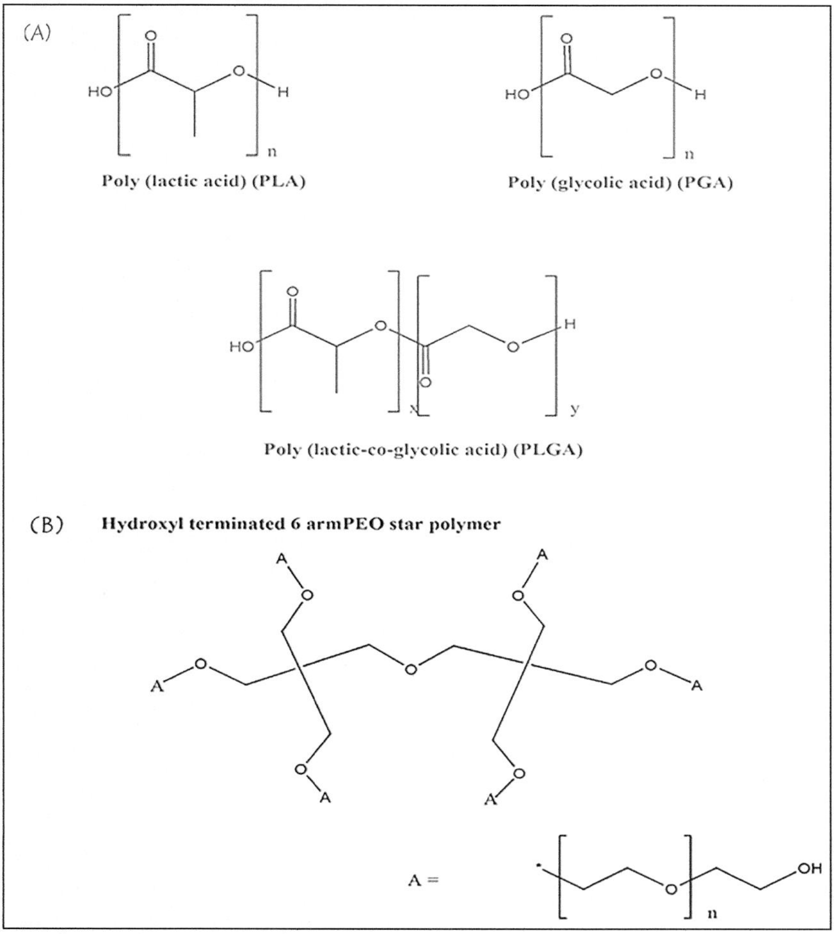

FIGURE 3.2 (a) Structure of PLA, PGA and their copolymerization product PLGA, here "n" characterizes No of monomeric unit existing in PLA and PGA; In PLGA, 'x' and 'y' signifies No of monomeric units of PLA and PGA, respectively. (b) Structural form of hydroxyl-terminated 6-arm PEO star shaped polymer.

Due to the amphiphilic nature, PEO-PPO block copolymer tends to aggregate in the presence of water, thus facilitating the formation of stable micelles in aqueous media. Such polymers are extensively used as hydro stabilizers for the increase of solubility of poorly water-soluble drugs [54]. Another ability of soluble block copolymers is to assemble themselves into supramolecular structures; these have been widely studied for drug, protein, and nucleic acid delivery. Such materials can facilitate effective drug targeting and controlled release profiles via impersonating biological transport systems [55]. A schematic display of self-assembled ligand-adhered block copolymers along with drugs or bio-based molecules and the consequent formation of micelles [56] is depicted in Figure 3.3.

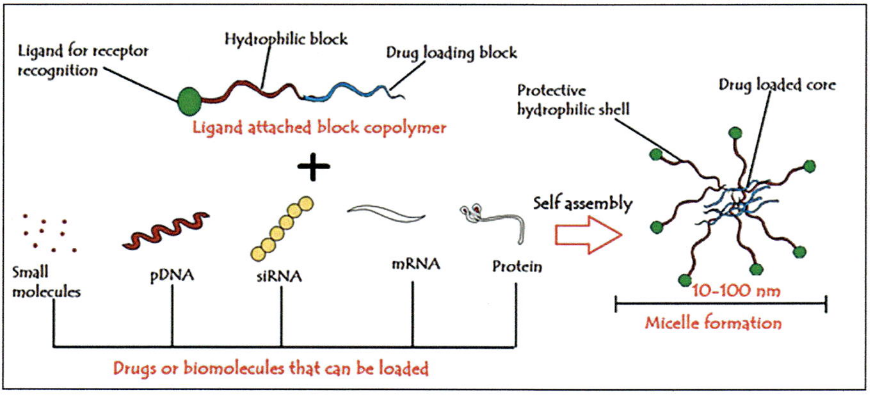

FIGURE 3.3 Self-assembled structure and formation of micelle adhered ligand and drug consisting block copolymers.

3.4.2 POLY (E-CAPROLACTONE) (PCL)

It is a type of polyester that is acquired via the ring-opening type of polymerization reaction of ε-caprolactone via metal alkoxides (tin octoate) – catalyst [56]. Attributable to its awfully sluggish degradation in physiological fluids, it has expanded its use in the advancement of implantable drug release systems [57] as well as a scaffold matrix media in tissue engineering [29]. In contrast, the sluggish rate of degradation and poor water solubility constrict its use to be in particulate delivery systems [58]. Though the incorporation of block copolymers enhances the rate of degradation [59]. Hydrophilic-based polymers can also be combined with a hydrophobic part (PCL) for the development of micelles. The ratio of polymer in the PCL block copolymer may be altered to acquire the required structure having diverse physio-mechanical characteristics [60].

3.4.3 POLYPHOSPHAZENE

The polymer consists of phosphorus atoms connected to nitrogen atoms via alternate double-single bonds [61]. It has a unique structure that is composed of two substitutional locations (two side groups attached to phosphorus) that allow the addition of side groups to influence the degradation [33]. Moreover, the coupling of targeting ligands to the polyphosphazene may alter the efficacy of the drug release profile [62]. Owing to its ease of modification, scientists have established controlled drug release systems such as insulin [63] and various other proteins [63]. Advanced research has revealed the immunologically assisted characteristics of polyphosphazene, and it can be used for the fabrication of particulate-based delivery systems for the release of antigenic materials [64].

3.4.4 BIODEGRADABLE BLOCK COPOLYMER

Such polymers are fabricated with the plan of *in vivo* demolition into suitable biocompatible monomer or oligomer units accepted as common metabolic types for clearance from the body system. Furthermore, the rate of degradation and possible side products formed during the process should be considered for the anticipated use in the drug delivery field. The purpose of biodegradable polymers is the continual transitory breakdown of the polymer, thus avoiding long-term habitation *in vivo* (common with the case of biostable implants) or intra-cellular isolation (macromolecular syndrome).

3.4.5 POLY ANHYDRIDES

Bucher and Slade in 1909 [65] stated the case of isophthalic acid and terephthalic acid anhydride synthesis employing a high temperature range. After that, advancements in the synthesis of anhydrides have been noted via various techniques that include dehydrochlorination, melt condensation, dehydrative coupling [66], and ring-opening polymerization [67].

Domb and Langer [68] developed a method for the synthesis of high molecular weight polyanhydride (PAH), using dehydration of diacid monomers to form mixed acetic anhydrides, followed by additional acetic anhydride reflux. Advanced synthesis of PAHs has led to two main alternate species, one having anhydride bonds in the polymeric backbone chain, while the second one has anhydrides as side chains.

PAHs are considered the most studied biodegradable polymeric class, owing to their low-cost nature, ease of synthesis, and flexibility of reaction. In the late 90s, Langer and his coworkers [69] recognized highly accountable anhydride linkages for hydrolytically biodegradable polymer DDS by exhibiting the zero-order discharge of cholic acid. Another study [69] demonstrated that the rate of degradation can be controlled via the hydrophobic groups present in the poly [bis(p-carboxyphenoy) alkane anhydrides]. The rising pH for the biocompatibility studies indicates that no corneal inflammation was observed for 6 weeks, while minor subcutaneous inflammation was shown for over 6 months.

3.5 PREPARATION OF DELIVERY DEVICES BY MEANS OF BIODEGRADABLE POLYMERS

Various procedures have been developed primarily for the fabrication of microscale and nanoscale delivery equipment, but the selection of procedure is mostly dependent on the nature of the biomolecules or drugs that have to be loaded, the physical and chemical properties of the polymer, the intended usage, and the needed time span of therapy [70, 71]. Procedures used for the encapsulation of biomolecules or drugs such as peptides, proteins, or any other cellular constituents have been discussed in further sections.

3.5.1 IONIC GELATION METHOD

For the release of micro or nano-formulations (such as microcapsules, microparticles, nanoparticles) through sustained or controlled methods, the ionic gelation method is often used. In this procedure, polyelectrolyte solutions (such as chitosan, carboxymethylcellulose, and alginates) are added drop by drop under constant agitation to the counterion solutions (e.g., $BaCl_2$, tripolyphosphate, $MgCl_2$, $CaCl_2$, pyrophosphate). Due to the presence of oppositely charged species, electrostatic interactions exist that subsequently lead to the formation of a cross-linked matrix that produces the anticipated controlled release of active constituents from the polymer media[72, 73]. The advantages of this method are the ease of operation and inexpensive nature, yet it has some limitations, such as the optimization of parameters [74]. Ji and coworkers used the ionic gelation procedure for the fabrication of nanoparticles by means of carboxymethyl small chain amylose and chitosan for the enclosure of the protein-based drug insulin. The fabricated nanoparticles exhibited more than 80% enclosure efficacy, and the model showed the sustained discharge of insulin [75].

3.5.2 SPRAY DRYING METHOD

This method comprises the fabrication of a water/oil/water emulsion by blending the organic solvent and aqueous phase, proceeding to the atomization and then vaporization of the resulting emulsion media in the presence of a jet stream of inert gas. The organic phase is composed of solvents like dichloromethane or acetone in which the polymer is soluble, while the aqueous phase consists of a dispersion of the drug [76]. By means of this method, particles have a lean size distribution and high encapsulation efficacy [76]. Moreover, this method is prompt, effortlessly scalable, requires mild conditions, and the solubility factor of the drug or any other additives added does not influence this method [70]. Arrighi and coworkers fabricated polyclonal immunoglobulin G encapsulated PLGA microparticles via the spray drying method for sustained release. The microparticles produced have a mean diameter of $< 10\mu m$, and the encapsulation efficacy was found to be greater than 85% [77]. For the last few decades, the nano spray drying method has been gaining worldwide attention; some modifications in technology have been made for the mass-scale production of nanoparticles [78].

3.5.3 COACERVATION (PHASE SEPARATION) METHOD

The coacervation method involves the fabrication of the super dense liquid phase from the aqueous dispersion of a macromolecular drug solution into the organic solvent solution of a polymer. Incorporation of the organic non-solvent into the arrangement with continuous stirring can gradually eradicate the polymeric solvent, leading to phase separation and the creation of microspheres (coacervate drops) that coat the drug [79]. In this case, the concentration of the polymer is critical, as a high concentration can cause swift phase separation that leads to the formation of incomplete encapsulation of the drug. The most common problem seen in this method is agglomeration, due to the absence of an emulsion stabilizer [79]. Saravanan et al. encapsulated metronidazole hydrochloride, indomethacin, and diclofenac sodium via the coacervation procedure along with the use of pectin and alginate with gelatin. Indomethacin exhibited higher encapsulation efficacy compared to metronidazole hydrochloride and diclofenac sodium. The aggregation of microparticles has been reduced by the incorporation of sodium carboxymethyl cellulose. The fabricated microparticles show an *in vitro* sustained release profile. It was studied that the incorporation of alginate was preferable over pectin for the coacervation method with gelatin, owing to its ease of dispersion and small particle size [80].

3.5.4 SOLVENT EVAPORATION METHOD

It is the most often used method for the fabrication of nanoparticles and microparticles by means of a biodegradable method. Primarily, the polymeric solution should be volatile; thus, solvents like ethyl acetate, chloroform, and dichloromethane are employed for the preparation of the polymer solution. The drug is then incorporated into that solution. The addition of the polymer solution and dispersion into aqueous media consists of an emulsifying agent, and then the whole system is subjected to stirring for the development of an emulsion (oil in water). The evaporation of the organic solvent results in the formation of a suspension consisting of particles [71]. The size of the prepared particles is greatly influenced by the concentration or the types of stabilizers, temperature, polymeric concentration, stirring rate, and viscosity of both the aqueous and organic phases [81]. However, this method can be applied solely for lipid-soluble drugs, and upgrading is quite problematic [82]. Polymers that can be employed for the fabrication of particulate systems via the solvent evaporation method include PLA [83], PLGA [84], ethyl cellulose [85], poly(β-caprolactone) (PCL) [86], and so forth.

3.5.5 SALTING OUT METHOD

This is considered a modification of the emulsion method but with reduced usage of unsafe organic solvents and emulsifiers. A polymeric solution was formed in a miscible solvent like acetone, and then emulsification was done in aqueous media that comprises a salting-out agent, which may include sucrose, magnesium chloride, and calcium chloride. More dilution of the fabricated emulsion with aqueous media facilitates the motion of solvent particles to the aqueous media, causing the development of nanospheres [71]. This process may be utilized for heat-sensitive specimens, as such procedures do not require an elevated temperature range [86]. The procedure studied for the fabrication of drug or bio-based molecules consists of nano-based particles employing polymers like PLA [87], ethyl cellulose [88], and PLGA [88]. The salting-out method offers extraordinary efficacy and ease of upgrade probability; yet, it is solely restricted to lipophilic drugs, and the formation of nanoparticles requires numerous washings [89].

3.6 POLYMERIC-BASED DRUG DELIVERY SYSTEMS (DDS)

There are three distinct types of polymeric drug delivery systems: colloidal carriers (e.g., nano/microparticles, micelles, nano or microgels), hydrogels or implantable networks, and polymer-drug conjugates (PDCs) [58].

Sadly, there is no magic bullet for the successful delivery of a wide range of therapeutics. The choice of the drug release system is totally governed by the type of drug and the inherent characteristics of the drug delivery system. Furthermore, the section of the system regulates the loading capacity, duration of release, and the route best suited for administration. For any kind of polymer carrier, drug release is influenced by complex interactions between drug characteristics, polymer properties, and the environment (*in vivo* conditions) [13].

Depending on the mechanism of action, polymeric drug release systems can be categorized as solvent-activated systems, diffusion-controlled systems, chemically controlled systems, and externally activated or modulated systems. In the case of improved DDS, various mechanisms are intricate, even though one can be leading in contrast to the other [9].

Diffusion-based controlled systems can be further fractionated into matrix and reservoir systems. The reservoir system is established on the basis of a polymeric membrane that covers the core structure constituting the drug. The release of the drug is governed by the membrane of biodegradable nature. Mostly, polymers with non-biodegradable nature are employed in this system. In contrast, the matrix is the polymeric media that has the drug dispersed homogeneously. The release of the drug is controlled via erosion of the polymer, diffusion of the drug, or the combination of both [90]. Figure 3.4 represents the matrix and reservoir systems.

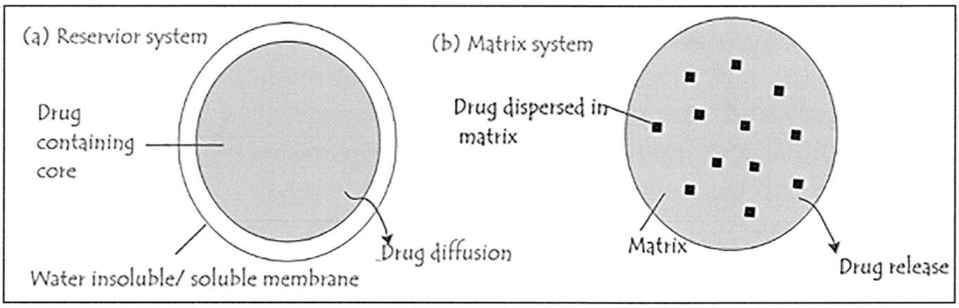

FIGURE 3.4 Pictorial illustration of reservoir (a) and matrix (b) systems.

Solvent-activated systems can be influenced by the osmosis and swelling processes. Osmosis-controlled systems depend on a device consisting of a semipermeable membrane that allows the flow of a solvent containing a drug or a simple solvent that flows in the direction of a cavity containing the drug. The pressure inside the cavity increases with the flow of the solvent, which allows the drug to flow through a small opening inside the cavity. The systems controlled by means of swelling depend on hydrophilic polymers that have cross-linking chains, allowing the absorption of water molecules without dissolving. The absorption of water facilitates the drug present in the system to diffuse towards the outside at a velocity determined by the amount of water moving into the polymeric media [43]. The scheme representing both the swelling and osmotically controlled systems is shown in Figure 3.5.

Chemically activated-based systems can be categorized further into pendant chain systems and biodegradable polymer systems. Both consist of biodegradation and erosion phenomena of polymeric media or membranes.

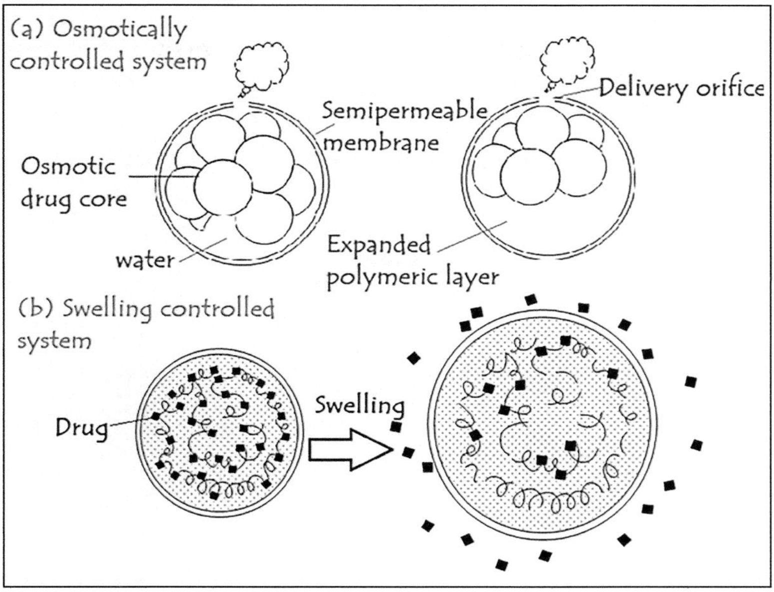

FIGURE 3.5 Pictorial illustration of osmotically (a) and swelling (b) controlled systems.

The chemical linkage of drug molecules to the polymeric backbone exists in the pendant chain system. Due to the presence of physiological fluid in the body, chemical hydrolysis or enzymatic bond breaking occurs with the drug release at a controlled rate. There can be a direct linkage of the drug to the polymer or by the presence of a spacer group. Various types of hydrolysable chemicals or biodegradable groups can be employed to adhere the drug to the polymer.

The conjugates of the drug and polymer normally hold a transport method that is accountable for guiding the polymeric chains to the targeted area (organ or tissue). In the case of biodegradable polymer systems, the controlled drug release rate encompasses biodegradable polymers that slowly disintegrate. The uniform dispersion of the drug into the polymeric media allows for the gradual release of it as the polymer erodes. Before the drug release, the time is considered as zero (t=0), when the drug is distributed into the polymeric media homogeneously. While at time t=t, partially the drug is released or the disintegration of the polymer occurs. In most cases of biodegradable polymer-based DDS, they follow this model [91]. The pictorial presentation of biodegradable polymer and pendant chain systems is shown in Figure 3.6.

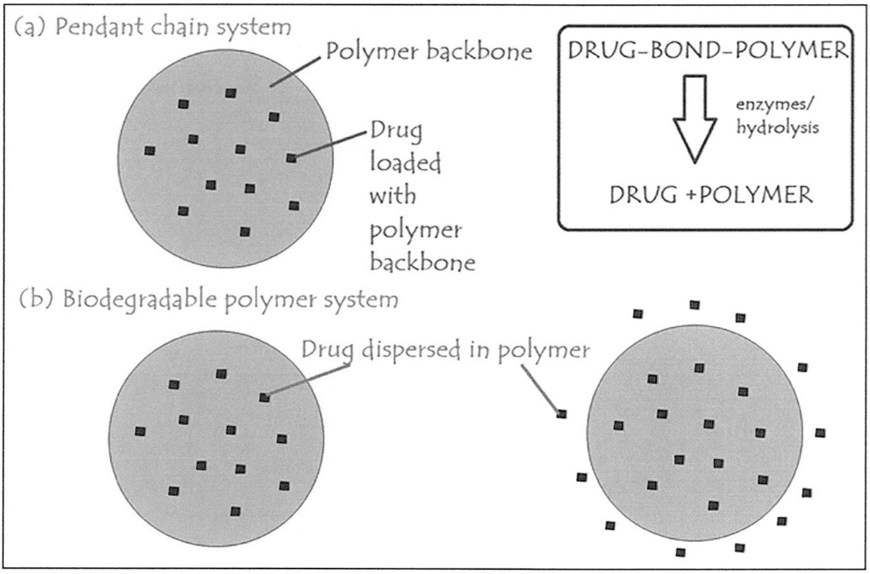

FIGURE 3.6 Pictorial illustration of (a) pendant chain and (b) biodegradable polymer systems.

3.7 POLYMER BIO-DEGRADATION AND EROSION

Erosion of polymer can be recounted as the mixture of both chemical erosion or biodegradation and physical erosion or dissolution. The diffusion of minor fragments (oligomers or monomers) results from chemical degradation (Figure 3.7).

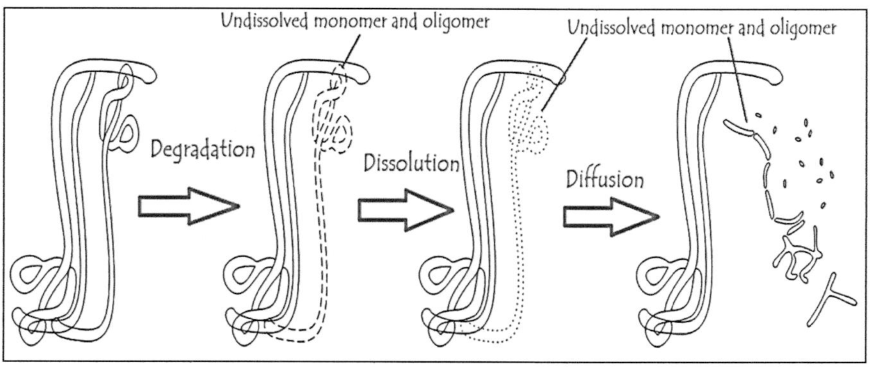

FIGURE 3.7 Schematic representation of polymer bio-degradation and erosion.

3.7.1 CHEMICAL EROSION

It is also termed biodegradation, which is the cleavage of polymeric chains chemically into minor fragments (i.e., oligomers) that occurs in polymeric media. The degradation can be an enzymatic or hydrolytic process. Even though the use of enzymes *in vivo* for biodegradable polymers is controversial, specifically in the case of parental conditions, enzymes are considered bulky in nature and cannot easily enter the drug delivery system. The probability that enzymes influence the rate of degradation of polymers at an advanced stage of *in vivo* degradation is more likely on the surface, not in the bulk of the drug delivery system [92].

In the 1980s, Heller elucidated three mechanisms of polymeric bio-erosion [93]. The first mechanism, also termed crosslinked degradation, mainly involves crosslinked macromolecules that are water-insoluble and constitute a hydrolytically unstable crosslinked network. Such polymers can be employed for the release of drugs that are sparingly soluble in water. The second mechanism (side chain degradation) involves macromolecules that are insoluble in water; they are solubilized via the protonation or ionization process of a pendant group without the breakdown of the backbone chain (Figure 3.8).

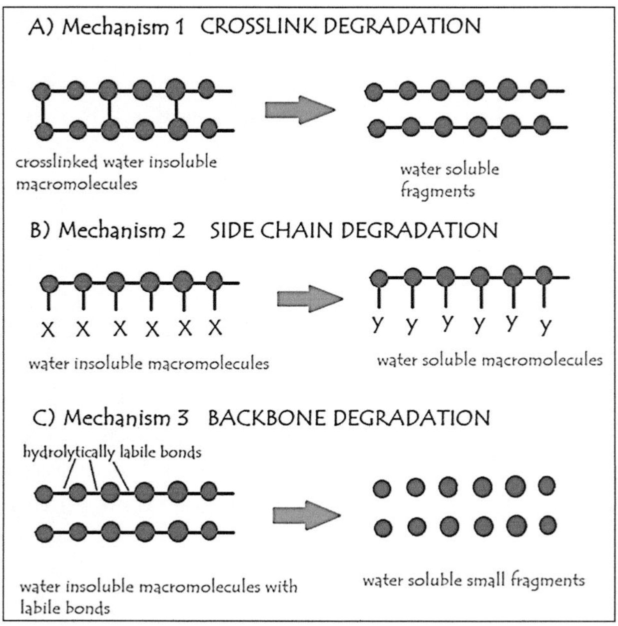

FIGURE 3.8 Pictorial illustration of three pathways of polymer breakdown: a) crosslink degradation, b) side chain degradation and c) backbone degradation.

The side chain cleavage (transformation) results in the creation of charged groups (polar). The third mechanism, also termed as backbone breakdown, states that hydrophobic macromolecules have hydrolytically unstable bonds that can easily be converted to minor soluble fragments via the cleavage of the main backbone chain, resulting in repeating units. This type of mechanism is most commonly observed in biodegradable synthetic polymers (Figure 3.8).

3.7.2 PHYSICAL EROSION

Physical erosion, also known as bio-erosion, can be categorized into two patterns: surface erosion and bulk erosion [94]. In the case of bulk erosion, the whole area of the polymer media is involved in enzymatic or chemical reactions; therefore, homogeneous erosion occurs throughout the entire polymer. Through bulk erosion, polymers degrade completely to their cross-section, exhibiting a nonlinear kinetic of erosion that is normally elucidated by a discontinuity. The mass of the device will remain constant for a substantial period of time throughout the course of its application.

In contrast, surface erosion comprises polymer degradation restricted only to its surface that is exposed to the reaction media. Thus, the erosion initiates from the exposed area and occurs layer by layer. The main benefit of this type of erosion in polymers is the predictability of the erosion process. Therefore, the drug dispersed homogeneously in such a media implant, whose surface is irregular over time, exhibits a constant drug release throughout the implant period.

3.8 FACTORS THAT AFFECTS POLYMER DEGRADATION RATE

Factors that affect the polymer degradation rate include the most common chemical factors such as the chemical stability of the bonds present among monomeric units, the hydrophobic character of the polymer, and the structural arrangement mainly of side groups and their steric effects. Significant physical factors involved are crystallinity and the production of fragments (autocatalytic), mostly in bulk eroding systems [95].

3.8.1 CHEMICAL FACTORS

The bonding present between the monomers of biodegradable-based synthetic polymers can be classified based on their stability during hydrolytic reactions [96]. Figure 3.9 (a) depicts the ortho-ester and anhydride links, which are less stable in contrast to the amide or ester bonds. Based on these inclinations, DDS based on polyorthoester or PAH erode via a surface erosion process due to rapid mass loss and a higher polymer hydrolysis rate in comparison to bulk erosion. In contrast, DDS based on polyester polymers undergo bulk erosion, as the penetration of water molecules is higher than the degradation rate [97].

The structure of the polymer has a significant influence on the arrangement and size of the side groups attached to the polymeric chain. Through the steric effect, side groups can lessen the hydrolysis reaction; that's why lactic acid in the case of PLA is more reactive than glycolic acid in PGA. The methyl group is much bulkier than a single atom of hydrogen (Figure 3.9 b) [98].

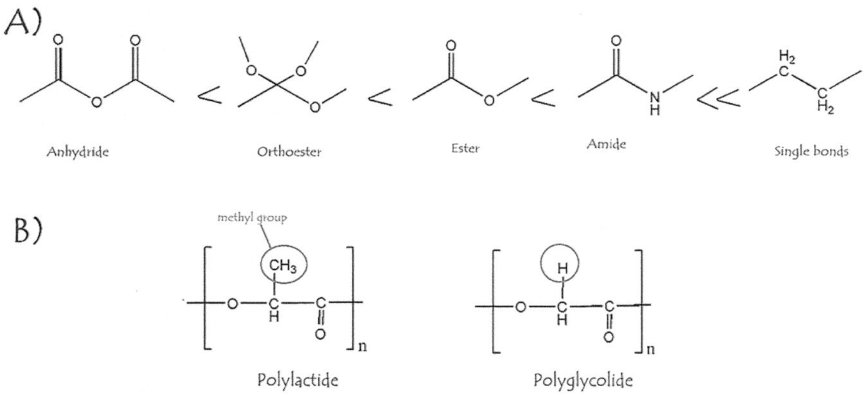

FIGURE 3.9 (a) Kind of chemical bonds and their stability against hydrolysis of the biodegradable synthetic polymers (b) Impact of local structure of the polymers on the hydrolysis rate on lactic acid unit in polylactide (PLA) versus glycolic acid unit in polyglycolide (PGA).

The vital concept of the design of biodegradable drug systems is the solubility of monomers. It has a great impact on the mechanism of erosion of polymers and the drug release rate. It mostly depends on the structure, composition, and degree of crystallinity present in the polymer. The use of the hydrophobic nature of the polymer in drug delivery causes the release of the drug via surface erosion. On the other hand, if there is an equilibrium between hydrophobic and hydrophilic groups in the polymer, degradation happens from within the bulk. Moreover, the addition of hydrophilic groups to hydrophobic polymers enhances the formation of pores that increase the rate of drug release and degradation of the polymer [22, 99].

3.8.2 PHYSICAL FACTORS

Throughout the hydrolytic reaction of biodegradable polymers, carboxylic end group byproducts are formed, and they are capable of facilitating ester hydrolysis. This process is more dominant in DDS where the agglomeration of byproducts occurs, similar to bulk erosion systems. As a result, a rapid rate of degradation happens in the polymeric media, in contrast to the surface, because of autocatalysis. The penetration of water molecules into the polymer media leads the way to the hydrolytic breakdown of ester bonds, and degradation occurs in the bulk matrix (STEP 1). The byproducts of degradation agglomerate in large amounts in the internal media (STEP 2). Byproducts present at the surface can diffuse out from the media, while agglomeration inside roots the spurt of internal degradation (STEP 3). As a result of these circumstances, a hollow structure is developed when the internal side is transformed into soluble oligomers that solubilize in water. Only amorphous polymers exhibit a hollow structure; crystalline polymers do not depict this as crystallization of byproducts occurs (STEP 4) [98, 100, 101].

Depending on the structural arrangements of monomeric units and side groups present along the macroradical chain, synthetic polymers can be categorized into semi-crystalline or amorphous polymers. The rate of degradation and physical characteristics depend on the degree of crystallinity of the polymer. It is well established that crystalline areas can hinder hydrolytic reactions in contrast to amorphous areas, as water molecules can enter amorphous areas easily [102].

3.9 CONCLUSION

During the last few decades, the significance of advanced drug delivery has multiplied, and substantial advancements have been made in the development of new technologies that are based on biodegradable polymers as drug carriers. The broad range of applicability of polymers for advanced drug delivery has been recognized, as the polymers propose distinctive characteristics that have not been achieved by any other kind of material. Polymers (macromolecules) are composed of lengthy chains that consist of varying functional groups, which can be easily blended with high or low molecular weight compounds and have flexibility in tailoring for a wide range of applications. Improving the therapeutic efficiency of drugs via the use of synthetic and natural biodegradable polymers is the prime aim of DDS. Future advancements of biodegradable polymers will be based on determining the macromolecules that not only have suitable physicochemical and mechanical characteristics but also possess distinctive biological characteristics.

KEYWORDS

- **biodegradable drug systems**
- **biodegradable polymers**
- **hyaluronic acid**
- **polyethylene glycol**
- **polymeric bio-erosion**
- **polymeric drug delivery systems**
- **protein-based polymers**

REFERENCES

1. Chen, V., et al. (1997). Particle deposition during membrane filtration of colloids: Transition between concentration polarization and cake formation. *Journal of Membrane Science*, *125*(1), 109–122.
2. Hu, X. J., et al. (2011). Adsorption of chromium (VI) by ethylenediamine-modified cross-linked magnetic chitosan resin: Isotherms, kinetics and thermodynamics. *Journal of Hazardous Materials*, *185*(1), 306–314.
3. Rajesha, B. J., et al. (2019). Effective composite membranes of cellulose acetate for removal of benzophenone-3. *Journal of Water Process Engineering*, *30*, 100419.
4. Criscuoli, A., & Figoli, A. (2018). Pressure-driven and thermally-driven membrane operations for the treatment of arsenic-contaminated waters: A comparison. *Journal of Hazardous Materials*, *370*.

5. Figoli, A., Criscuoli, A., & Hoinkis, J. (2010). Review of membrane processes for arsenic removal from drinking water: Challenges for safe water production. pp. 131–145.
6. Lalia, B. S., et al. (2013). A review on membrane fabrication: Structure, properties and performance relationship. *Desalination*, *326*, 77–95.
7. Ulbricht, M. (2006). Advanced functional polymer membranes. *Polymer*, *47*(7), 2217–2262.
8. Salehi, E., Daraei, P., & Arabi Shamsabadi, A. (2016). A review on chitosan-based adsorptive membranes. *Carbohydrate Polymers*, *152*, 419–432.
9. Liu, Y. L., Chen, W. H., & Chang, Y. H. (2009). Preparation and properties of chitosan/carbon nanotube nanocomposites using poly (styrene sulfonic acid)-modified CNTs. *Carbohydrate Polymers*, *76*(2), 232–238.
10. Ji, Y. L., et al. (2014). Fabrication of chitosan/PDMCHEA blend positively charged membranes with improved mechanical properties and high nanofiltration performances. *Desalination*, *357*.
11. Choi, H. S., et al. (2020). Development of Co-hemin MOF/chitosan composite based biosensor for rapid detection of lactose. *Journal of the Taiwan Institute of Chemical Engineers*, *113*, 1–7.
12. Rol, F., et al. (2019). Recent advances in surface-modified cellulose nanofibrils. *Progress in Polymer Science*, *88*, 241–264.
13. Radzyminska-Lenarcik, E., & Ulewicz, M. (2019). The application of polymer inclusion membranes based on CTA with 1-alkylimidazole for the separation of zinc (II) and manganese (II) ions from aqueous solutions. *Polymers*, *11*(2), 242.
14. Ritchie, S., et al. (1999). Surface modification of silica- and cellulose-based microfiltration membranes with functional polyamine acids for heavy metal sorption. *Langmuir*, *15*.
15. Ibrahim, Y., et al. (2019). Synthesis of super hydrophilic cellulose-alpha zirconium phosphate ion exchange membrane via surface coating for the removal of heavy metals from wastewater. *Science of the Total Environment*, *690*, 167–180.
16. Alnaief, M., Obaidat, R., & Mashaqbeh, H. (2018). Effect of processing parameters on preparation of carrageenan aerogel microparticles. *Carbohydrate Polymers*, *180*, 264–275.
17. Mola Ali Abasiyan, S., Dashbolaghi, F., & Mahdavinia, G. R. (2019). Chitosan cross-linked with κ-carrageenan to remove cadmium from water and soil systems. *Environmental Science and Pollution Research*, *26*(25), 26254–26264.
18. Campo, V. L., et al. (2009). Carrageenans: Biological properties, chemical modifications and structural analysis–A review. *Carbohydrate Polymers*, *77*(2), 167–180.
19. Piculell, L., Nilsson, S., & Ström, P. (1989). On the specificity of the binding of cations to carrageenans: Counterion N.M.R. spectroscopy in mixed carrageenan systems. *Carbohydrate Research*, *188*, 121–135.
20. Liew, J., et al. (2017). Synthesis and characterization of modified κ-carrageenan for enhanced proton conductivity as polymer electrolyte membrane. *PLOS ONE*, *12*, e0185313.
21. Nogueira, L. F. B., et al. (2016). Formation of carrageenan-$CaCO_3$ bioactive membranes. *Materials Science and Engineering: C*, *58*, 1–6.

22. Prasannan, A., et al. (2020). Robust underwater superoleophobic membranes with bio-inspired carrageenan/laponite multilayers for the effective removal of emulsions, metal ions, and organic dyes from wastewater. *Chemical Engineering Journal, 391*, 123585.
23. Wang, B., et al. (2018). Alginate-based composites for environmental applications: A critical review. *Critical Reviews in Environmental Science and Technology, 49*, 1–39.
24. Wang, M., et al. (2019). Efficient removal of heavy metal ions in wastewater by using a novel alginate-EDTA hybrid aerogel. *Applied Sciences, 9*(3), 547.
25. Wang, Z., et al. (2018). Bioavailability of wilforlide A in mice and its concentration determination using an HPLC-APCI-MS/MS method. *Journal of Chromatography B, 1090*, 65–72.
26. Lee, K. Y., & Mooney, D. J. (2012). Alginate: Properties and biomedical applications. *Progress in Polymer Science, 37*(1), 106–126.
27. Aburabie, J. H., Puspasari, T., & Peinemann, K. V. (2020). Alginate-based membranes: Paving the way for green organic solvent nanofiltration. *Journal of Membrane Science, 596*, 117615.
28. Dudek, G., & Turczyn, R. (2018). New type of alginate/chitosan microparticle membranes for highly efficient pervaporative dehydration of ethanol. *RSC Advances, 8*, 39567–39578.
29. Chen, J. H., et al. (2010). Cr (III) ionic imprinted polyvinyl alcohol/sodium alginate (PVA/SA) porous composite membranes for selective adsorption of Cr (III) ions. *Chemical Engineering Journal, 165*(2), 465–473.
30. Esmaeili, A., & Aghababai Beni, A. (2015). Novel membrane reactor design for heavy-metal removal by alginate nanoparticles. *Journal of Industrial and Engineering Chemistry, 26*, 122–128.
31. Googerdchian, F., Moheb, A., & Emadi, R. (2012). Lead sorption properties of nanohydroxyapatite–alginate composite adsorbents. *Chemical Engineering Journal, 200–202*, 471–479.
32. Kochameshki, M. G., et al. (2017). Grafting of diallyl dimethylammonium chloride on graphene oxide by RAFT polymerization for modification of nanocomposite polysulfide membranes using in water treatment. *Chemical Engineering Journal, 309*, 206–221.
33. Ghaemi, N., Zereshki, S., & Heidari, S. (2017). Removal of lead ions from water using PES-based nanocomposite membrane incorporated with polyaniline modified GO nanoparticles: Performance optimization by central composite design. *Process Safety and Environmental Protection, 111*, 475–490.
34. Gholami, A., et al. (2014). Preparation and characterization of polyvinyl chloride-based nanocomposite nanofiltration membrane modified by iron oxide nanoparticles for lead removal from water. *Journal of Industrial and Engineering Chemistry, 20*(4), 1517–1522.
35. Daraei, P., et al. (2012). Novel polyether sulfone nanocomposite membrane prepared by PANI/Fe_3O_4 nanoparticles with enhanced performance for Cu(II) removal from water. *Journal of Membrane Science, 415–416*, 250–259.
36. Hebbar, R. S., Isloor, A. M., & Ismail, A. F. (2014). Preparation and evaluation of heavy metal rejection properties of polyetherimide/porous activated bentonite clay nanocomposite membrane. *RSC Advances, 4*(88), 47240–47248.

37. Mukhopadhyay, M., et al. (2018). Removal of arsenic from aqueous media using zeolite/chitosan nanocomposite membrane. *Separation Science and Technology*, *54*, 1–7.
38. Gohari, R. J., et al. (2015). Arsenate removal from contaminated water by a highly adsorptive nanocomposite ultrafiltration membrane. *New Journal of Chemistry*, *39*(11), 8263–8272.
39. Zinadini, S., et al. (2014). Preparation of a novel antifouling mixed matrix PES membrane by embedding graphene oxide nanoplates. *Journal of Membrane Science*, *453*, 292–301.
40. Zhu, J., et al. (2015). Fabrication of a novel "loose" nanofiltration membrane by facile blending with chitosan–montmorillonite nanosheets for dyes purification. *Chemical Engineering Journal*, *265*, 184–193.
41. Wang, C., et al. (2017). Covalent organic framework modified polyamide nanofiltration membrane with enhanced performance for desalination. *Journal of Membrane Science*, *523*, 273–281.
42. Liu, F., Abed, M. R. M., & Li, K. (2011). Preparation and characterization of poly (vinylidene fluoride) (PVDF) based ultrafiltration membranes using nano γ-Al_2O_3. *Journal of Membrane Science*, *366*(1), 97–103.
43. Zhang, Z. B., et al. (2015). Layer-by-layer assembly of graphene oxide on polypropylene macroporous membranes via click chemistry to improve antibacterial and antifouling performance. *Applied Surface Science*, *332*, 300–307.
44. Li, Z., et al. (2011). Removal of arsenic from water using Fe-exchanged natural zeolite. *Journal of Hazardous Materials*, *187*(1), 318–323.
45. Khan, A. A. P., et al. (2016). Conventional surfactant-doped poly(o-anisidine)/GO nanocomposites for benzaldehyde chemical sensor development. *Journal of Sol-Gel Science and Technology*, *77*(2), 361–370.
46. An, D., et al. (2016). Separation performance of graphene oxide membrane in aqueous solution. *Industrial & Engineering Chemistry Research*, *55*(17), 4803–4810.
47. He, L., et al. (2015). Promoted water transport across graphene oxide–poly(amide) thin film composite membranes and their antibacterial activity. *Desalination*, *365*, 126–135.
48. Sophia, C., et al. (2016). Application of graphene-based materials for adsorption of pharmaceutical traces from water and wastewater–A review. *Desalination and Water Treatment*, *57*, 1–14.
49. Xia, S., et al. (2015). Preparation of graphene oxide modified polyamide thin film composite membranes with improved hydrophilicity for natural organic matter removal. *Chemical Engineering Journal*, *280*, 720–727.
50. Chang, X., et al. (2014). Exploring the synergetic effects of graphene oxide (GO) and polyvinylpyrrolidone (PVP) on poly (vinylidene fluoride) (PVDF) ultrafiltration membrane performance. *Applied Surface Science*, *316*, 537–548.
51. Zhang, Y., Zhang, S., & Chung, T. S. (2015). Nanometric graphene oxide framework membranes with enhanced heavy metal removal via nanofiltration. *Environmental Science & Technology*, *49*(16), 10235–10242.
52. Xu, Z., et al. (2014). Organ silane-functionalized graphene oxide for enhanced antifouling and mechanical properties of polyvinylidene fluoride ultrafiltration membranes. *Journal of Membrane Science*, *458*, 1–13.

53. Zhang, C., et al. (2017). Graphene oxide quantum dots incorporated into a thin film nanocomposite membrane with high flux and antifouling properties for low-pressure nanofiltration. *ACS Applied Materials & Interfaces*, *9*(12), 11082–11094.
54. Zhang, A., et al. (2017). *In situ* formation of copper nanoparticles in carboxylate chitosan layer: Preparation and characterization of surface modified TFC membrane with protein fouling resistance and long-lasting antibacterial properties. *Separation and Purification Technology*, *176*, 164–172.
55. Zhang, P., et al. (2017). Cross-linking to prepare composite graphene oxide-framework membranes with high-flux for dyes and heavy metal ions removal. *Chemical Engineering Journal*, *322*, 657–666.
56. Abdi, G., et al. (2018). Removal of dye and heavy metal ion using a novel synthetic polyethersulfone nanofiltration membrane modified by magnetic graphene oxide/metformin hybrid. *Journal of Membrane Science*, *552*, 326–335.
57. Wei, Y., et al. (2018). Multilayered graphene oxide membranes for water treatment: A review. *Carbon*, *139*, 964–981.
58. Chang, C., et al. (2010). Superabsorbent hydrogels based on cellulose for smart swelling and controllable delivery. *European Polymer Journal*, *46*(1), 92–100.
59. Pourjavadi, A., Ayyari, M., & Amini-Fazl, M. S. (2008). Taguchi optimized synthesis of collagen-g-poly (acrylic acid)/kaolin composite superabsorbent hydrogel. *European Polymer Journal*, *44*(4), 1209–1216.
60. Argin, S., Kofinas, P., & Lo, Y. M. (2014). The cell release kinetics and the swelling behavior of physically crosslinked xanthan–chitosan hydrogels in simulated gastrointestinal conditions. *Food Hydrocolloids*, *40*, 138–144.
61. Ibrahim, M., Abd-Eladl, M., & Abou-Baker, N. (2015). Lignocellulosic biomass for the preparation of cellulose-based hydrogel and its use for optimizing water resources in agriculture. *Journal of Applied Polymer Science*, *132*.
62. Guilherme, M., et al. (2007). Superabsorbent hydrogel based on modified polysaccharide for removal of Pb^{2+} and Cu^{2+} from water with excellent performance. *Journal of Applied Polymer Science*, *105*, 2903–2909.
63. Ma, J., Li, X., & Bao, Y. (2015). Advances in cellulose-based superabsorbent hydrogels. *RSC Advances*, *5*.
64. Rodríguez, R. A., Alvarez-Lorenzo, C., & Concheiro, A. (2003). Cationic cellulose hydrogels: Kinetics of the cross-linking process and characterization as pH-/ion-sensitive drug delivery systems. *Journal of Controlled Release*, *86*(2), 253–265.
65. Ng, L. Y., et al. (2013). Polymeric membranes incorporated with metal/metal oxide nanoparticles: A comprehensive review. *Desalination*, *308*, 15–33.
66. Wieszczycka, K., & Staszak, K. (2017). *Polymers in Separation Processes*, 235–275.
67. Qin, Z., et al. (2013). Synthesis of positively charged polyelectrolyte multilayer membranes for removal of divalent metal ions. *Journal of Materials Research*, *28*(11), 1449–1457.
68. Zhu, W. P., et al. (2014). Dual-layer polybenzimidazole/polyether sulfone (PBI/PES) nanofiltration (NF) hollow fiber membranes for heavy metals removal from wastewater. *Journal of Membrane Science*, *456*, 117–127.
69. Khulbe, K. C., & Matsuura, T. (2018). Removal of heavy metals and pollutants by membrane adsorption techniques. *Applied Water Science*, *8*(1), 19.

70. Javed, R., et al. (2018). Uptake of heavy metal ions from aqueous media by hydrogels and their conversion to nanoparticles for generation of a catalyst system: Two-fold application study. *RSC Advances*, *8*, 14787–14797.
71. Bello, K., et al. (2018). A study on adsorption behavior of newly synthesized banana pseudo-stem derived superabsorbent hydrogels for cationic and anionic dye removal from effluents. *Carbohydrate Polymers*, *181*, 605–615.
72. Maciel, V., et al. (2017). Electrostatic self-assembled chitosan–pectin nano- and microparticles for insulin delivery. *Molecules*, *22*, 1707.
73. Demir, D., et al. (2021). Extraction of pectin from albedo of lemon peels for preparation of tissue engineering scaffolds. *Polymer Bulletin*, *78*.
74. Zhou, W., et al. (2015). Removal of copper ions from aqueous solution by adsorption onto novel polyelectrolyte film-coated nanofibrous silk fibroin non-wovens. *Applied Surface Science*, *345*.
75. Petersen, H., et al. (2002). Synthesis, characterization, and biocompatibility of polyethyleneimine-graft-poly (ethylene glycol) block copolymers. *Macromolecules*, *35*(18), 6867–6874.
76. Wang, Y., et al. (2021). Nanocellulose aerogel for highly efficient adsorption of uranium (VI) from aqueous solution. *Carbohydrate Polymers*, *267*, 118233.
77. Rafiee, J., et al. (2012). Wetting transparency of graphene. *Nature Materials*, *11*(3), 217–222.
78. Mittal, H., et al. (2021). Graphene oxide crosslinked hydrogel nanocomposites of xanthan gum for the adsorption of crystal violet dye. *Journal of Molecular Liquids*, *323*, 115034.
79. Wanyonyi, W. C., Onyari, J. M., & Shiundu, P. M. (2014). Adsorption of Congo Red dye from aqueous solutions using roots of *Eichhornia crassipes*: Kinetic and equilibrium studies. *Energy Procedia*, *50*, 862–869.
80. Cheruiyot, G. K., et al. (2019). Adsorption of toxic crystal violet dye using coffee husks: Equilibrium, kinetics and thermodynamics study. *Scientific African*, *5*, e00116.
81. Peighambardoust, S. J., et al. (2020). Removal of malachite green using carboxymethyl cellulose-g-polyacrylamide/montmorillonite nanocomposite hydrogel. *International Journal of Biological Macromolecules*, *159*, 1122–1131.
82. Pashaei-Fakhri, S., et al. (2021). Crystal violet dye sorption over acrylamide/graphene oxide bonded sodium alginate nanocomposite hydrogel. *Chemosphere*, *270*, 129419.
83. Shoukat, S., et al. (2017). Mango stone bio composite preparation and application for crystal violet adsorption: A mechanistic study. *Microporous and Mesoporous Materials*, *239*, 180–189.
84. Mushtaq, M., et al. (2016). *Eriobotrya japonica* seed bio composite efficiency for copper adsorption: Isotherms, kinetics, thermodynamic and desorption studies. *Journal of Environmental Management*, *176*, 21–33.
85. Rashid, A., et al. (2016). Fungal biomass composite with bentonite efficiency for nickel and zinc adsorption: A mechanistic study. *Ecological Engineering*, *91*, 459–471.
86. Cui, S., et al. (2017). Effects of pectin structure and crosslinking method on the properties of crosslinked pectin nanofibers. *Carbohydrate Polymers*, *157*, 766–774.
87. Kochkodan, V. M., et al. (2006). Effect of the surface modification of polymer membranes on their microbiological fouling. *Colloid Journal*, *68*(3), 267–273.

88. Feng, X., et al. (2018). Facile fabrication of graphene oxide–polyethyleneimine composite and its application for the Cr (VI) removal. *Separation Science and Technology*, *53*, 1–12.
89. Geng, J., et al. (2019). Polyethyleneimine cross-linked graphene oxide for removing hazardous hexavalent chromium: Adsorption performance and mechanism. *Chemical Engineering Journal*, *361*, 1497–1510.
90. Nan, Q., Li, P., & Cao, B. (2016). Fabrication of positively charged nanofiltration membrane via the layer-by-layer assembly of graphene oxide and polyethylenimine for desalination. *Applied Surface Science*, *387*, 521–528.
91. Han, Y., Xu, Z., & Gao, C. (2013). Ultrathin graphene nanofiltration membrane for water purification. *Advanced Functional Materials*, *23*.
92. Liu, G., et al. (2016). Graphene oxide for high-efficiency separation membranes: Role of electrostatic interactions. *Carbon*, *110*, 56–61.
93. Ding, M., et al. (2020). 2D laminar maleic acid-crosslinked MXene membrane with tunable nanochannels for efficient and stable pervaporation desalination. *Journal of Membrane Science*, *600*, 117871.
94. Ding, L., et al. (2017). A two-dimensional lamellar membrane: MXene nanosheet stacks. *Angewandte Chemie International Edition*, *56*.
95. Kang, K., et al. (2017). Selective molecular separation on $Ti_3C_2T_x$-graphene oxide membranes during pressure-driven filtration: Comparison with graphene oxide and MXenes. *ACS Applied Materials & Interfaces*, *9*.
96. Xu, D., et al. (2021). MXene nanosheet templated nanofiltration membranes toward ultrahigh water transport. *Environmental Science & Technology*, *55*(2), 1270–1278.
97. Pandey, R. P., et al. (2018). Ultrahigh-flux and fouling-resistant membranes based on layered silver/MXene ($Ti_3C_2T_x$) nanosheets. *Journal of Materials Chemistry A*, *6*(8), 3522–3533.
98. Xing, Y., et al. (2020). Crumpled two-dimensional $Ti_3C_2T_x$ MXene lamellar membranes for solvent permeation and separation. *ACS Applied Nano Materials*, *3*(2), 1526–1534.
99. Liu, T., et al. (2020). Two-dimensional MXene incorporated graphene oxide composite membrane with enhanced water purification performance. *Journal of Membrane Science*, *593*, 117431.
100. Wang, J., et al. (2020). Ion sieving by a two-dimensional $Ti_3C_2T_x$ alginate lamellar membrane with stable interlayer spacing. *Nature Communications*, *11*(1), 3540.
101. Jiang, F., et al. (2008). Thermoelectric performance of poly(3,4-ethylenedioxythiophene): Poly(styrenesulfonate). *Chinese Physics Letters*, *25*, 2202–2205.
102. Yao, H., et al. (2018). Recent development of thermoelectric polymers and composites. *Macromolecular Rapid Communications*, *39*, 1700727.

CHAPTER 4

Supramolecular Polymers in Drug Delivery and Biomedical Applications

ADITYA DAM,[1,*] MOHD. ARHAM KHAN,[2] and MOHD. FARHAN KHAN[3]

[1]*Department of Applied Chemistry, Delhi Technological University, New Delhi, Delhi, India*

[2]*Interdisciplinary Nanotechnology Centre, Faculty of Engineering and Technology, Aligarh Muslim University, Aligarh, Uttar Pradesh, India*

[3]*Department of Science, Gagan College of Management and Technology, Aligarh, Uttar Pradesh, India*

*Corresponding author

ABSTRACT

Supramolecular polymers (SPs) lie in the field between supramolecular chemistry and polymer chemistry. Over recent years, the research and development based on SPs have increased significantly. SPs employ comparatively weak interactions between small monomers to produce better 2D or 3D structures. Most of the non-covalent interactions in SPs are weaker than the covalent interactions, resulting in a dynamic nature. With the development of SPs, an emphasis on artificial water-compatible SPs (WCSPs) began to appear, having unique properties and the ability to undergo stimulus-promoted reversible changes in structure and morphology. The combination of SPs with biological hydrogels, which are soft, water-soluble 3D polymer networks, has produced great uses in complex tissue engineering, cancer therapy, and drug delivery. Tissue engineering involves the transcription of biological tissues for various reasons such as drug discovery, identification of diseases, biomaterials,

Polymer Applications in Medicine: Revolutionizing Treatment and Therapeutics.
Mohd. Imran Ahamed, Faheem Ahmad, and Ishaat M. Khan (Eds.)

DOI: 10.1201/9781779640871-4

and replacement of organs. Polymer hydrogels, including SPs based on amphiphiles, peptides, peptide-amphiphiles, and ureido pyrimidinone self-assembly, have been extensively investigated for regenerative medicine and other medical applications. In this chapter, we summarize the modern and promising progress made in the biomedical and drug delivery areas of various SPs.

4.1 INTRODUCTION

Self-assembly can be explained as the unconscious and reversible connection of molecules or ions to form larger, more complex supramolecular structures, as stated by the characteristic data accommodated in the molecules. Supramolecular self-assembly is the procedure of a system's components where its molecules, polymers, colloids, or macroscopic particles assemble into adjustable or operational structures or patterns as a consequence of specific local interactions among the components themselves, without external orientation, under the intermolecular control of relatively unsettled, noncovalent interactions such as coordination interactions, hydrogen bonds, dipolar interactions, and so forth. It can be defined in two types: static and dynamic. Most of the research is based on the static type component. The changeable capability of supramolecular self-assembly is the answer to the outgoing system's capability to convey through the accessible components to form the most thermodynamically favorable structure [1–4].

Supramolecular chemistry may be expressed as the 'chemistry beyond the molecule.' Basically, it is defined as the non-covalent interaction between a 'host' and a 'guest' molecule using a variety of non-covalent interactions, and some possess a remarkable covalent component (e.g., metal–ligand interactions). If we look upon supramolecular chemistry in its simplest form, we generally consider a molecule ('host') binding another molecule ('guest') to produce a 'host–guest' complex or supermolecule [5]. The host is a larger molecule than the guest molecule. The guest may be a cation, an anion, an ion pair, or a molecule, and the host can be the molecular entity possessing intersecting binding sites (i.e., Lewis donors, hydrogen bond donors, etc) (Figure 4.1). The host–guest relationship has been defined by Donald, who shared the 1987 Nobel Prize in Chemistry with Jean-Marie Lehn and Charles J. Pedersen.

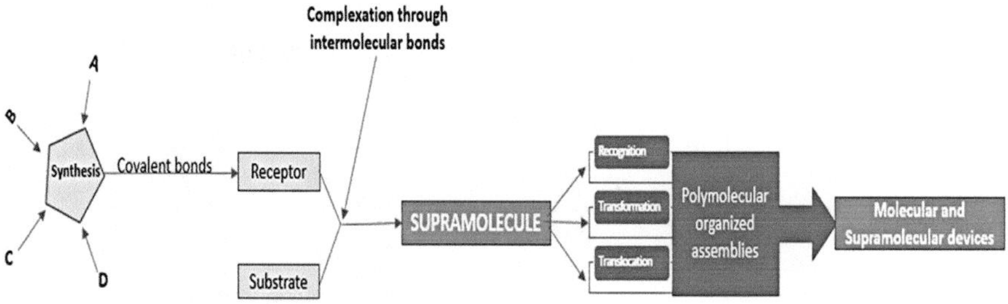

FIGURE 4.1 Molecular and supramolecular chemistry according to Lehn.
Source: Adapted from Ref. [5].

SPs are polymeric demonstrations of monomeric particles, embraced jointly by changeable and highly orientational secondary interactions. The produced particles thus retain their polymeric characteristics in solution. SPs are repeatedly developed under conditions of thermodynamic equilibrium, and thus the lengths of the chains are connected to the robustness of the bond. They can be randomly twisted with the mechanical properties of plastics and elastomers and have considerable efficiency for manufacturability and self-healing owing to their reversible monomer-polymer interactions [6].

4.2 HISTORY OF SUPRAMOLECULAR POLYMERS (SPS)

In many interactions, such as hydrogen bonding, all unprocessed polymeric substances are optimized for appearing in a practical state. In polysaccharides and polypeptides, it is often a mixture of both intermolecular and intramolecular interactions, where the latter plays an important role in folding polymer chains into the correct conformations. For engineering plastics, the nature of non-covalent interactions is used for further improvement of the useful properties at high temperatures. Some of the earliest cases of applying supramolecular concepts in polymer science were introduced by Fréchet in 1989 and Stadler in 1990. Fréchet and coworkers demonstrated the formation of a mesophase in a dual combination of polymers and small molecules via hydrogen bonding interactions. Jean-Marie Lehn, using this polymeric approach, synthesized a "liquid crystalline supramolecular polymer" using complementary triple hydrogen bonding motifs in bulk. [7–10] (Figure 4.2).

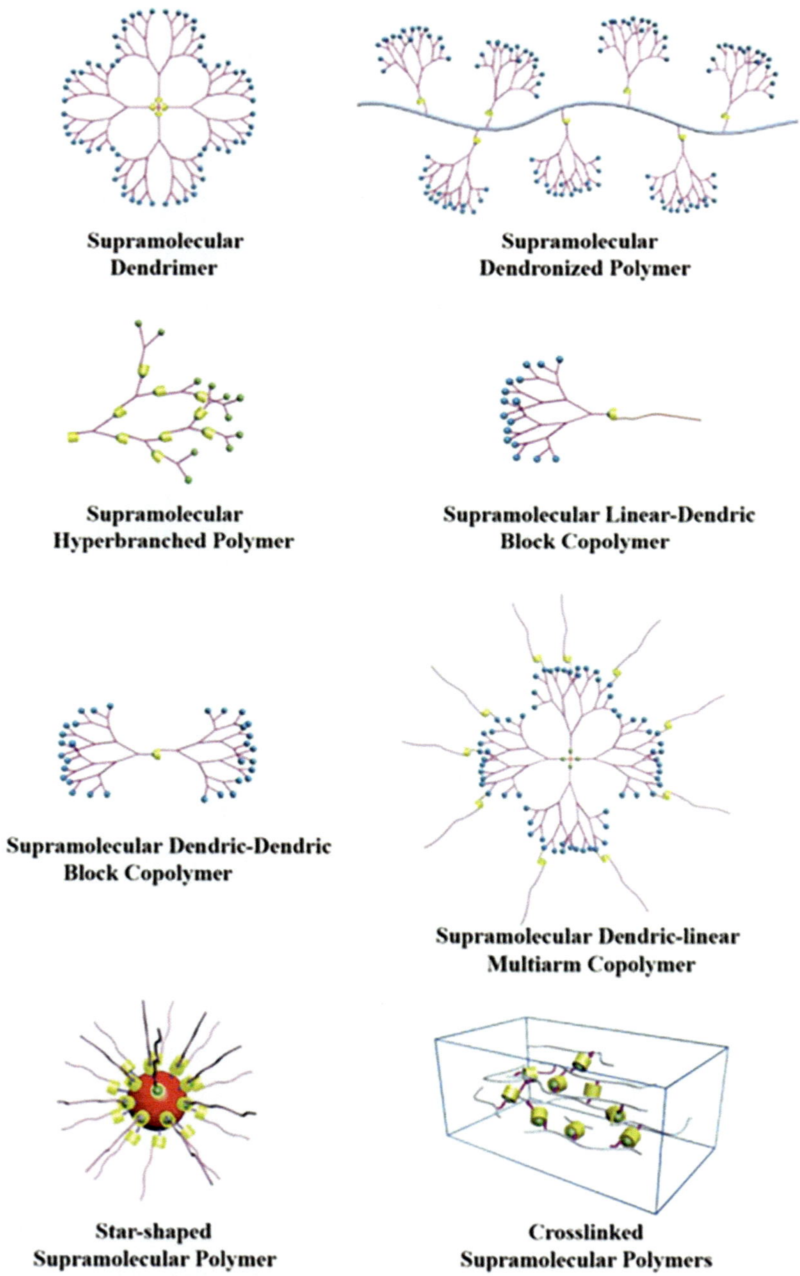

FIGURE 4.2 Different types of supramolecular polymers.

Source: Adapted from Ref. [7].

Later, Ghadiri et al. demonstrated a nanotubular SP where a β-sheet-forming macrocyclic peptide monomer convened together through miscellaneous hydrogen bonding between neighboring macrocycles. In 1997, E.W. Meijer showed a SP assembled by 2-ureido-4-pyrimidone units via quadruple hydrogen bonding (Figure 4.3). These are of concentration and temperature-dependent viscoelastic properties, which make them great candidates for material science applications. These polymers, self-assembled by notable dimerization of the quadruple hydrogen-bonded ureido-pyrimidone functionality, have distinctive characteristics that differentiate them from existing structures [11–13]. Because of their outrageous association constant, these linear polymers have DPs far more significant than those of existing self-assembled structures based on fewer than four hydrogen bonds.

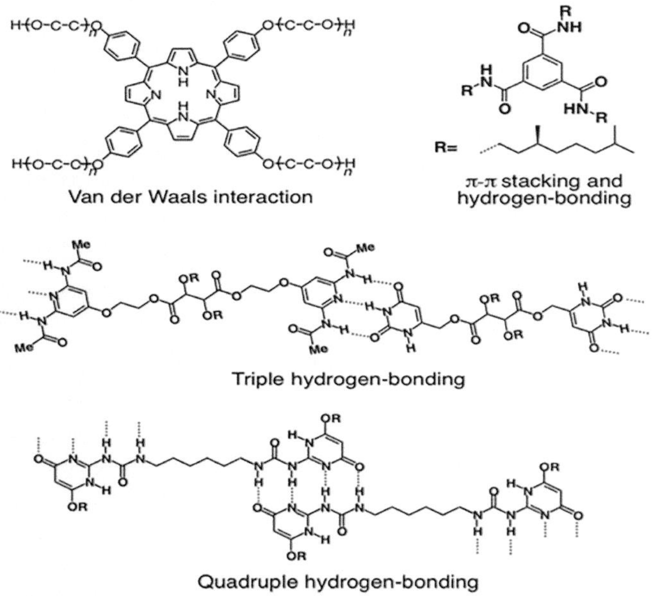

FIGURE 4.3 Improvement of supramolecular polymers in the via various hydrogen bonding. *Source*: Reprinted with permission from Ref. [4]. Copyright © 2019 WILEY-VCH Verlag GmbH & Co. KGaA, Weinheim.

4.3 APPLICATIONS OF SPS

4.3.1 APPLICATIONS IN DRUG DELIVERY

There are different types of SPs having different characteristics and applications (Figure 4.3). Drug delivery is a large field of research for the development of novel materials or transportable materials for remarkable therapeutic delivery of drugs. It may involve stable, dominant, or selective drug delivery and is commonly used. Drug delivery with metal nanoparticles is an efficient strategy in medicine to treat various diseases. It is the method of administering a pharmaceutical compound to bring about therapeutic effects in humans or animals. Transdermal drug delivery (TDD) is an effective way of controlling the release rate of drugs. It aims to alter the pharmacokinetics of drugs. A large number of SPs are promising drug carriers; with improved water solubility, they preferentially accumulate at the targeted site through the EPR effect, thereby lowering side effects. In recent progress, drug delivery techniques based on non-covalent self-assembly mainly include complexation, hydrogen-bonded polymeric interactions, and host–guest polymeric interactions, and they show unique advantages in drug delivery as they are able to control the release of encapsulated drugs into the system. [14–18].

Hydrogen-bonded SPs are highly preferable candidates in anti-cancer and anti-inflammatory drug deliveries. Dankers and his co-partners in 2011 made advancements in supramolecular hydrogels for intrarenal drug delivery. In their work, they synthesized three different supramolecular hydrogelators based on PEG chains and UPy moieties. Two chain-extended hydrogelators possessing UPy units in the main chain, and one bifunctional hydrogelator with UPy groups at the chain end, were produced. The chain-extended hydrogelators are shape-persistent, while the biofunctional hydrogelators are weak and elastic in nature. The properties and behavior of the biofunctionalized hydrogel *in vivo* make it a great candidate for intrarenal drug delivery in the short term, while the properties of one of the chain-extended hydrogels make it suitable for long-term intrarenal organic drug delivery. This type of SP provides a new way for intrarenal therapy (Figure 4.4) [8, 19–21].

In recent years, a new type of peptide-containing supramolecular nanostructures, including supramolecular micelles and supramolecular bio-membranes, has been developed. In a study, Tirrell et al. showed that a cylindrical micelle, diC16-OVA, without any additional adjuvant, offers *in vivo* protection from tumors by stimulating OVA-specific Tc-cells. This diC16-OVA does not stimulate the pathogen recognition receptor TLR2. This type of cylindrical micelle was very effective in inhibiting the growth of tumors by producing the tumor antigen [22].

Later, Stupp and his co-workers reported that the nanoscale supramolecular morphology of PAs in solution could detect the outgoing

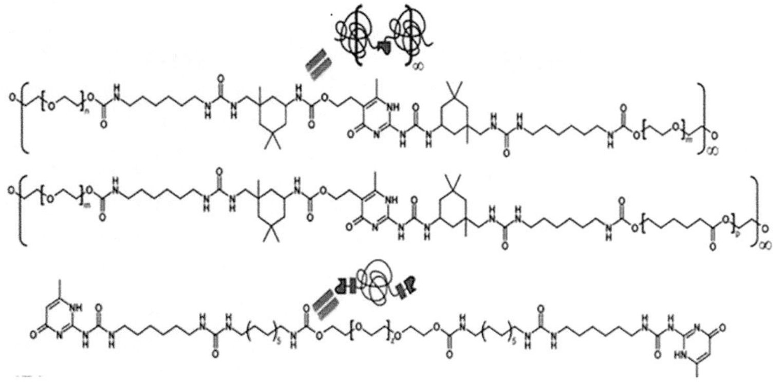

FIGURE 4.4 UPy modified chain-extended and end-functionalized hydrogelator synthesized by Danker et al. [8].

Source: Reprinted with permission from Ref. [8]. Copyright © 2012 Elsevier Ltd.

microstructure and functions of hierarchically gathered membranes. They also showed that this hierarchical self-assembled action could be utilized to assimilate anti-cancer bioactivity via particular PAs into membranes. The membranes developed by the non-covalent interactions of hyaluronic acid (HA) and positively charged peptide-based amphiphiles with a KLAKLAK-KLAKLAK peptide sequence can behave as reservoirs for a sustainable supply of cytotoxic drugs upon enzymatic degradation with strongly confined surface cytotoxicity (Figure 4.5). This is an excellent perspective for the study of anti-tumor therapeutics [19, 22–27].

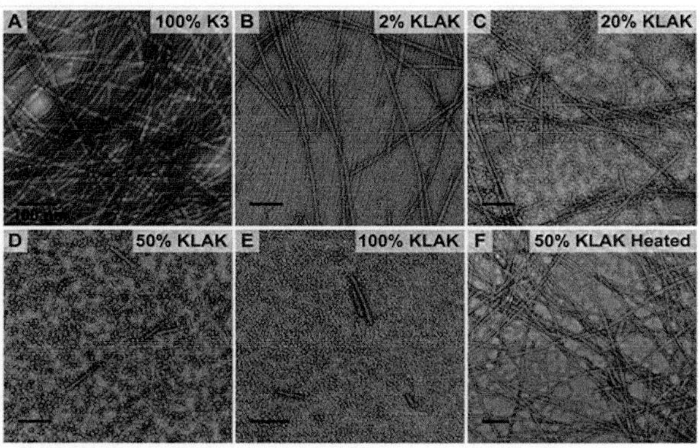

FIGURE 4.5 Transmission electron micrograph diagram of PA nanostructures at various co-assembled compositions.

Source: Reprinted with permission from Ref. [23]. Copyright © 2013 WILEY-VCH Verlag GmbH & Co. KGaA, Weinheim.

Furthermore, cyclodextrin-based (CDs) SPs have been great candidates for drug delivery due to their complexation ability, notable insertion property, and strong functionalization capacity. Nanoscaled supramolecular polymeric systems have been considered promising carriers for drug and gene delivery, as well as for other biomedical uses. Researchers enhanced the supramolecular polymeric flexibility and biocompatibility towards drug delivery by inducing CDs into it. CDs are easily scaled up with supramolecular interactions but still require advancement to yield small molecule CD derivatives with high purity and a better yield for future perspectives, and also to give rise to CD-containing polymers with sharply controlled topology [28, 29].

4.3.2 APPLICATIONS IN CANCER THERAPY

Cancer is a disease caused by the uncontrolled division of abnormal cells in a part of the body. For several decades, anticancer treatment has been a broad research topic throughout the world. The economic impact of cancer is significant and increasing. The total annual economic cost of cancer in the previous decade was estimated in trillions. When cancer cells break away from a tumor, they travel to other parts of the body through either the bloodstream or the lymph system; this process is called metastasis. The agents of chemotherapy (CT) have many drawbacks because it is an indispensable method for cancer treatment; thus, SPs need to improve their efficiency for better drug delivery [30–32].

A number of SPs are used in cancer treatment. For the improvement of cervical cancer treatment, Zhao et al. reported a theragnostic drug pustule with host–guest interactions. These pustules transport camptothecin along with siRNA to battle various types of cancer. The assembled structure can be synthesized very easily by the combination of disulfide bond cleavage in response to excessive concentrations of intracellular glutathione in the targeted area. After a few years, they developed a GSH-responsive AB-type supramolecular monomer CD-SS-CPT, in which the anticancer drug CPT behaved as the guest and β-CD as the host, which improved the solubility of CPT by a factor of 232. This nanomedicine shows excellent anti-tumor efficacy and anti-metastasis effect without major side effects, opening up a new approach to polymers for anti-cancer treatment. [33] Curcumin is renowned for its resistance to cancer properties via inhibiting the STAT3 phosphorylation process. It has poor solubility in water.

To solubilize curcumin in water, Stang also described an approach combining organoplatinum (II) Z pyridyl coordination-operated interaction and a cucurbit [8] CB [8]-mediated heteroternary to result in a successful delivery system via host-guest interactions (Figure 4.6) [34–36].

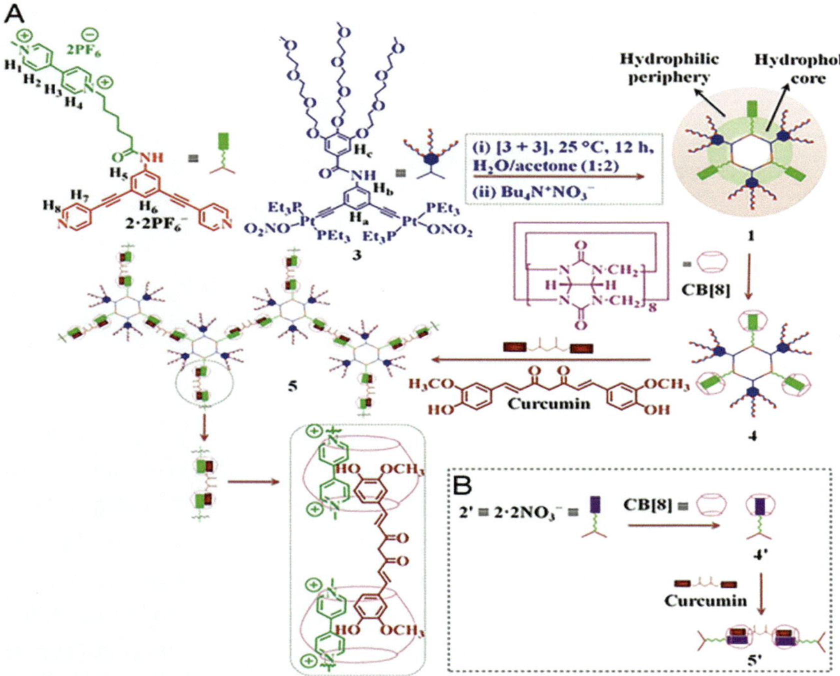

FIGURE 4.6 (A) Graphical portrayal of the generation of host–guest complex 5 from the hierarchical self-assembly of 1, CB [8], and Curcumin. (B) Host–guest complexation of 2′ with CB [8] and Curcumin [34] Tang in 2012, reported an anticancer drug system introducing Ad-DOX to the β-CD chains for the improvement of ovarian cancer treatment.

Source: Reprinted from Ref. [34]. https://creativecommons.org/licenses/by/4.0/

Later, Li reported a new PEG detachable gene vector aimed at the fibroblast growth factor receptor (FGFR), cultivated through self-assembly between MPC and Ad-SS-PEG. This vector establishes a PEG layer under *in vivo* conditions to provide equivalent defensive potential and stability to MPC/Ad-SS-PEG polyplexes against extracellular salt. The disconnection of PEG in intracellular depletive situations could be more impactful in prompting DNA rescue from the MPC matrix through the model polyanion (Figure 4.7). This end-functionalized FGFR-aimed ornament developed therapeutic productivity for ovarian cancer cells [37].

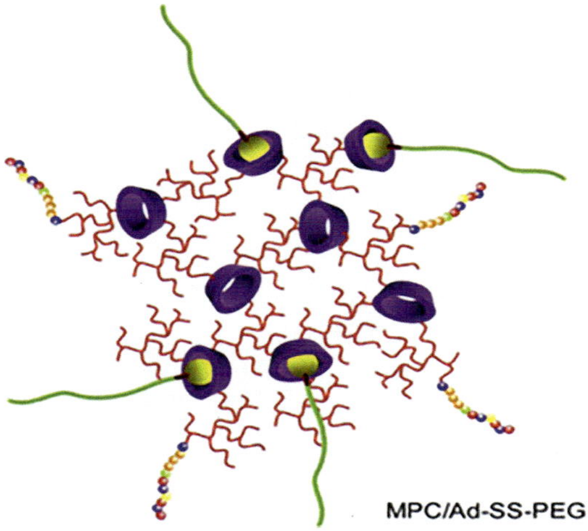

FIGURE 4.7 Li et al. reported multi-arm dendritic supramolecular polymer structure.

Source: Reprinted from Ref. [37]. Copyright © 2013 Elsevier Ltd.

Some of the Au (III) complexes of porphyrin rings were found to show phototoxicity. Zhang and his co-workers showed that Au (III) porphyrins and complexes are potent for anticancer therapy via *in vitro* and *in vivo* processes. They reported a dual-functionalized SP produced through an Au (III) complex of 2,6-diphenylpyridine and a 2,4-diamino-6-(4-pyridyl)-1,3,5-triazine (4-dpt) SP from a cyclometalated Au (III) complex accommodating a hydrogen-bonded design, which shows inherent properties in the treatment of cancer therapy (Figure 4.8). This polymer showed sustainably and selectively cytotoxic nature towards cancerous cells. It can also abbreviate immunosuppressive representatives like [Au(III)(TPP)]Cl to attain its sustainable-released nature [38, 39].

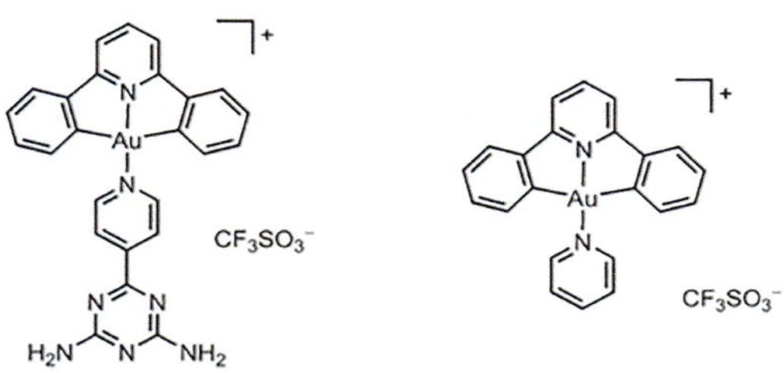

FIGURE 4.8 Structure of Au (III) complexes designed by Zhang.

Source: Reprinted from Ref. [38]. Copyright © 2012 WILEY-VCH Verlag GmbH & Co. KGaA, Weinheim

In the 21st century, breast cancer is an extremely prominent cancer diagnosed in women worldwide. In 2020, there were 2.3 million women diagnosed with breast cancer. In recent years, there has been a rapid development of hydrogel networks for breast cancer surgery. Yuanhao Wu and his coworkers in 2018 demonstrated a SP, namely poly [N-acryloyl glycinamide-co-acrylamide] (PNAm) nanocomposite hydrogel containing gold nanoparticles (AuNPs) and doxorubicin (DOX) through a one-step synthesis of the monomers NAGA and AAm, with the inclusion of PDA-AuNPs (Figure 4.9). Due to the photothermal effect of the nanocomposite with the hydrogels, this is an excellent candidate for controlled drug delivery under 808 nm Near-Infrared irradiations [40–46].

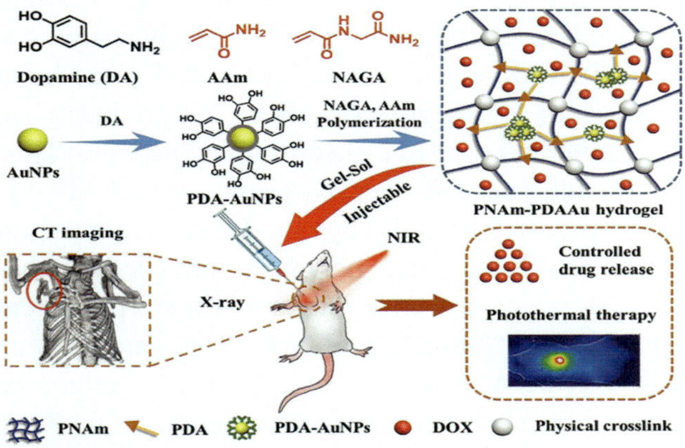

FIGURE 4.9 Synthesis of the nanocomposite hydrogel polymer and its applicable graphical diagram as a liner of breast cancer.

Source: Reprinted from Ref. [41]. Copyright © 2018 WILEY-VCH Verlag GmbH & Co. KGaA, Weinheim

4.3.3 APPLICATIONS IN TISSUE ENGINEERING

Tissue engineering is a biochemical method using a combination of cells, engineering, and biomaterials to improve or regenerate different biological tissues. It is an expeditiously progressing discipline that aims to repair, replace, regenerate, or form tissues or organs by translating fundamental knowledge in physics, chemistry, and biology into experimental and effective materials, devices, and clinical strategies (Figure 4.10) [47]. The outcome of tissue engineering on society is admirable. It holds the approach of sustainable development in the quality of human life, with a reduction in the societal and economic costs associated with healthcare and life expectancy. Nowadays, tissue engineering, with the use of microfabrication and 3D bioprinting, has the ability to regenerate many tissues in the body. In several years, with the help of SPs, researchers have been able to generate new tissues much more efficiently [25, 48].

Recently, it was observed that electrospinning of bioactive materials is a significant, low-cost proficiency for creating long fibers in solution. The supramolecular structure of the fibers could verify that certain overages, like bio-epitopes, are portrayed on the surface even after processing, which could furnish a suitable set of circumstances for tissue engineering applications because of the electrospinning of peptide-functionalized bioactive materials. Bioorganic chemistry allows the generation of supramolecular units like SBPs that can be applicable for novel applications in tissue engineering (TE). Hauser and his coworkers recently analyzed three types of SBP: peptide-derived, nucleic acid-derived, and oligosaccharide-derived for tissue engineering. Zhang and co-workers, for producing supramolecular nanofiber scaffolds, reported β-sheet-forming peptides. This nanofiber could be used for adhesion and extensive growth of cells [49–51].

Danker and his co-workers, through the fabrication of supramolecular bioactive materials, showed that polymers formed through quadruple hydrogen bonding ureido-pyrimidinone moieties are prominently appropriate enough to bring out low-temperature handling capacities and compatible behaviors by the combination of UPy-altered oligocaprolactones with UPy-operationalized cell-adhesion-promoting UPy-Gly-Arg-Gly-Asp-Ser and synergistic UPy-Pro-His-Ser-Arg-Asn peptide series. This UPy-modified bioactive material has a great tendency in tissue repairing applications both *in vivo* and *in vitro* because of the reversible nature of quadruple bonding (Figure 4.10). *In vitro* processes result in specific and strong binding of fibroblast cells, and *in vivo* results in triggered tissue by the production of giant cells on the material's surface [2, 52–55].

Bian and his coworkers developed the HGM approach using HA adjusted with adamantane particles for cartilage regeneration to produce self-assembled hydrogels induced by *in situ* comprised polyvalent nanoclusters as the cross-linking intersections of biopolymers. This type of HGM proposal, through the combination of well-organized noncovalent entanglement and *in situ* gathering of the host–guest complexes, produced durable HGM hydrogels and could control mechanical properties more efficiently than previous ones. They could slacken the constrictive strain quickly via rapid and reversible host-guest separation and bear successive shielding on the summarized stem cells throughout the contraction

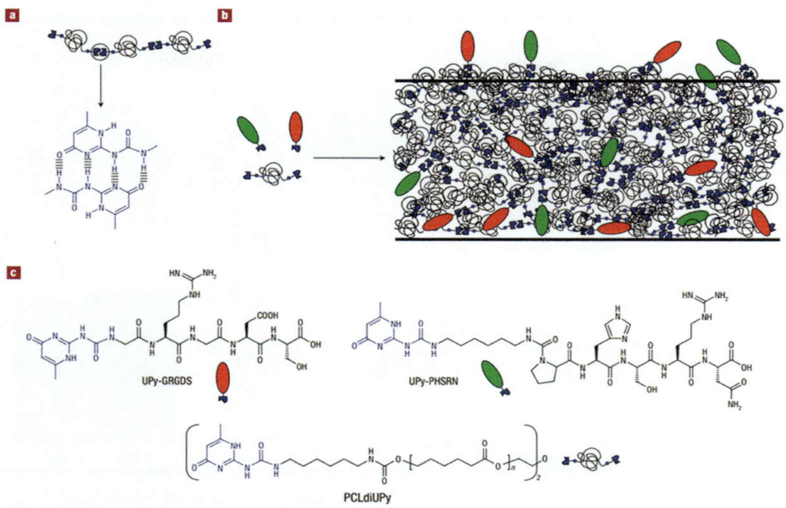

FIGURE 4.10 (a) The self-supportive H-bonding UPy moiety in the polymer. (b) Construction of bioactive materials with various holdings by the combination of different UPy-functionalized biomolecules with UPy-polymers. (c) Use of UPy-GRGDS and UPy-PHSRN as constituent in combination with an oligocaprolactones with UPy-unit (PCLdiUPy) for these materials.

Source: Reprinted from Ref. [52]. Copyright © 2005, Springer Nature Limited

modification, which made them good biomaterials for targeting defects in surrounding tissues quickly. Thus, the hydrogels are auspicious transporting substances for stem cells and curative negotiators for tissue repair and tissue adherent treatment (Figure 4.11) [56–58].

Tissue adhesion is also important in surgeries like fistulas and cardiothoracic surgery. A splendid muscle-prompt viscous material could adhere well to the interface of a wet bone and be organized to lay in an acceptable way for sternal closure uses. For this purpose, Wang and his co-workers demonstrated a mussel-inspired, catechol-altered hyperbranched nanopolymeric material adhesive consisting of a poly (b-amino ester) (polydopamine-co-acrylate) matrix fortified with hydroxyapatite nanoparticles as a sternal bone closure approach. The cross-linked reagent Fe^{3+} was found to be gummy. With the process, tri-acrylates, when synthesized with dopamine via Michael addition, yield a majorly functionalized component with a 3D structure and abundant catechol end groups. Due to the poor contacts between Fe^{3+} and Dihydroxyphenylalanine, when the coordination linker Fe^{3+} is applied, it provides strong and reversible interaction within a short time (less than or equal to 100 min). This PDA nanocomposite is observed to showcase excellent adhesive and mechanistic properties via oxidation to

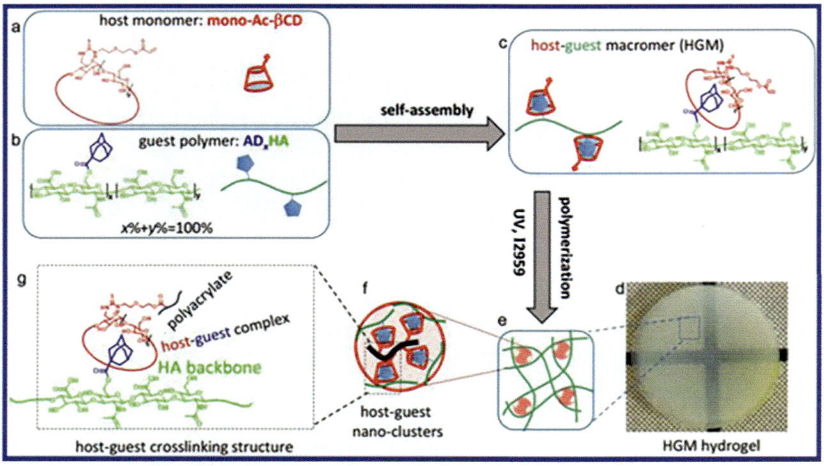

FIGURE 4.11 Structures and graphical representation of (a) host monomer, (b) guest polymer, and their step-by-step polymerization process(c>e>f) via host-guest crosslinking. (d) clear aspect of the HGM hydrogel under microscope.

Source: Reprinted from Ref. [56]. Copyright © 2016, American Chemical Society.

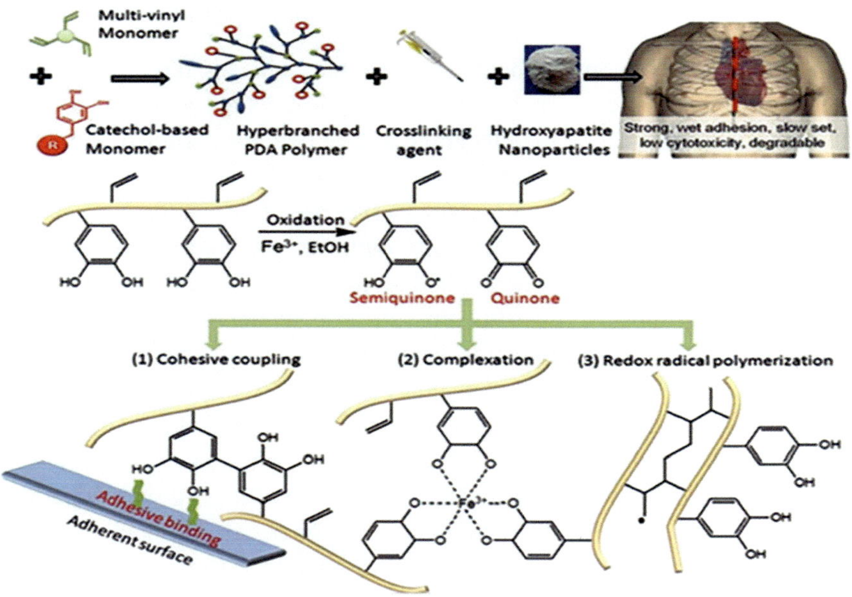

FIGURE 4.12 Cross-linking graphical representation of Polydopamine with Fe^{3+} via 1) Cohesive coupling, 2) complexation process. 3) Redox radical process.

Source: Reprinted from Ref. [63]. Copyright 2013. Royal Society of Chemistry.

semi-quinone or quinone forms by Fe^{3+}. This approach developed the curing speed of tissues by improving the adhesion effect (Figure 4.12) [10, 59–64].

Recently, Huang and his co-workers described non-covalent crosslinking glass-like polymers with slow, tunable dissociation kinetics (kd < 1 s^{-1}) that enable high compressibility in SP networks, achieving compressive strengths of up to 100 MPa with no fracture, even when compressed at 93% strain over 12 cycles of compression and relaxation [65]. This innovation could have a tremendous impact on fast and high-performance tissue engineering.

4.4 CONCLUSION

The purpose of this review is to summarize some of the important research on polymers and materials based on supramolecular polymeric interactions from the past few years, which have shown and demonstrated a tremendous impact in the applications of drug delivery and biomedical approaches. Moreover, some of the materials, like UPy modified hydrogelators, SBM-, CD-, HGM-based, and metal-centered supramolecular polymeric materials discussed in this chapter, have great potential for cancer therapy, tissue regeneration, and so forth [66–68].

KEYWORDS

- **biopolymers**
- **cancer therapy**
- **drug delivery**
- **hyaluronic acid**
- **hydrogel networks**
- **polymer chemistry**
- **supramolecular polymers**
- **tissue engineering**

REFERENCES

1. Park, T., Zimmerman, S. C., & Nakashima, S. (2015). A highly stable quadruply hydrogen-bonded heterocomplex useful for supramolecular polymer blends. *Journal of the American Chemical Society*, *127*, 6520–6521.

2. Yang, L., Tan, X., Wang, Z., & Zhang, X. (2015). Supramolecular polymers: Historical development, preparation, characterization, and functions. *Chemical Reviews, 115*, 7196–7239.
3. Yu, X., Chen, L., Zhang, M., & Yi, T. (2014). Low-molecular-mass gels responding to ultrasound and mechanical stress: Towards self-healing materials. *Chemical Society Reviews, 43*, 5346–5371.
4. Chen, W., Kretzschmann, A., Tian, W., & Wu, S. (2018). Nonlinear supramolecular polymers for therapeutic applications. *Advanced Therapeutics, 2.*
5. Steed, J. W., & Atwood, J. L. (2009). Concepts. In *Supramolecular Chemistry.*
6. Yu, G., Yan, X., Han, C., & Huang, F. (2013). Characterization of supramolecular gels. *Chemical Society Reviews, 42*, 6697–6722.
7. Sijbesma, R. P., Beijer, F. H., Brunsveld, L., Folmer, B. J., Hirschberg, J., Lange, R. F., Lowe, J., & Meijer, E. W. (1997). Reversible polymers formed from self-complementary monomers using quadruple hydrogen bonding. *Science, 278*, 1601–1604.
8. Dankers, P. Y., van Luyn, M. J., Huizinga-van der Vlag, A., van Gemert, G. M., Petersen, A. H., Meijer, E. W., Janssen, H. M., Bosman, A. W., & Popa, E. R. (2012). Development and *in-vivo* characterization of supramolecular hydrogels for intrarenal drug delivery. *Biomaterials*, 5144–5155.
9. Han, L., Yan, L., Wang, K., Fang, L., Zhang, H., Tang, Y., Ding, Y., Weng, L. T., Xu, J., Weng, J., Liu, Y., Ren, F., & Lu, X. (2017). Tough, self-healable and tissue-adhesive hydrogel with tunable multifunctionality. *NPG Asia Materials, 9*, e372.
10. Bastús, N. G., Comenge, J., & Puntes, V. (2011). Kinetically controlled seeded growth synthesis of citrate-stabilized gold nanoparticles of up to 200 nm: Size focusing versus Ostwald ripening. *Langmuir, 27*, 11098–11105.
11. Cheng, J., Amin, D., Latona, J., Heber-Katz, E., & Messersmith, P. B. (2019). Supramolecular polymer hydrogels for drug-induced tissue regeneration. *ACS Nano, 13*, 5493–5501.
12. Li, J., & Loh, X. J. (2008). Cyclodextrin-based supramolecular architectures: Syntheses, structures, and applications for drug and gene delivery. *Advanced Drug Delivery Reviews, 60*, 1000–1017.
13. Dong, R. J., Zhou, Y. F., & Zhu, X. Y. (2014). Supramolecular dendritic polymers: From synthesis to applications. *Accounts of Chemical Research, 47*, 2006–2016.
14. Kotcherlakota, R., Das, S., & Patra, C. R. (2019). Therapeutic applications of green synthesized silver nanoparticles. *Elsevier BV*, 389–428.
15. Yan, J. T., Li, W., & Zhang, A. (2014). Dendronized supramolecular polymers. *Chemical Communications, 50*, 12221–12233.
16. Tan, X., Li, B. B., Lu, X., Jia, F., Santori, C., Menon, P., Li, H., Zhang, B., Zhao, J. J., & Zhang, K. (2015). Light-triggered, self-immolative nucleic acid-drug nanostructures. *Journal of the American Chemical Society, 137*, 6112–6115.
17. Leung, K. C. F., Mendes, P. M., Magonov, S. N., Northrop, B. H., Kim, S., Patel, K., Flood, A. H., Tseng, H. R., & Stoddart, J. F. (2006). Supramolecular self-assembly of dendronized polymers: Reversible control of the polymer architectures through acid–base reactions. *Journal of the American Chemical Society, 128*, 10707–10715.
18. Chen, H., Jia, H., Tham, H. P., Qu, Q., Xing, P., Zhao, J., Phua, S. Z. F., Chen, G., & Zhao, Y. (2019). Theragnostic prodrug vesicles for imaging guided codelivery

of calprotectin and siRNA in synergistic cancer therapy. *ACS Applied Materials & Interfaces*, *9*, 23536–23543.
19. Dong, R., Zhou, Y., Huang, X., Zhu, X., Lu, Y., & Shen, J. (2015). Functional supramolecular polymers for biomedical applications. *Advanced Materials*, *27*, 498–526.
20. Hu, Q., Li, W., Hu, X., Hu, Q., Shen, J., Jin, X., Zhou, J., Tang, G., & Chu, P. K. (2012). Synergistic treatment of ovarian cancer by co-delivery of survivin shRNA and paclitaxel via supramolecular micellar assembly. *Biomaterials*, *33*, 6580–6591.
21. Rodell, C. B., Dusaj, N. N., Highley, C. B., & Burdick, J. A. (2016). Injectable and cytocompatibility tough double-network hydrogels through tandem supramolecular and covalent crosslinking. *Advanced Materials*, *28*, 8419–8424.
22. Black, M., Trent, A., Kostenko, Y., Lee, J. S., Olive, C., & Tirrell, M. (2012). Self-assembled peptide amphiphile micelles containing a cytotoxic T-cell epitope promote a protective immune response *in vivo*. *Advanced Materials*, *24*, 3845–3849.
23. Zha, R. H., Sur, S., & Stupp, S. I. (2012). Self-assembly of cytotoxic peptide amphiphiles into supramolecular membranes for cancer therapy. *Advanced Healthcare Materials*, *2*, 126–133.
24. Han, W., Xiang, W., Li, Q., Zhang, H., Yang, Y., Shi, J., Ji, Y., Wang, S., Ji, X., Khashab, N. M., & Sessler, J. L. (2021). Water compatible supramolecular polymers: Recent progress. *Chemical Society Reviews*, *50*, 10025–10043.
25. Pekkanen, A. M., Mondschein, R. J., Williams, C. B., & Long, T. E. (2017). 3D printing polymers with supramolecular functionality for biological applications. *Biomacromolecules*, *18*(9), 2669–2687.
26. Goor, O. J. G. M., Hendrikse, S. I. S., Dankers, P. Y. W., & Meijer, E. W. (2017). From supramolecular polymers to multi-component biomaterials. *Chemical Society Reviews*, *46*(21), 6621–6637.
27. Zhao, F., Yin, H., & Li, J. (2014). Supramolecular self-assembly forming a multifunctional synergistic system for targeted co-delivery of gene and drug. *Biomaterials*, *35*, 1050–1062.
28. Tu, C. L., Zhu, L. J., Li, P. P., Chen, Y., Su, Y., Yan, D. Y., Zhu, X. Y., & Zhou, G. Y. (2011). Supramolecular polymeric micelles by the host–guest interaction of star-like calix [4] arene and chlorin e6 for photodynamic therapy. *Chemical Communications*, *47*, 6063–6065.
29. Zhang, J., & Ma, P. X. (2013). Cyclodextrin-based supramolecular systems for drug delivery: Recent progress and future perspective. *Advanced Drug Delivery Reviews*, *65*, 1215–1233.
30. Dankers, P. Y. W., Boomker, J. M., Huizinga-van der Vlag, A., Wisse, E., Appel, W. P. J., Smedts, F. M. M., Harmsen, M. C., Bosman, A. W., Meijer, E. W., & van Luyn, M. J. A. (2011). Bioengineering of living renal membranes consisting of hierarchical, bioactive supramolecular meshes and human tubular cells. *Biomaterials*, *32*, 723–733.
31. Peng, C., Zheng, L., Chen, Q., Shen, M., Guo, R., Wang, H., Cao, X., Zhang, G., & Shi, X. (2012). PEGylated dendrimer-entrapped gold nanoparticles for *in vivo* blood pool and tumor imaging by computed tomography. *Biomaterials*, *33*, 1107–1119.
32. Shi, X., Gao, H., Dai, F., Feng, X., & Liu, W. (2016). A thermoresponsive supramolecular copolymer hydrogel for the embolization of kidney arteries. *Biomaterials Science*, *4*, 1673–1681.

33. Yu, G., Zhao, X., Zhou, J., Mao, Z., Huang, X., Wang, Z., Hua, B., Liu, Y., Zhang, F., He, Z., Jacobson, O., Gao, C., Wang, W., Yu, C., Zhu, X., Huang, F., & Chen, X. (2018). Supramolecular polymer-based nanomedicine: High therapeutic performance and negligible long-term immunotoxicity. *Journal of the American Chemical Society*, *140*, 8005–8019.
34. Datta, S., Misra, S. K., Saha, M. L., Lahiri, N., Louie, J., Pan, D., & Stang, P. J. (2018). Orthogonal self-assembly of an organoplatinum (II) metallacycle and cucurbit [8] uril that delivers curcumin to cancer cells. *Proceedings of the National Academy of Sciences*, *115*(32), 8087–8092.
35. Yu, G., Zhang, M., Saha, M. L., Mao, Z., Chen, J., Yao, Y., Zhou, Z., Liu, Y., Gao, C., Huang, F., Chen, X., & Stang, P. J. (2017). Antitumor activity of a unique polymer that incorporates a fluorescent self-assembled metallacycle. *Journal of the American Chemical Society*, *139*, 15940–15949.
36. Zhang, P., Qian, X., Zhang, Z., Li, C., Xie, C., Wu, W., & Jiang, X. (2017). Supramolecular amphiphilic polymer-based micelles with seven-armed polyoxazoline coating for drug delivery. *ACS Applied Materials & Interfaces*, *9*, 5768–5777.
37. Ping, Y., Hu, Q., Tang, G., & Li, J. (2013). FGFR-targeted gene delivery mediated by supramolecular assembly between β-cyclodextrin-crosslinked PEI and redox-sensitive PEG. *Biomaterials*, *34*(27), 6482–6494.
38. Zhang, J. J., Lu, W., Sun, R. W. Y., & Che, C. M. (2012). Organogold (III) supramolecular polymers for anticancer treatment. *Angewandte Chemie International Edition*, *51*(20), 4882–4886.
39. Hu, C., Liu, X., Ran, W., Meng, J., Zhai, Y., Zhang, P., Yin, Q., Yu, H., Zhang, Z., & Li, Y. (2017). Regulating cancer associated fibroblasts with losartan-loaded injectable peptide hydrogel to potentiate chemotherapy in inhibiting growth and lung metastasis of triple negative breast cancer. *Biomaterials*, *144*, 60–72.
40. Astolfo, A., Qie, F., Kibleur, A., Hao, X., Menk, R. H., Arfelli, F., Rigon, L., Hinton, T. M., Wickramaratna, M., Tan, T., & Hughes, T. C. (2014). A simple way to track single gold-loaded alginate microcapsules using X-ray CT in small animal longitudinal studies. *Nanomedicine*, *10*, 1821–1828.
41. Wu, Y., Wang, H., Gao, F., Xu, Z., Dai, F., & Liu, W. (2018). An injectable supramolecular polymer nanocomposite hydrogel for prevention of breast cancer recurrence with theragnostic and mammoplasty functions. *Advanced Functional Materials*, *28*.
42. Torre, L. A., Siegel, R. L., Ward, E. M., & Jemal, A. (2016). Global cancer incidence and mortality rates and trends—An update. *Cancer Epidemiology, Biomarkers & Prevention*, *25*, 16–27.
43. Aida, T., Meijer, E. W., & Stupp, S. I. (2012). Functional supramolecular polymers. *Science*, *335*, 813–817.
44. Jemal, A., Bray, F., Center, M. M., Ferlay, J., Ward, E., & Forman, D. (2011). Global cancer statistics. *CA: A Cancer Journal for Clinicians*, *61*, 69–90.
45. Liu, Y., Chen, Y., & Zhang, H. Y. (2020). *Handbook of Macrocyclic Supramolecular Assembly*.
46. Liu, K., Kang, Y. T., Wang, Z. Q., & Zhang, X. (2013). 25th anniversary article: Reversible and adaptive functional supramolecular materials: "Noncovalent interaction" matters. *Advanced Materials*, *25*, 5530–5548.

47. Silvio, L. D. (2007). Bone tissue engineering and biomineralization. In *Tissue Engineering Using Ceramics and Polymers* (pp. 319–331). Woodhead Publishing.
48. Bambole, V., & Yakhmi, J. V. (2016). Tissue engineering: Use of electrospinning technique for recreating physiological functions. *Elsevier BV*, 387–455.
49. Cheetham, A. G., Chakroun, R. W., Ma, W., & Cui, H. (2017). Self-assembling prodrugs. *Chemical Society Reviews*, *46*, 6638–6663.
50. Huang, D., Wang, Y. Q., Yang, F., Shen, H., Weng, Z. Q., & Wu, D. C. (2017). Charge-reversible and pH-responsive biodegradable micelles and vesicles from linear-dendritic supramolecular amphiphiles for anticancer drug delivery. *Polymer Chemistry*, *8*, 6675.
51. Webber, M. J., & Langer, R. (2017). Drug delivery by supramolecular design. *Chemical Society Reviews*, *46*, 6600–6620.
52. Dankers, P. Y. W., Harmsen, M. C., Brouwer, L. A., van Luyn, M. J. A., & Meijer, E. W. (2005). A modular and supramolecular approach to bioactive scaffolds for tissue engineering. *Nature Materials*, *4*(7), 568–574.
53. Bakota, E. L., Wang, Y., Danesh, F. R., & Hartgerink, J. D. (2011). Injectable multidomain peptide nanofiber hydrogel as a delivery agent for stem cell secretome. *Biomacromolecules*, *12*, 1651–1657.
54. Guo, M. Y., Pitet, L. M., Wyss, H. M., Vos, M., Dankers, P. Y. W., & Meijer, E. W. (2014). Tough stimuli-responsive supramolecular hydrogels with hydrogen-bonding network junctions. *Journal of the American Chemical Society*, *136*, 6969–6977.
55. Li, J., Wang, W., Zhao, L., Rong, L., Lan, S., Sun, H., Zhang, H., & Yang, B. (2015). Hydroquinone-assisted synthesis of branched Au–Ag nanoparticles with polydopamine coating as highly efficient photothermal agents. *ACS Applied Materials & Interfaces*, *7*, 11613–11623.
56. Wei, K., Zhu, M., Sun, Y., Xu, J., Feng, Q., Lin, S., Wu, T., Xu, J., Tian, F., Li, G., & Bian, L. (2016). Robust biopolymeric supramolecular "host–guest macromer" hydrogels reinforced by *in situ* formed multivalent nanoclusters for cartilage regeneration. *Macromolecules*, *49*(3), 866–875.
57. Yanagisawa, Y., Nan, Y., Okuro, K., & Aida, T. (2018). Mechanically robust, readily repairable polymers via tailored noncovalent cross-linking. *Science*, *359*, 72–76.
58. Moulin, E., Armao, J. J., IV, & Giuseppone, N. (2019). Triarylamine-based supramolecular polymers: Structures, dynamics, and functions. *Accounts of Chemical Research*, *52*, 975–983.
59. Mtangi, W., Tassinari, F., Vankayala, K., Vargas Jentzsch, A., Adelizzi, B., Palmans, A. R. A., Fontanesi, C., Meijer, E. W., & Naaman, R. (2017). Control of electrons' spin eliminates hydrogen peroxide formation during water splitting. *Journal of the American Chemical Society*, *139*(7), 2794–2798.
60. Vantomme, G., ter Huurne, G. M., Kulkarni, C., ten Eikelder, H. M. M., Markvoort, A. J., Palmans, A. R. A., & Meijer, E. W. (2019). Tuning the length of cooperative supramolecular polymers under thermodynamic control. *Journal of the American Chemical Society*, *141*, 18278–18285.
61. Venkata Rao, K., Mabesoone, M. F. J., Miyajima, D., Nihonyanagi, A., Meijer, E. W., & Aida, T. (2020). Distinct pathways in "thermally bisignate supramolecular polymerization": Spectroscopic and computational studies. *Journal of the American Chemical Society*, *142*, 598–605.

62. Wagner, W., Wehner, M., Stepanenko, V., & Würthner, F. (2019). Supramolecular block copolymers by seeded living polymerization of perylene bisimides. *Journal of the American Chemical Society*, *141*, 12044–12054.
63. Zhang, H., Bre´, L., Zhao, T., Newland, B., Da Costa, M., & Wang, W. (2014). A biomimetic hyperbranched poly (amino ester)-based nanocomposite as a tunable bone adhesive for sternal closure. *Journal of Materials Chemistry B*, *2*(26), 4067–4071.
64. Ma, X., & Zhao, Y. (2015). Biomedical applications of supramolecular systems based on host–guest interactions. *Chemical Reviews*, *115*(15), 7794–7839.
65. Huang, Z., Chen, X., O'Neill, S. J. K., Wu, G., Whitaker, D. J., Li, J., McCune, J. A., & Scherman, O. A. (2022). Highly compressible glass-like supramolecular polymer networks. *Nature Materials*, *21*, 103–109.
66. Aida, T., & Meijer, E. W. (2020). Supramolecular polymers–we've come full circle. *Israel Journal of Chemistry*, *60*, 33–47.
67. Rutz, A. L., Hyland, K. E., Jakus, A. E., Burghardt, W. R., & Shah, R. N. (2015). A multimaterial bioink method for 3D printing tunable, cell-compatible hydrogels. *Advanced Materials*, *27*(9), 1607–1614.
68. Hung, K. C., Tseng, C. S., Dai, L. G., & Hsu, S. H. (2016). Water-based polyurethane 3D printed scaffolds with controlled release function for customized cartilage tissue engineering. *Biomaterials*, *83*, 156–168.
69. Bajaj, P., Schweller, R. M., Khademhosseini, A., West, J. L., & Bashir, R. (2014). 3D bio fabrication strategies for tissue engineering and regenerative medicine. *Annual Review of Biomedical Engineering*, *16*, 247–276..

CHAPTER 5

Recent Advancements in Cancer Therapy by Using Polymers and Their Nanocomposites

M. RAMESH,[1,*] K. SAKTHISHOBANA,[2] and M. S. KAMALI[3]

[1]*Department of Mechanical Engineering, Mahendra Engineering College, Mallasamudram, Namakkal, Tamil Nadu, India*

[2]*Department of Biotechnology, Bannari Amman Institute of Technology, Sathyamangalam, Tamil Nadu, India*

[3]*Department of Biotechnology, Kalaignarkarunanidhi Institute of Technology (KIT), Coimbatore, Tamil Nadu, India*

*Corresponding author

ABSTRACT

The biggest challenge in tumor therapy is identified as hydrophobicity of drugs, clearance of drug by first pass metabolism, bioavailability of the drug at the target site, drug uptake efficiency, non-specific distribution of drug. The latest development in the cancer therapy exhibits commendable progress in improvement of drug dissolubility in water by using a carrier. This carrier can be based on a polymer in conjugation with the drug or encapsulation of drug within a scaffold/micelle. The creation of nanoparticle provides a feasible solution in evading the hydrophobic character of drug. The different types of nano-structures like nano-shell type, nano-core type and nano-scaffolds can provide a sophisticated hydrophobic region inside them making the drug to be placed comfortably. In addition to solving water dissolution problem, creating nanoparticles can increase bioavailability of drugs at the target site.

Polymer Applications in Medicine: Revolutionizing Treatment and Therapeutics.
Mohd. Imran Ahamed, Faheem Ahmad, and Ishaat M. Khan (Eds.)

DOI: 10.1201/9781779640871-5

5.1 INTRODUCTION

Cancer is the second leading cause of death worldwide and a major hindrance to increasing life expectancy globally. The WHO carried out an analysis and reported that cancer is the first or second cause of death before the age of 70 in 112 out of 183 countries and has gained third or fourth rank in another 23 countries. The global cancer burden was estimated by the International Agency for Research on Cancer using GLOBOCAN 2020, which reported that 19.3 million new cancer cases and 10 million deaths due to cancer were recorded in the year 2020 amidst the COVID-19 pandemic [1]. Cancer is the uncontrolled proliferation of cells leading to the formation of a tumor. Conventional cancer therapies are available; despite this, deaths due to cancer are increasing day by day. Chemotherapy (CT) and radiotherapy are the classic treatment methodologies being followed in cancer management. However, these treatments are not effective for malignant tumors due to tumor metastasis, recurrence, and cancer cell resistance to CT [2]. The scientific community is continuously exploring effective and economical drugs for the treatment of different cancer types. Regardless, every drug has its limitations in being brought from bench to bed. The major challenges in using drugs are their poor bioavailability because of nonspecific drug distribution, and they are barely soluble in body fluids, getting eliminated from the system rapidly [3].

Certain drugs used for CT are toxic chemicals capable of inhibiting cancer cell proliferation. These drugs are very useful in suppressing the disease, but their poor solubility and inability to act specifically on tumor cells make them unsuitable candidates for CT [4]. Therapeutic genes are also being studied to inhibit cancer cell proliferation. However, the internalization of these genes exclusively into tumor cells hampers successful treatment [5]. All these limitations can be addressed by developing a novel method to deliver drugs or therapeutic genes. One such strategy is using nanocomposites as a delivery vehicle for cancer treatment. Nanocomposites made of polymers have gained much attention in recent times as they can be procured from natural sources, are economical and eco-friendly, can be modified with targeting moieties, and can be made responsive specifically to the tumor microenvironment (TME). Nanocomposites can be synthesized in different forms, and using one or more than one polymer, they can be functionalized as per the demand [6, 7]. In this chapter, we have discussed the recently synthesized polymer nanocomposites and their novelty in cancer management.

Figure 5.1 shows the organic and bioorganic polymers available for nano-composite tailoring, the application of these nano-fabrications, and the most commonly employed strategies to treat cancer.

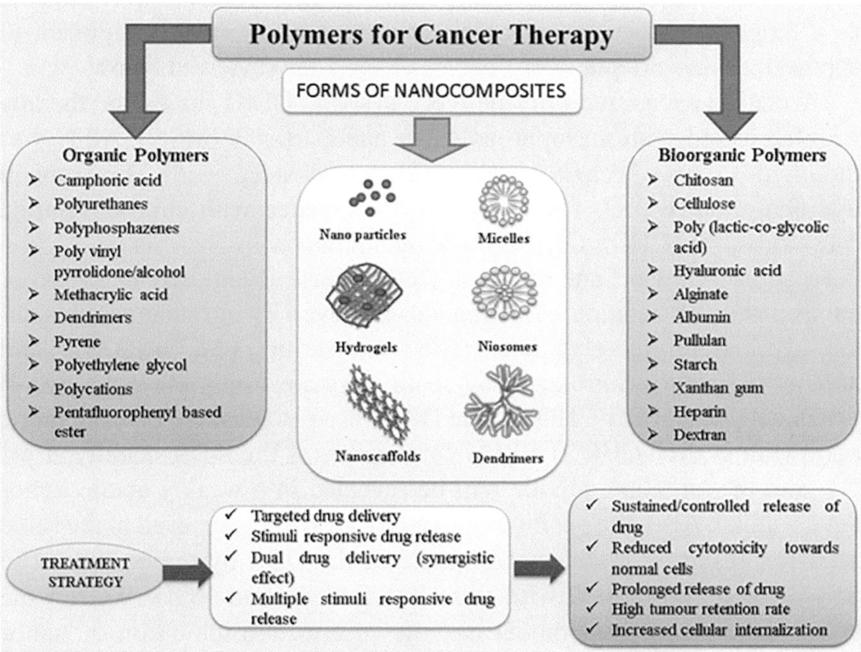

FIGURE 5.1 Schematic representation of recent advancement in cancer therapy by polymer nanocomposites.

5.2 BIOORGANIC POLYMERS

Polymers that are naturally available are biodegradable, biocompatible, and mostly non-toxic or less toxic. Some of these bioorganic polymers possess antimicrobial, antioxidant, and even a few polymers render anti-cancer properties as well [8]. The following section provides a summary of studies that have utilized some of the bioorganic polymers for tailoring nano-vehicles to deliver therapeutic agents for treating different cancers.

5.2.1 CHITOSAN

A derivative of chitin, chitosan is the second most abundant biopolymer and is widely used in the fabrication of nano-drug delivery moieties.

Biodegradability and abundant availability are the major reasons for exploiting chitosan as a biopolymer in various biopharmaceutical applications. In addition, properties such as biodegradability, biocompatibility, low toxicity, antibacterial, and antifungal activities make it more suitable as a biopolymer. Studies using chitosan as an important component to synthesize nano-drug delivery systems have been reviewed below.

A dual-pH-sensitive drug delivery system (DDS) for tumor therapy was fabricated with mesoporous silica nanoparticles (MSN). MSN was modified to have benzimidazole (Bz) and loaded with Doxorubicin hydrochloride (DOX). The MSN was then coated with chitosan-grafted β-cyclodextrin (CHI-g-CD) through interaction with Bz; this interaction is sensitive to low pH and results in DOX release specifically in the tumor environment. In addition, targeting was achieved by introducing adamantine-glycine-arginine-glycine-aspartic acid-serine (Ad-GRGDS), and another trigger was introduced by coating methoxy poly(ethylene glycol) benzaldehyde (mPEG-CHO) on the DDS via a pH-sensitive benzoic imine bond with grafted CHI. The PEG coating makes the DDS stealthy at pH 7.4, and the targeting peptide will be revealed in a weakly acidic tumor environment. Also, the positive charge of CHI will be exposed in the same scenario, resulting in enhanced uptake of the DDS by tumor cells. The *in vivo* study performed with this DOX@MSN-CHI-RGD-PEG on the breast cancer xenograft model has shown effective inhibition of tumor growth and enhanced drug uptake with significantly fewer side effects on bystander cells [9].

A multi-functional superparamagnetic iron oxide core-gold shell nanoparticle was coated with chitosan to make it suitable for DOX delivery and folate for enhancing cellular uptake. The fabricated SPION@Au-CS-DOX-FA NPs, upon evaluation, were found to be a remarkable nanomedicine for delivering DOX with low cytotoxicity and showed a significant therapeutic effect against cancer cells [10]. Ellagic acid (EA), a polyphenol present in pomegranate, green tea, and berries, is known for its anticancer and antiproliferative properties against various cancer cells. The usage of EA as a chemotherapeutic agent is challenging due to its poor water solubility, low bioavailability, and its elimination through first-pass metabolism. These limitations can be nullified by delivering EA through nanoparticles, which provide a sustained release of EA and make it available in circulation for a prolonged time. One such strategy to use EA as a drug was by entrapping the drug in Tween 80-coated chitosan nanoparticles. *In vitro* and *in vivo* evaluation of this formulation has shown good encapsulation efficiency and tumor regression rate; its efficiency as a therapeutic moiety was improved by the synergistic effect of EA and chitosan [11]. Another study reported the use of PEG-coated chitosan nanoparticles (CSNPs) for obtaining a sustained release of DOX selectively in the tumor environment. PEG coating seems to increase the circulation time in blood, and drug selectivity and cellular uptake were enhanced by functionalizing the nanoparticles with two different breast cancer-specific monoclonal antibodies, namely anti-human mammaglobin (Anti-hMAM) and anti-human epidermal growth factor (Anti-HER2). The two nanoformulations having different targeting mAbs have shown significant cytotoxicity towards tumor cells compared to normal cells [12].

5.2.2 POLY (LACTIC-CO-GLYCOLIC ACID) (PLGA)

Poly (lactic-co-glycolic acid) (PLGA), an FDA and EMA approved biopolymer for synthesizing drug delivery nanoparticles, has gained wide attention from the scientific community for its biodegradability and biocompatibility [13, 14]. Apart from these, PLGA is known to render controlled and sustained release of payload. It has the ability to accumulate in the tumor environment by the EPR effect, which can also be enhanced by decorating the nano-carrier with targeting ligands [15]. PLGA nanoparticles were used as a delivery vehicle to efficiently utilize the properties of curcumin to treat cancer. The curcumin-loaded PLGA NPs showed good encapsulation efficiency, and the drug was released in a sustained manner. The efficiency of curcumin-loaded NPs was evaluated against MDA-MB231 cells, and they showed a significant reduction in cell viability, cell invasion, and migration. This makes them an efficient anti-metastatic agent and a promising therapeutic moiety to combat cancer-like diseases [16].

Paclitaxel, a drug used to treat different types of cancer, has many disadvantages such as low bioavailability, high toxicity, low metabolic stability, and can result in liver damage, neutropenia, and bone marrow suppression when injected. A study performed to evaluate PLGA NPs for delivering paclitaxel to neuroblastoma cells (SH-SY5Y) has proven them to be a promising candidate to treat cancer, as they have shown higher efficacy in managing cancer than free paclitaxel [17]. The biodegradability and safety of PLGA NPs make them an advanced drug delivery system; however, PLGA NPs require certain functionalization to be more efficient. PLGA NPs must be functionalized in such a way as to improve cell selectivity, cellular uptake, and to enhance slow drug release specifically in the TME. Star PLGA nanoparticles were coated with HA (HA-sPLGA-XNPs) for the targeted delivery of docetaxel (DTX) and were studied on the A549 cell line. It was reported that these robust HA-sPLGA-XNPs showed improvement in cellular uptake, and the drug release profile was also significantly improved [18].

PLGA NPs have been utilized for the delivery of hesperidin, an anti-inflammatory and anti-carcinogenic flavanone glycoside present abundantly in citrus fruits. The fabricated Hes-PLGA nano vehicle was characterized to be spherical with an average size of 4 to 30 nm. *In vitro* evaluation of these NPs has shown a reduction in cell viability and has enhanced mitochondrial-mediated apoptosis. Altogether, these Hes-PLGA NPs have proven to be a promising nano vehicle for efficient, sustained, and targeted delivery of hesperidin [19]. Afatinib (AFA), an FDA-approved drug for treating non-small cell lung cancer (NSCLC), has a major disadvantage in its use for treatment due to its low bioavailability resulting from its poorly soluble nature. A study performed to improve the efficient utilization of AFA has used PLGA NPs to deliver AFA. AFA NPs formulated using PLGA were designed for non-invasive inhalation of AFA deep into the lungs to treat NSCLC. The AFA NPs have proven to be a good inhalable formulation with a mass median aerodynamic diameter of 4.7 ± 0.1 μm and a fine-particle fraction of $77.8 \pm 4.3\%$; moreover, they have the ability to be deposited in deep lung regions. The study of these NPs on tumor spheroids has shown efficient tumor penetration ability and has significantly reduced the growth of tumors [20].

5.2.3 HYALURONIC ACID (HA)

Hyaluronic acid (HA) is a bioorganic polymer that has the ability to target CD44 receptors present on tumor cells, making it an effective ingredient in drug delivery systems (DDS). Chitosan nanoparticles (NPs) were coated with HA to deliver siRNA for treating bladder cancer, and they were synthesized and studied. Although gene therapy is effective in managing bladder cancer, the major shortcoming is the lack of targeted therapy.

This issue is addressed by giving HA coating to the aforementioned NPs to deliver siRNA that can downregulate Bcl2. *In vitro* and *in vivo* studies performed using T24 cells showed that siRNA@CS-HAD is a stable system with good bioavailability, encapsulation efficiency, and less cytotoxicity, which can accumulate specifically in the tumor environment to show a significant reduction in tumor development [21].

MSN were coated with HA to deliver curcumin (C) specifically to tumor cells. This nano formulation, MSN-HA-C, was fabricated to be approximately 75 nm and had around 14.76% drug loading efficiency. This nanosized therapeutic agent significantly reduced tumor volume and increased the bioavailability of curcumin effectively compared to free curcumin [22]. HA nanoparticles were induced with amphiphilicity using dexamethasone (DEX) and then loaded with doxorubicin (DOX) for treating cancer. This approach was strategized to reduce the cytotoxicity of DOX. The effects of HA-DEX-DOX and free DOX have shown that free DOX activated complement proteins and the coagulation cascade, whereas the other group did not show such deleterious effects. DEX, being an anti-inflammatory agent, has suppressed the cytotoxic effect of DOX, and both DEX and DOX have rendered a synergistic effect to kill cancer cells. This nano formulation was also reported to polarize bone marrow-derived anti-inflammatory M2 macrophages to a pro-inflammatory M1 phenotype with the upregulation of TNF-α, iNOS, and IL-1β [23].

In another study, HA was conjugated with cysteine to introduce a disulfide bond (SS) and then conjugated with tetraphenyl ethylene (TPE) to create a self-assembling polymer. This conjugate HA-SS-TPE can self-assemble, target CD44-positive cells, and release the payload only in glutathione-rich regions. DOX was introduced during the self-assembly of HA-SS-TPE micelles and was evaluated both *in vitro* and *in vivo*. The results show that these DOX-loaded micelles can target CD44-positive cancer cells and can dissociate quickly in the tumor environment due to the presence of glutathione, unloading DOX [24].

5.2.4 ALBUMIN

Albumin is a natural biomaterial with good biocompatibility, is biodegradable, and is also non-immunogenic. One important feature of using albumin in nano drug formulation is that it can be efficiently internalized by tumor cells as a nutrient through a glycoprotein-mediated pathway; thereby, albumin can activate the respective receptor in the tumor region [25]. Albumin-based nanoparticles were fabricated to treat both tumors and tumor metastasis by photothermal therapy. In this study, human serum albumin (HSA) was used after conjugating it with a P-selectin-targeting peptide (PSN) or with IR780. By using a disulfide reprogramming method, the HSA-IR780 and HSA-PSN were mixed to form nanoparticles. The strategy behind this neoformation is that after administration, the nanoparticles will accumulate in the tumor. When excited with an 808 nm LASER, the tumor will be injured due to the photothermal effect of IR780. This will lead to increased infiltration of platelets into the tumor region, which in turn leads to increased accumulation of nanoparticles as the PSN can target P-selectin-positive platelets. Together, this novel fabrication effectively inhibits tumors and tumor metastasis by inducing a "platelet bridge" [26].

A novel drug delivery system was designed using albumin nanoparticles by Nab™ technology to deliver paclitaxel palmitate (PTX-PA). The DDS has shown a longer retention time in the tumor region and has significantly reduced tumor growth compared to the commercial PTX-loaded albumin NP (Abraxane®). The study reported that the toxicity of PTX in normal organs was reduced, an increase in animal weight was also observed, and the release of PTX was sustained. In addition, Nab-PTX-PA remained in the tumor for more than 40 days with fewer adverse effects [27].

The same PTX-loaded albumin NPs by Nab™ were pooled with an anti-PD-L1 monoclonal antibody through a pH-sensitive linker for combination therapy. These PD-L1/PTX@HSA NPs are designed to target immune checkpoints such as programmed cell death ligand-1 and cytotoxic T-lymphocyte antigen-4. This formulation showed increased cellular internalization due to the targeting ligand, and the drug release was higher in the acidic TME. Overall, this combinatorial therapy has proven to be an efficient strategy to treat cancer [28]. Bovine serum albumin (BSA) is used in the formulation of nanoparticles to treat ovarian cancer. In this study, they encapsulated carboplatin (CRB) as a therapeutic agent, and the NPs were characterized to be spherical with a negative charge, with a particle size of 253 nm. The *in vitro* study reported that CRB-loaded albumin NPs showed an enhanced anti-cancer effect compared to free CRB [29].

5.2.5 ALGINATE

Alginate (Alg) is yet another natural biopolymer, present abundantly in brown algae, consisting of repeated units of β-D-mannuronic acid and α-L-guluronic acid linked by a 1,4 linkage. It has shown good biocompatibility, biodegradability, and in addition, it is non-toxic, making alginate a better option for synthesizing nanocarriers [30]. Mucoadhesive NPs were fabricated using two mucoadhesive moieties, such as catechol-bearing alginate (Cat-Alg) and maleimide-bearing chitosan (Mal-CS), for intravesical CT. These dual-functional mucoadhesive NPs (Mal-CS-Cat-Alg) were then loaded with DOX and characterized and evaluated for their efficacy in treating bladder cancer. The NPs were retained in the bladder mucosa for an extended period due to excellent mucoadhesive properties and were reported to release DOX in a sustained manner for more than 24 hours. Additionally, the cellular internalization was efficient, effectively targeting tumor cells with a low IC50 [31].

pH-sensitive and redox-responsive NPs were fabricated for the targeted delivery of DOX by mounting fluorescein-labeled wheat germ agglutinin (fWGA) on disulfide cross-linked alginate NPs (fDTP2). This formulation is reported to have a 19.3% drug loading efficiency and releases DOX by stimulation into gastrointestinal conditions only. Cellular internalization of this therapeutic moiety was found to be good, as shown by fluorescence and confocal imaging [32]. A multi-responsive nanocomposite hydrogel was synthesized, composed of poly(N-isopropyl acrylamide) (PNIPAM) and alginate interpenetrating polymer and GO-Fe_3O_4 nanomaterials, to be used as a DOX delivery system. The composition makes this hydrogel responsive to near-infrared light, altering magnetic fields, and also acidic pH, resulting in the controlled release of the drug specifically in the tumor environment. The pH responsiveness is rendered by the alginate, which also provides the gelation and mechanical properties. The study outcome has shown that this novel DOX delivery system holds great promise for managing tumors [33].

Hydrogels of alginate and sodium carboxymethyl cellulose were synthesized by crosslinking with Ca^{2+} for delivering two drugs: aspirin (Asp) for pain relief and $CaCO_3$-loaded methotrexate ($CaCO_3$/MTX) for treating colorectal cancer. The pH-responsive nature of the as-formulated hydrogel prevents the absorption of drugs in the stomach and small intestine. The drug release profile proved this hydrogel to be an effective strategy to deliver drugs selectively in the target regions of the colorectum, triggered by the gastrointestinal fluid pH [34].

5.2.6 PULLULAN

A natural polymer obtained from the fermentation medium of *Aureobasidium pullulans* (black yeast) is non-toxic, non-mutagenic, tasteless, and odorless, and is a water-soluble polymer with high thermal stability. The hydrophobic derivative of pullulan is widely used in the synthesis of nanocarriers for drug and gene delivery [35]. Gold nano-hybrids (GNHs) were functionalized with folate-hydrophobic-quaternized pullulan (FHQ-PUL) for the delivery of the hydrophobic anticancer drug camptothecin (CPT). The spherical CPT-GNHs@FHQ-PUL was approximately 10.97 nm and can release the drug in response to acidic pH. This nano formulation has enhanced cellular internalization by folate receptor-mediated endocytosis and increases cell death by inducing apoptosis. The cytotoxicity study revealed that the delivery of CPT by GNHs@FHQ-PUL has enhanced toxicity towards cancer cells compared to free CPT; in addition, the toxicity of CPT towards normal cells was also prevented [36].

A carboxymethyl pullulan-based nano scaffold was tailored to improve the chemosensitivity of erlotinib (ERL) on hypoxic cancer cells. For this nano scaffold, carboxymethyl pullulan (CMP) was conjugated with 6-(2-nitroimidazole) hexylamine (HA-NI), a hydrophobic hypoxia-responsive moiety. This highly negative scaffold (CMP-HA-NI) was then grafted with polyethyleneimine (PEI) after being modified with nitrobenzoic acid (NBA) to make it biocompatible. The CMP-HA-NI and PEI-NBA were self-assembled to form a nano micelle for the efficient delivery of ERL. The evaluation study has proven this nano formulation to be a successful method to improve the therapeutic efficiency of ERL by surpassing hypoxia-induced ERL resistance. Additionally, this formulation has been confirmed to induce apoptosis significantly and has exhibited good antiproliferative properties against HeLa cells [37].

A similar strategy was verified again to ensure the integrity of the pullulan-based co-polymer to deliver ERL. Herein, succinyl pullulan (Pull-SA) was conjugated with (HA-NI), and then they self-assembled to form nanocarriers. Finally, ERL was loaded into the hydrophobic core of (Pull-SA-HA-NI) NPs. The NI in this nano formulation is sensitive to the hypoxic tumor environment and will dissociate, resulting in the release of the payload. In addition to the inhibition of drug resistance, these nanocarriers have significantly enhanced apoptosis [38].

5.2.7 CELLULOSE

Cellulose is the principal component of plant cell walls. It is present in any plant; also, algae and some bacteria synthesize cellulose. The solubility of cellulose is a major concern for using it to fabricate nanosystems, which has been well addressed by synthesizing the derivatives of cellulose [39]. A bio-nanocomposite (BNC) was synthesized using 5-Fluorouracil (5-FU) encapsulated cellulose fiber (CF) from rice straw and chitosan (CS-CF / 5FU BNCs) by the ionic gelation method and sodium tripolyphosphate as a cross-linker. The formulated BNCs have enhanced the thermal stability of 5-FU compared to free 5-FU, and the nano composition has shown triggered drug release at collateral fluid pH (pH 7.4) compared to gastric fluid pH (pH 1.0). The drug encapsulation efficiency was around 86%, and the outcome of the cytotoxicity study has illustrated these BNCs as a reliable and eco-friendly candidate for treating colorectal cancer [40].

A DDS based on nano-cellulose was fabricated to deliver curcumin in a controlled manner and specifically to cancer cells by targeting. The nanocellulose synthesized by the acid-alkali method was first conjugated with folic acid (NC-FA). Using ceric ammonium sulfate (CAS) as an initiator and ethyl glycol dimethacrylate (EGDMA) as a cross-linker, the NC-FA was polymerized with glycidyl methacrylate (GMA) and hydroxyethyl methacrylate (HEMA). The final formulation FA-NC/GMA-HEMA/EGDMA was then loaded with curcumin, and performance was evaluated *in vitro*. It was concluded that the novel DDS has shown good drug loading efficiency, and it has also released the payload in a sustained manner for an extended period. Moreover, this nano-therapeutic moiety has released the drug only in response to low pH and has transported curcumin specifically to cancer cells with the help of FA receptors. In summary, this curcumin-loaded FA-NC/GMA-HEMA/EGDMA has proven to be an essential candidate in cancer management [41].

Cellulose nanoparticles were prepared from waste cotton using the acid hydrolysis method for delivering DOX, which was reported for the first time. The waste cotton was first hydrolyzed using HCl to prepare cellulose, and then it was used to synthesize cellulose nanoparticles. The as-formed cellulose NPs were spherical and 300 nm in size. The DOX was loaded during NP synthesis, and the entrapment efficiency was approximately 99%. *In vitro* analysis showed that the payload was released in a controlled manner at pH 7.4, and DOX release was observed for about 34 days. The therapeutic efficiency was also significant. Altogether, these NPs were proven to be economical, environmentally friendly, and a promising nano vehicle for drug delivery [42].

5.3 SYNTHETIC POLYMERS

5.3.1 CAMPHORIC ACID (CA)

Camphoric acid (CA), a derivative of camphor, is used in medical applications. It is non-toxic and antiseptic. It is assumed to paralyze nerve terminals within the sweat glands and is thus used in the treatment of tuberculosis-associated night sweats. Polyester derived from CA and group IVB metallocene dichloride's demonstrated a remarkable ability for tumor suppression in a pancreatic cancer cell line. The EC50 shown by this polyester was 100 to 1000 times lower than the concentration required by the model cancer drug cisplatin. Its requirement is just in the amount of nanograms/mL[43].

5.3.2 POLYURETHANES (PUR)

The active transport of a molecule into a cell requires specific signals/receptors to recognize a particular cell type. Polyurethane is an amphiphilic synthetic polymer that exhibits biocompatibility and biodegradability within living cells. Assisted with polyethylene glycol (PEG) and polycaprolactone, it can be tailor-made for a specific particle size and can synthesize pH and temperature-sensitive nanoparticles[44]. The PUR, with the correct amount of hydrophobic to hydrophilic ratio, can be derivatized with a specific surface ligand. Due to the presence of the ligand, this can identify a particular cell type, especially cancer cells, to boost its remission. The ligand employed in this study is the monoclonal antibody trastuzumab, marketed as Herceptin. It binds to the human epidermal receptor-2 (HER-2) displayed on the surface of breast cancer cells, thereby blocking the signaling pathway essential for their growth and division. The binding of Herceptin to the receptor induces an intracellular signaling cascade that can lead to cell cycle blocking, inducing apoptosis, preventing the reception of growth signals, or inhibiting DNA repair. Any or all of these actions will lead to the death of the cancer cell. This was confirmed by the reduction of half the amount of cancer-specific carbohydrate antigen usually expressed on the surface of cancer cells (ca50%) [45].

The polyurethane-based pH-sensitive carrier nanoparticle was synthesized for delivering the cancer drug doxorubicin (DOX) to human breast cancer (MCF-7) cells. The PU-DOX nanoparticle showed a greater drug loading capacity of 14.1 wt %, and the pH-dependent drug release was effective at pH 4.0, pH 5.0, and almost none of the DOX was released at pH 7.4. *In vitro* tests revealed elevated PU-DOX nanoparticle internalization and a greater arrest of cancer cell proliferation than the pure DOX[44].

5.3.3 POLYPHOSPHAZENE

Phosphazenes are a hybrid of inorganic and organic molecules having a backbone of inorganic (-P=N-) and organic molecules/monomers as side groups. These molecules are primarily securing attention in tissue engineering as well as in the controlled release of drug delivery. A Poly(cyclotriphosphazene-co-dopamine) (PCTD) microsphere is synthesized in a single step by one-pot synthesis through the precipitation polymerization technique. This microsphere contains dopamine, a neurotransmitter, as the monomer. The PCTD was used as an agent to control the release of the anticancer model drug acriflavine. The drug loading capacity of PCTD is 19.5 mg/g, and the drug release profile at pH 5.0 is 29%, while at pH 7.0 it is 47% during 7 days [46].

5.3.4 METHACRYLIC ACID

Methacrylic acid, a synthetic polymer with the brand name Eudragit®, is a pH-sensitive molecule. It is used along with a porous/matrix-forming compound termed Sylysia® 350 in developing a nanoparticulate formulation. A nano-matrix is used for effective dissolution and absorption of the sorafenib drug in the gastrointestinal tract. The bioavailability determinant AUC0–36 h for the nano-matrix was 13–33 times that of the drug's suspension, but only 16.8% to 40.8% that of Eudragit® S100 nanoparticles [47].

5.3.5 POLYVINYL ALCOHOL (PVA)

The synergistic effect of cancer drugs like doxorubicin and sorafenib can help in effective and targeted liver cancer therapy. However, the use of nanoparticles helps in increasing their bioavailability. A nano-shell type nanoparticle was formulated for sorafenib, and it was attached to a nano-core type nanoparticle containing doxorubicin and aimed at the transferrin protein receptor present in the cancer cells. The combinatorial effect of these drugs, effectively released at the specific site, resulted in uniform cell death of more than 75% of the tumor. Targeting transferrin ligands contributed to achieving 92% of synergistic cytotoxicity of cancer cells in the iron-deficient region [47].

5.3.6 CALCIUM CARBONATE/CALCIUM PHOSPHATE

Cancer occurs mostly due to mutations in DNA, especially the p53 gene. Normally, the DNA repair process is very active in removing any kind of mutation, but in the case of cancer, it is not removed, thus leading to cancer. So, in addition to CT, co-therapy with gene modification or gene therapy can arrest cancer cell formation. In order to achieve this mission, the anticancer drug doxorubicin and the p53 gene were encapsulated in a novel multifunctional nanoparticle. It is a hybrid made of inorganic and biopolymers termed heparin–biotin/heparin/$CaCO_3$/calcium phosphate/DNA/DOX (HPB/HP/$CaCO_3$/CaP/DNA/DOX). The inorganic moiety $CaCO_3$/CaP imparts pH sensitivity due to its dissolution inside the cellular pH, whereas the biotin helps in achieving tumor targeting potential for the synthesized nanoparticle. The cellular growth inhibition assay gave a positive result in repressing cancer HeLa cell growth and effectively delivering the therapeutic gene inside cells [48].

5.3.7 POLY LACTIDE-CO-GLYCOLIC ACID (PLGA) AND POLY HYDROXYBUTYRATE (PHB)

Most cancer drugs are hydrophobic and thus face a similar issue of poor dissolution in water. On account of their hydrophobicity, effective delivery into the target cell becomes difficult. The use of nanoparticles has minimized this issue and can provide moderate efficiency. However, there is always room for improvement. To enhance the blood retention time of the anticancer drugs and also to address the poor dissolution in water, spherical polymeric nano-constructs (SPNs) were developed with a hydrophobic core. The anticancer drug docetaxel (DTXL) will be present in the core and will be enclosed by the synthetic biodegradable poly (D, L-lactide-co-glycolic) acid (PLGA). Even though the degradation products of PLGA are biocompatible, they are acidic molecules that can create inflammation in the nearby tissues. So, PLGA is swapped with poly (3-hydroxybutyrate) (PHB) in SPNs. The comparison of these two types of SPNs demonstrated that PHB has a slower drug release rate than PLGA. PHB SPNs also displayed a higher drug loading rate in nanoparticles and better internalization and toxicity [49].

5.3.8 DENDRIMERS

Dendrimers are globular-shaped, nano-sized synthetic polymers having a regularly branched tree-like construction formed by step-by-step progressive growth. Due to their uniform size, they can be used as scaffolds for encapsulating anticancer drugs using non-covalent interactions. They can be internally conjugated to drugs by covalent bonds. Dendrimer drug conjugates are used for carrying methotrexate for targeted cancer cell therapy [50]. DOX-encapsulated polyamidoamine dendrimers with a covalently bonded 2,3-dimethylmaleic anhydride (DMA) were used for tumor therapy as nanoaggregates. It is based on proton-induced drug release, in other words, at lower pH in the cancer cell environment [51].

5.3.9 OLIGO (ETHYLENE GLYCOL) METHYL ETHER METHACRYLATE

Mesoglobules are stable colloids that form above the transition temperature of any thermo-reactive polymers. These are nanoaggregates that can carry drugs conjugated with them. A terpolymer of diethylene glycol methyl methacrylate, oligoethylene glycol methyl methacrylate, and 2-aminoethylmethacrylate hydrochloride was manufactured. The drug DOX was linked using a carbamate linkage to the mesoglobules [52].

5.3.10 POLYVINYL PYRIDINE (PVP)

A stimuli-responsive drug release nanoparticle can be synthesized using many external factors like pH, temperature, magnetic field, and sensitivity to light. Among these factors, pH-based drug release response is mostly studied because endosomes (pH 5.5) and cancer cells (pH 6.8) have higher acidity than the near-neutral normal cells (pH 7.2). Magnetite-based mesoporous silica nanoparticles (MMSN) were synthesized and attached externally with polyethylene glycol-co-polyvinyl pyridine (PEG-co-PVP) to act as a controlled release pH-responsive carrier. The prepared DOX-carrying nanoparticle is a core-shell type nanocarrier and showed complete release at pH 5.5 inside the cellular endosomes [53].

In another study, the DOX-carrying MMSN was secured with β-cyclodextrin and enveloped within poly N-isopropyl acrylamide. It displayed stimuli-responsive drug release under both pH and temperature factors. The experiment resulted in the release of the drug at pH 5.5 inside endosomes and furthermore observed the crumbling of the carrier shell above the lower critical temperature of the solution [54]. A core-shell type nanofiber was formulated with PVP as the shell material while hyperbranched poly (butylene adipate) forms as the core material. This was allowed to carry the anticancer drug sesquiterpene doperoxide Artemisinin. In addition to tumor therapy, it is also employed in malarial treatment approved by WHO. The drug has a natural peroxide group in its structure, which, upon reaction with metal ions, can release free radicals. They can, in turn, destroy tumor cells [55].

An FDA-approved hepatocellular carcinoma (HCC) drug called sorafenib has serious difficulties in being utilized as a full-scale drug for tumor therapy. The reason is its poor dissolution in water and inadequate bioavailability due to hepatic first-pass metabolism. A nanoparticle based on synthetic polymers like polyvinylpyrrolidone-vinyl acetate and sodium lauryl sulfate (SLS) was developed to improve its solubility and bioavailability of the drug in systemic circulation. An experiment to test the drug-releasing capacity of the aforementioned nanoparticles was conducted with individual components as well as in combination of both PVP-VP and SLS. The results indicated a 1.85-fold increase in Cmax bioavailability and a 1.79-fold increase in the area under the curve (AUC) by PVP-VP compared to the SLS counterpart. The results also indicated that the combination of both polymers provided improvement only in intermittent bioavailability[47].

5.3.11 POLY METHACRYLIC ACID

One of the mesoporous structures, MCM41, is found to have biodegradability, biocompatibility, and porosity due to its unique properties like adjustable pore diameter, pore distribution, and large surface-to-pore volume. It was used to produce a nanocomposite along with methacrylic acid (MMA). The produced nanocomposite has sustained release characteristics; however, it shows poor drug loading capacity. Thus, it is surface modified by polymers and converted into nanocapsules by treatment with hydrofluoric acid (HF). The prepared nanocapsule carried naproxen as a model drug. It was identified as a pH-responsive capsule that can effectively release the drug at pH 7.4 [56].

5.3.12 PYRENE

Pyrene is a photosensitive molecule that exhibits photogenotoxicity under UV irradiation and can produce reactive oxygen species (ROS). These ROS are toxic to cells as they oxidize cellular molecules. A novel material based on the release of photosensitive pyrene under reducing conditions was synthesized and designated as d-PEG-ss-Py (Figure 5.2). This molecule displays a disulfide bond that can be reduced in a reducing environment. Normally, a reducing environment is present inside cancer cells, thus releasing the pyrene. It can subsequently self-aggregate *in situ*, and upon activation under UV light, can produce ROS and induce cancer cell apoptosis [57].

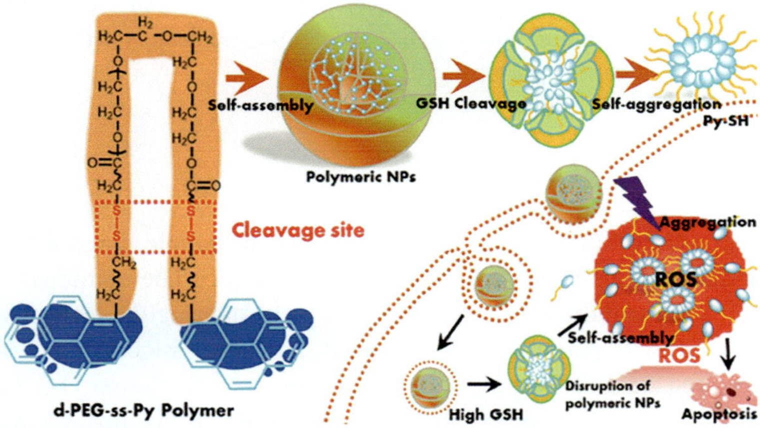

FIGURE 5.2 Illustrative diagram of mechanism followed by d-PEG-ss-Py NPs in cancer therapy.

Source: Reprinted with permission from Ref. [57]

5.3.13 POLYETHYLENEIMINE

In a shell core type nanoparticle structure, the shell is created using polyethyleneimine, a polymer responsive to pH modification, and magnetic iron oxide as the core particle. This nanoparticle carries DOX as the anticancer drug. The loading capacity of DOX was found to be 85.19% and it was found to possess a higher drug releasing capacity at acidic pH [58].

5.3.14 POLYETHYLENE GLYCOL (PEG)

To boost the drug uptake capacity of any nanoparticle, the hydrophobicity of the drug has to be masked by the encapsulating molecule. The use of a polymer-small molecule conjugate can increase the hydrophobicity of the nanoparticle and can help load the highest concentration of drug in its core. The use of biodegradable synthetic polymer PEG conjugated to coumarin from plants can showcase the highest cancer drug loading capacity of 17% DOX. It has the additional characteristic of pH stimuli-based controlled release [59].

5.3.15 DIMETHYL MALEIC ANHYDRIDE

A pH responsive nanoparticle was custom made into a polymer 2,3-dimethylmaleic-anhydride-poly(ethylene glycol)-ε-poly-L-lysine-doxorubicin/lapatinib. The DOX and lapatinib are antineoplastic drugs used synergistically for breast cancer therapy [60].

5.3.16 PFBT

The recent advancement in cancer therapy is to couple diagnostics and therapeutics in a single go, termed as theragnostic. The combination of identification and drug therapy emerged by considering the humanitarian aspects of cancer patients. In this process, a polymer bioconjugate molecule termed as PFBT (poly [9,9-bis(6-bromohexyl)-fluorenyl-2,7-diyl-co-4,7-(2,1,3-benzothiadiazole)], which has inherent diagnostic capacity and produces greenish-yellow fluorescence, was used as a theranostic agent for supplying the anticancer drug 5-fluorouracil (5FU). PFBT-B is coated onto a magnetite nanoparticle which displays the cancer-specific biotin moieties. The thickness of the nanoparticle shell was found to be 1.88 nm, with a drug loading capacity of approximately 6.64 μg/μg of PFBT-B, which was found to discharge its cargo at acidic pH. It was found to accumulate in HeLa cancer cells more than in normal HEK293T cells (Figure 5.3) [61].

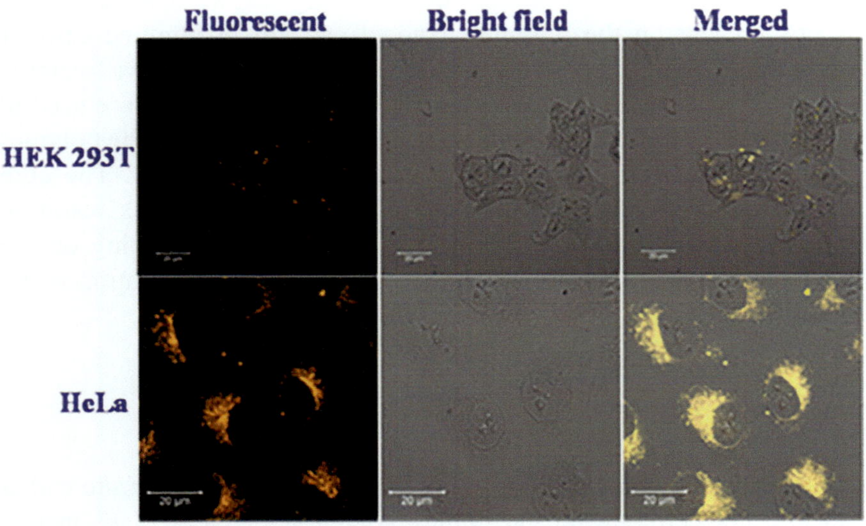

FIGURE 5.3 Comparison of accumulated PFBT-B nanoparticles at the HeLa cells and HEK293T cells by a) fluorescent b) bright filed microscopy and c) merged images.

Source: Reprinted with permission from Ref. [61]

5.3.17 POLYCATIONS

Polycations are used for gene delivery with the sole purpose of condensing nucleic acid inside the nanoparticle. The nanoparticle is synthesized by copolymerization of methacryloylchloroquine (MACQ) and 2-(dimethyl-amino)ethyl methacrylate (DMAEMA). This copolymer has an inherent capacity to inhibit autophagy and carries a gene for TRAIL (tumor necrosis factor-related apoptosis-inducing ligand). The plasmid-encoded gene can sensitize tumor cells for apoptosis in an autophagy-dependent way. This study demonstrated that the therapeutic outcome can be enhanced by the chosen delivery vehicle [62].

5.3.18 PENTAFLUOROPHENYL-BASED ESTER

With the recent advancements in cancer studies, it was found from the 2018 Nobel Prize-winning research of Allison and Honjo that immune checkpoints are critical for cancer formation. The research revealed that the attenuation of the immune system over time and the curbing of T cell function can induce tumor growth and metastasis. The polymer-based nanogels are the newest trend in cancer therapy. The polymer cross-linking helps in reversible drug loading/release. The functional groups present on the polymer nanogel can aid in immune cellular targeting. Polymer nanogels based on pentafluorophenyl reactive esters synthesized by the method of RAFT polymerization are used in cancer therapy as drug carriers. They permit fine-tuning of the polymer carrier to design an individualized cancer immunotherapy. The core reactive esters modified with functional amino molecules result in immune-stimulating IMDQ. Disulfide and ketal cross-linking on the precursor micelles demonstrate carrier integrity and dissolution at the target site [63].

5.4 CONCLUSION

The latest progress is targeting the nanoparticle at a particular site with a cancer cell-specific ligand and stimuli-based drug delivery. Many factors can trigger the release of drugs under the cancer cell environment, such as pH, temperature, magnetic field, and light activation. Major research focuses on pH-based stimuli since there is a clear differentiation of the internal environment inside cancer cells. Dual-responsive stimuli nanoparticles are also being developed, and synergistic approaches are gaining attention. Research focusing on the delivery of dual drugs or the delivery of a drug and a gene for gene therapy is also in progress. The most recent expansion is the introduction of a new field entitled theragnostics, a combination of diagnostics coupled with therapeutics. At the time of diagnostics, the anticancer drug will be equipped. Though there are many studies focused on the targeted delivery of drugs to cancer cells, further insight into drug delivery and cell interactions is mandatory to take this to the clinical level.

KEYWORDS

- **cancer cell-specific ligand**
- **cancer therapy**
- **cellulose**
- **dendrimers**
- **hepatocellular carcinoma**
- **nanocomposites**
- **nano-scaffolds**
- **polymers**
- **synthetic polymers**
- **tumor therapy**

REFERENCES

1. Sung, H., et al. (2021). Global cancer statistics 2020: GLOBOCAN estimates of incidence and mortality worldwide for 36 cancers in 185 countries. *CA: A Cancer Journal for Clinicians*, *71*, 209–249.
2. Sun, Y. (2015). Translational horizons in the tumor microenvironment: Harnessing breakthroughs and targeting cures. *Medicinal Research Reviews*, *35*, 1–29.
3. Yahya, E. B., & Alqadhi, A. M. (2020). Recent trends in cancer therapy: A review on the current state of gene delivery. *Life Sciences*, *269*, 119087.
4. Feldman, D. (2019). Polymers and polymer nanocomposites for cancer therapy. *Applied Sciences*, *9*.
5. Dunbar, C. E., High, K. A., Joung, J. K., Kohn, D. B., Ozawa, K., & Sadelain, M. (2018). Gene therapy comes of age. *Science*, *359*.
6. Sahayaraj, A. F., Muthukrishnan, M., Ramesh, M., & Rajeshkumar, L. (2021). Effect of hybridization on properties of tamarind (*Tamarindus indica* L.) seed nano-powder incorporated jute-hemp fibers reinforced epoxy composites. *Polymer Composites*, *42*, 6611.
7. Ramesh, M., Deepa, C., Niranjana, K., Rajeshkumar, L., Bhoopathi, R., & Balaji, D. (2022). Influence of Haritaki (*Terminalia chebula*) nano-powder on thermo-mechanical, water absorption and morphological properties of Tindora (*Coccinia grandis*) tendril fiber reinforced epoxy composites. *Journal of Natural Fibers*, *19*, 6452–6468.
8. Ramesh, M., Sakthisobana, K., & Suriya, S. B. (2021). Microbial polysaccharides as cell/drug delivery systems. In *Polysaccharides of Microbial Origin*.

9. Liao, T., et al. (2021). A chitosan/mesoporous silica nanoparticle-based anticancer drug delivery system with a 'tumor-triggered targeting' property. *International Journal of Biological Macromolecules*, *183*, 2017–2029.
10. Al-Musawi, S., Albukhaty, S., Al-Karagoly, H., & Almalki, F. (2021). Design and synthesis of multi-functional superparamagnetic core-gold shell coated with chitosan and folate nanoparticles for targeted antitumor therapy. *Nanomaterials*, *11*, 1–14.
11. Kaur, H., Ghosh, S., Kumar, P., Basu, B., & Nagpal, K. (2021). Ellagic acid-loaded, Tween 80-coated, chitosan nanoparticles as a promising therapeutic approach against breast cancer: *In-vitro* and *in-vivo* study. *Life Sciences*, *284*, 119927.
12. Helmi, O., Elshishiny, F., & Mamdouh, W. (2021). Targeted doxorubicin delivery and release within breast cancer environment using PEGylated chitosan nanoparticles labeled with monoclonal antibodies. *International Journal of Biological Macromolecules*, *184*, 325–338.
13. Deepa, C., & Ramesh, M. (2021). Bio composites for prosthesis. In *Green Bio Composites for Biomedical Engineering* (pp. 339–351).
14. Ramesh, M., & Deepa, C. (2021). Bio composites for biomedical devices. In *Green Bio Composites for Biomedical Engineering.*
15. Chiu, H. I., Samad, N. A., Fang, L., & Lim, V. (2021). Cytotoxicity of targeted PLGA nanoparticles: A systematic review. *RSC Advances*, *11*, 9433–9449.
16. Sharma, A., et al. (2021). Effects of curcumin-loaded poly (lactic-co-glycolic acid) nanoparticles in MDA-MB231 human breast cancer cells. *Nanomedicine*, *16*, 1763–1773.
17. Bacanlı, M., Eşim, Ö., Erdoğan, H., Sarper, M., Erdem, O., & Özkan, Y. (2021). Evaluation of cytotoxic and genotoxic effects of paclitaxel-loaded PLGA nanoparticles in neuroblastoma cells. *Food and Chemical Toxicology*, *154*.
18. Wang, X., Cheng, R., & Zhong, Z. (2021). Facile fabrication of robust, hyaluronic acid-surfaced and disulfide-crosslinked PLGA nanoparticles for tumor-targeted and reduction-triggered release of docetaxel. *Acta Biomaterial*, *125*, 280–289.
19. Balakrishnan, K., Casimeer, S. C., Ghidan, A. Y., Ghethan, F. Y., Venkatachalam, K., & Singaravelu, A. (2021). Bio formulated hesperidin-loaded PLGA nanoparticles counteract the mitochondrial-mediated intrinsic apoptotic pathway in cancer cells. *Journal of Inorganic and Organometallic Polymers and Materials*, *31*, 331–343.
20. Elbatanony, R. S., et al. (2021). Afatinib-loaded inhalable PLGA nanoparticles for localized therapy of non-small cell lung cancer (NSCLC)—development and *in-vitro* efficacy. *Drug Delivery and Translational Research*, *11*, 927–943.
21. Liang, Y., et al. (2021). Self-crosslinkable chitosan-hyaluronic acid dialdehyde nanoparticles for CD44-targeted siRNA delivery to treat bladder cancer. *Bioactive Materials*, *6*, 433–446.
22. Ghosh, S., Dutta, S., Sarkar, A., Kundu, M., & Sil, P. C. (2021). Targeted delivery of curcumin in breast cancer cells via hyaluronic acid modified mesoporous silica nanoparticle to enhance anticancer efficiency. *Colloids and Surfaces B: Bio Interfaces*, *197*, 111404.
23. Rangasami, V. K., et al. (2021). Harnessing hyaluronic acid-based nanoparticles for combination therapy: A novel approach for suppressing systemic inflammation and to promote antitumor macrophage polarization. *Carbohydrate Polymers*, *254*.

24. Yan, K., Feng, Y., Gao, K., Shi, X., & Zhao, X. (2022). Fabrication of hyaluronic acid-based micelles with glutathione-responsiveness for targeted anticancer drug delivery. *Journal of Colloid and Interface Science*, *606*, 1586–1596.
25. Lei, C., et al. (2020). Hyaluronic acid and albumin-based nanoparticles for drug delivery. *Journal of Controlled Release*, *331*, 416–433.
26. Zhao, W., et al. (2021). Self-promoted albumin-based nanoparticles for combination therapy against metastatic breast cancer via a hyperthermia-induced 'platelet bridge.' *ACS Applied Materials & Interfaces*, *13*, 25701–25714.
27. Chen, H., et al. (2021). Preparation and characterization of paclitaxel palmitate albumin nanoparticles with high loading efficacy: An *in vitro* and *in vivo* anti-tumor study in mouse models. *Drug Delivery*, *28*, 1067–1079.
28. Pham, L. M., et al. (2021). Combination chemotherapeutic and immune-therapeutic anticancer approach via anti-PD-L1 antibody conjugated albumin nanoparticles. *International Journal of Pharmaceutics*, *605*, 120816.
29. Esim, O., Gedik, M. E., Dogan, A. L., Gunaydin, G., & Hascicek, C. (2021). Development of carboplatin loaded bovine serum albumin nanoparticles and evaluation of its effect on an ovarian cancer cell line. *Journal of Drug Delivery Science and Technology*, *64*, 102655.
30. Lakkakula, J. R., Gujarathi, P., Pansare, P., & Tripathi, S. (2020). A comprehensive review on alginate-based delivery systems for the delivery of chemotherapeutic agent: Doxorubicin. *Carbohydrate Polymers*, *259*, 117696.
31. Sahatsapan, N., Rojanarata, T., Ngawhirunpat, T., Opanasopit, P., & Patrojanasophon, P. (2021). Doxorubicin-loaded chitosan-alginate nanoparticles with dual mucoadhesive functionalities for intravesical chemotherapy. *Journal of Drug Delivery Science and Technology*, *63*, 102481.
32. Chiu, H. I., & Lim, V. (2021). Wheat germ agglutinin-conjugated disulfide cross-linked alginate nanoparticles as a docetaxel carrier for colon cancer therapy. *International Journal of Nanomedicine*, *16*, 2995–3020.
33. Cao, Y., Cheng, Y., & Zhao, G. (2021). Near-infrared light-, magneto-, and pH-responsive GO-Fe_3O_4/poly(N-isopropylacrylamide)/alginate nanocomposite hydrogel microcapsules for controlled drug release. *Langmuir*, *37*, 5522–5530.
34. Sheng, Y., Gao, J., Yin, Z. Z., Kang, J., & Kong, Y. (2021). Dual-drug delivery system based on the hydrogels of alginate and sodium carboxymethyl cellulose for colorectal cancer treatment. *Carbohydrate Polymers*, *269*, 118325.
35. Ganie, S. A., Rather, L. J., & Li, Q. (2021). A review on anticancer applications of pullulan and pullulan derivative nanoparticles. *Carbohydrate Polymers: Technologies and Applications*, *2*, 100115.
36. Laksee, S., Supachettapun, C., Muangsin, N., Lertsarawut, P., Rattanawongwiboon, T., Sricharoen, P., Limchoowong, N., Chutimasakul, T., Kwamman, T., & Hemvichian, K. (2021). Targeted gold nanohybrids functionalized with folate-hydrophobic-quaternized pullulan delivering. *Polymers (Basel)*, *13*, 2670.
37. Bera, H., Abosheasha, M. A., Ito, Y., & Ueda, M. (2021). Etherified pullulan-polyethyleneimine based Nano scaffolds improved chemosensitivity of erlotinib on hypoxic cancer cells. *Carbohydrate Polymers*, *271*, 118441.

38. Bera, H., Abosheasha, M. A., Ito, Y., & Ueda, M. (2021). Hypoxia-responsive pullulan-based nanoparticles as erlotinib carriers. *International Journal of Biological Macromolecules*, *191*, 764–774.
39. Raghav, N., Sharma, M. R., & Kennedy, J. F. (2021). Nanocellulose: A mini-review on types and use in drug delivery systems. *Carbohydrate Polymers: Technologies and Applications*, *2*, 100031.
40. Yusefi, M., et al. (2021). 5-Fluorouracil encapsulated chitosan-cellulose fiber bio nanocomposites: Synthesis, characterization and *in vitro* analysis towards colorectal cancer cells. *Nanomaterials*, *11*, 11071691.
41. Anirudhan, T. S., Manjusha, V., & Chithra Sekhar, V. (2021). A new biodegradable nano cellulose-based drug delivery system for pH-controlled delivery of curcumin. *International Journal of Biological Macromolecules*, *183*, 2044–2054.
42. Gülsu, A., & Yüksektepe, E. (2021). Preparation of spherical cellulose nanoparticles from recycled waste cotton for anticancer drug delivery. *Chemistry Select*, *6*, 5419–5425.
43. Carraher, C. E., et al. (2018). Group IVB metallocene polyesters containing camphoric acid and preliminary cancer cell activity. *International Journal of Polymer Materials and Polymer Biomaterials*, *67*, 469–479.
44. Huang, D., et al. (2018). Polyurethane/doxorubicin nanoparticles based on electrostatic interactions as pH-sensitive drug delivery carriers. *Polymer International*, *67*, 1186–1193.
45. Mattu, C., et al. (2016). Surface-functionalized polyurethane nanoparticles for targeted cancer therapy. *Polymer International*, *65*, 770–779.
46. Metinoğlu Örüm, S., & Süzen Demircioğlu, Y. (2019). One-pot synthesis and characterization of crosslinked polyphosphate dopamine microspheres for controlled drug delivery applications. *Journal of Macromolecular Science, Part A: Pure and Applied Chemistry*, *56*, 854–859.
47. Khan, M. A., Raza, A., Ovais, M., Sohail, M. F., & Ali, S. (2018). Current state and prospects of nano-delivery systems for sorafenib. *International Journal of Polymer Materials and Polymer Biomaterials*, *67*, 1105–1115.
48. Liang, P., Wang, C. Q., Chen, H., Zhuo, R. X., & Cheng, S. X. (2015). Multi-functional heparin-biotin/heparin/calcium carbonate/calcium phosphate nanoparticles for targeted co-delivery of gene and drug. *Polymer International*, *64*, 647–653.
49. Di Mascolo, D., Basnett, P., Palange, A. L., Francardi, M., Roy, I., & Decuzzi, P. (2016). Tuning core hydrophobicity of spherical polymeric Nano constructs for docetaxel delivery. *Polymer International*, *65*, 741–746.
50. Li, X., & Kono, K. (2018). Functional dendrimer–gold nanoparticle hybrids for biomedical applications. *Polymer International*, *67*, 840–852.
51. Yuan, S., et al. (2018). Surface partially neutralized dendritic polymer demonstrating proton-triggered self-assembled aggregation for tumor therapy. *European Polymer Journal*, *103*, 59–67.
52. Lipowska-Kur, D., Szweda, R., Trzebicka, B., & Dworak, A. (2018). Preparation and characterization of doxorubicin nanocarriers based on thermoresponsive oligo (ethylene glycol) methyl ether methacrylate polymer-drug conjugates. *European Polymer Journal*, *109*, 391–401.

53. Pourjavadi, A., Tehrani, Z. M., & Bennett, C. (2015). PEG-co-polyvinyl pyridine coated magnetic mesoporous silica nanoparticles for pH-responsive controlled release of doxorubicin. *International Journal of Polymer Materials and Polymer Biomaterials*, *64*, 570–577.
54. Pourjavadi, A., & Tehrani, Z. M. (2017). *Poly(N-isopropylacrylamide)*-coated β-cyclodextrin–capped magnetic mesoporous silica nanoparticles exhibiting thermal and pH dual response for triggered anticancer drug delivery. *International Journal of Polymer Materials and Polymer Biomaterials*, *66*, 336–348.
55. Bonadies, I., et al. (2017). Electrospun core/shell nanofibers as designed devices for efficient Artemisinin delivery. *European Polymer Journal*, *89*, 211–220.
56. Abbaszad Rafi, A., Fakheri, F., & Mahkam, M. (2016). Synthesis and preparation of new pH-sensitive nanocomposite and nanocapsule based on 'MCM-41/poly methacrylic acid' as drug carriers. *Polymer Bulletin*, *73*, 2649–2659.
57. Su, T., et al. (2018). Reduction-induced decomposition and self-aggregation strategy to induce reactive oxygen species generation for cancer therapy. *ACS Applied Bio Materials*, *1*, 954–960.
58. Zaaeri, F., Khoobi, M., Rouini, M., & Akbari Javar, H. (2018). pH-responsive polymer in a core–shell magnetic structure as an efficient carrier for delivery of doxorubicin to tumor cells. *International Journal of Polymer Materials and Polymer Biomaterials*, *67*, 967–977.
59. Zhang, L., et al. (2020). pH responsive coumarin and imidazole grafted polymeric micelles for cancer therapy. *Journal of Drug Delivery Science and Technology*, *58*, 101789.
60. Guo, Z., et al. (2020). pH-responsive charge switchable PEGylated ε-poly-L-lysine polymeric nanoparticles-assisted combination therapy for improving breast cancer treatment. *Journal of Controlled Release*, *326*, 350–364.
61. Kalita, H., & Patowary, M. (2020). Fluorescent tumor-targeted polymer-bioconjugate: A potent theragnostic platform for cancer therapy. *European Polymer Journal*, *130*, 109661.
62. Wang, J., et al. (2020). Autophagy-inhibiting polymer as an effective nonviral cancer gene therapy vector with inherent apoptosis-sensitizing ability. *Biomaterials*, *255*, 120156.
63. Stickdorn, J., & Nuhn, L. (2020). Reactive-ester derived polymer nanogels for cancer immunotherapy. *European Polymer Journal*, *124*, 109481.

CHAPTER 6

Polymer-Based Nanocomposites in Clinical Diagnosis

ARSHI AMIN

Department of Chemistry, Noida International University, Greater Noida, Uttar Pradesh, India

ABSTRACT

The latest strict regulations and safety caveats related to clinical trials of new drugs have paved the way for finding synergistic combinations with advantages of dose reduction and improved efficacy. However, not many of such approaches are actually synergistic drugs. In lieu of that, the approaches to exploit nanomaterials in formulating drug delivery systems (DDS) with novel characteristics have gained prominence. The rise of nanotechnology enables the use of materials at nanoscale levels, eventually leading to the modification of the physical and chemical characteristics of the materials. Polymer nanocomposites comprising both natural and synthetic nanocomposites hold an integral part of the nanomaterials. The transition among the two phases of nanoscale compounds with large specific surface areas is beneficial in the fabrication of nanofiller composites. In this chapter, we will be focusing on a detailed study of polymer-based nanocomposites, their classification, synthesis, types, and applications in clinical diagnosis.

6.1 INTRODUCTION

Nanoscience and nanotechnology have made remarkable exponential progress worldwide in recent years, considering their new techniques,

Polymer Applications in Medicine: Revolutionizing Treatment and Therapeutics.
Mohd. Imran Ahamed, Faheem Ahmad, and Ishaat M. Khan (Eds.)

DOI: 10.1201/9781779640871-6

applications, and financially feasible impact [1–7]. The latest advancements in the field of synthesis and application of nanomaterials have paved a holistic path for both the diagnosis and treatment of diseases [8–14]. The primary focus of this innovative and promising field is the synthesis and characterization of new organic-inorganic materials with dimensions on the order of a few nanometers, generally described as nanocrystalline materials [15]. These newly synthesized nanosized materials have completely altered properties that are often significantly different from their parent organic-inorganic materials at bulk size. Nanomaterials find vast applications in the medical field, which has led to a new discipline mainly known as nanomedicine [16]. Nanomedicine covers numerous areas such as the processes of diagnosing, treating, curing, and preventing diseases, as well as dealing with traumatic injuries, relieving pain, and preserving/improving human health by using nanomaterials [17–20].

Polymers are one of the most widespread and crucial subjects for research study and industry [21–23]. They have various applications in several domains [24–27]. Ever since polymers were discovered, they have been employed to manufacture daily need products such as toys, containers, vessels, clothes, shoes, mattresses, etc. Over time, polymer nanocomposites have evolved significantly in the fields of food packaging, the pharmaceutical industry, and the medical industry. The properties of the newly synthesized polymer nanocomposites depend on the characteristics and properties of the components used and on the interaction between the polymer and the nanofiller [28–34]. These polymer-nanofillers comprise an organic polymer matrix and a mineral, organic, or metallic nanofiller. Polymer nanocomposites are a boon to modern medicine and offer new opportunities to generate products for antibacterial treatment, tissue engineering, cancer therapy, medical imaging, dental applications, drug delivery, and so forth [10, 35–40].

The chapter below deals with polymer-based nanocomposites and their usefulness in clinical diagnosis.

6.2 NANO COMPOSITE AND NANOTECHNOLOGY

Composite material is said to be a combination of materials that possess various physical and chemical properties on the macroscopic level. It showcases properties like high strength and stiffness at high temperatures, corrosion resistance, the potential to resist extreme temperature conditions, and the required thermal expansion coefficient. Composite material encompasses two stages: the continuous stage and the reinforcement stage. With the help of matrices (polymer, carbon, metal, ceramics) and reinforcement (particles, fibers, and layered materials), the synthesis of numerous composite and nanocomposite materials has been made possible [20, 28, 34, 41].

The polymer nanocomposites encompass materials such as nanoparticles or organic and inorganic substances as nanofillers diffused in a material matrix [21]. The features of polymer composites are based on numerous components, and the features can be expanded by altering the characteristics of the fillers. While preparing the polymer-based nanocomposites, difficulties arise in the dispersal of nanofillers in the matrix. To overcome this situation, mechano-chemical methods such as sonication by ultrasound can be incorporated. Polymer nanocomposites also have great physical and mechanical features due to the large interfacial area between the polymers and nanofillers. This large interfacial area is created because of the homogeneous and regular dispersal of nanofillers, which distinguishes polymer nanocomposites from traditional polymer composites.

Due to the novel features of silver nanoparticles, they have shown potential for medical applications like diagnostics, imaging, and drug delivery [42]. They require stabilization in different substrates, and the polymer matrices should be appropriate for medical use. Gold nanoparticles are also significant in the medical field. They have a wide range of usefulness, especially because of the biocompatibility of gold. They can be employed in producing wires for pacemakers and gold-plated stents used in the treatment of heart disease [43, 44].

There are two classes of molybdenum materials; the first class is transition metal oxides. MoO_2 and MoO_3 fall under this class. It has been found that molybdenum oxide nanomaterials have novelty for diagnosis and in treating cancer. In addition, many diagnostic methods are available to investigate cancer, and one of them is the optical method, which offers high efficiency and accuracy. Molybdenum sulfide (MoS_2) belongs to the second class of transition metal dichalcogenides. It has significant utilization in the biomedical sector [39]. They are inexpensive and have great physical and chemical features. With these features, they can be used as a sensing mechanism and help to detect particular biomolecules and gases.

The term "nanometer" was coined by Richard Zsigmondy, who won the title of Nobel Prize Laureate in Chemistry in 1925. He employed this term for characterizing particle size; he was also the first person to determine the size of particles, for instance, gold colloids, with the help of a microscope. In the International System of Units, "nanometer" (nm) is defined as 10^{-9} m in length. It is considered to be 80,000 times thinner than human hair and is equal to a billionth of a meter. Nanoparticles or nanofillers are counted as doping agents that are dispersed into the polymer matrix of composites, whose dimensions are in the nanoscale range [45–48]. Nanofillers derived from natural or synthetic origins are believed to be excellent materials due to their novel features compared to other bulky substances. In the year 1959, Richard Feynman, who won the Nobel Prize in Physics in 1965, delivered a lecture at the American Physical Society entitled "*There's Plenty of Room at the Bottom*," which demonstrated the idea of manipulating matter at the nanoscale level. 15 years after delivering the lecture, in 1974, a Japanese scientist, Norio Taniguchi, introduced the term "nanotechnology," illustrating it as the capability of exploiting a single nanoscale object. It can be stated as the fabrication and employment of materials, devices, and systems according to the range of nanometers. Nano diagnostics refer to the usage of nanobiotechnology in molecular diagnostics [49].

6.3 NANOTECHNOLOGY AS A TOOL IN DIAGNOSIS

This particular paragraph will enlighten nanotechnology in diagnosis. According to the United States Environmental Protection Agency, nanotechnology is the branch of science that deals with nanoscale particles to investigate their characteristics and utilize them for the further manufacturing of products in numerous fields such as engineering, medicine, agriculture, and pharmaceuticals. Particles whose size is less than 1µm are referred to as nanoparticles. Nanotechnology has great importance and imparts many techniques that can be used for the purpose of diagnosis, such as detecting biomolecules and analytes. It can be of immense advantage in medical diagnosis if we have an excellent knowledge of the features of nanoparticles [50]. Nanoparticles are useful in drug delivery, as they can aid in transporting the drug to the desired cell. When the desired amount of drug is carried to the desired place, drug consumption and its side effects are reduced. Nanotechnology is also beneficial in tissue engineering, as artificial implants and organ transplants can be substituted with tissue engineering [51]. Additionally, the chapter also states that gold has various applications in the Indian medical system, such as improving the mental fitness of babies and memory [52]. It deals with interdisciplinary areas such as chemistry, engineering, biology, and medical sciences. In nanomedicine, nanoparticles are the main factor, and there are many types of nanoparticles that exist [16]. Nanoparticles are small in size and have a large surface area and quantum tunneling effect. These features help them to appear in a wide range of application domains. With the help of unique chemical and physical features, they can be employed to create bulk counterparts. In medical science, they can be employed in areas like gene delivery, targeted drug delivery, imaging, artificial implants, and so forth [35, 36]. Currently, 3D printed nanocomposites are the new trend for the purpose of diagnostics and therapeutic devices [53, 54]. The purpose of this chapter is to discuss the application of polymer nanocomposites specifically in the arena of clinical diagnosis.

6.4 TYPES OF NANO COMPOSITES

Nano composites comprises of nano materials like nano particles, nano fibers and nano clays [55]. Based on the matrix material, nano composites are categorized into 3 parts as described in Table 6.1.

- Ceramic Matrix Nano Composites (CMNC).
- Polymer Matrix Nano Composites (PMNC).
- Metal Matrix Nanocomposites (MMNC).

Some of the advantages of nanocomposites other than traditional composites are described [55].

Lowered amounts of nanofiller materials can help improve the features of the matrix phase in nanocomposites.

In comparison with traditional composites, nanofiller-implanted nanocomposites have a low density-to-weight ratio. Based on the size and shape of nanomaterials, they can enhance their chemical, mechanical, thermal, magnetic, optical, and electrical features to a higher extent.

TABLE 6.1 Types of Nano-Composites Based on the Matrix Materials

Polymer Nanocomposites	Features	Examples	Applications	References
CMNC	Lower brittleness, increase durability	Al_2O_3, SiC, SiN	enhance the proliferation of osteoblasts (bone-forming cells).	[5, 7, 34, 55]
PMNC	high thermal stability, improved mechanical properties (high abrasion resistance) and lower gas permeability (higher barrier capacity), light weight, ductile nature	Thermoplastic/thermoset polymer/layered silicates, polyester/TiO_2, polymer/CNT, polymer/layered double hydroxides	packaging, power tool housing, fuel cell, solar cell, plastic containers, fuel tank	[5, 7, 34, 55]
MMNC	high ductility, toughness, strength and modulus	Fe-Cr/Al_2O_3, Ni/Al_2O_3, Co/Cr, Fe/MgO, Al/CNT, Mg/CNT	automotive, aerospace, electronics, military, biomedical applications and medical devices	[5, 7, 34, 55]

6.5 CLASSIFICATION OF NANO COMPOSITES

Classification of polymeric nanocomposites is sorted into three categories. It depends on the reinforcement materials: particles (silica, metal, and other organic and inorganic particles), layered materials (graphite, layered silicate, and other layered minerals), and fibrous materials (nanofibers and nanotubes) [55].

1. **Nano Clay-Reinforced Composites** – The clay is assumed to be comprised of small inorganic particles; a part of the soil fraction whose dimension is less than 2 mm. Each clay mineral includes two types of sheets: tetrahedral (T) and octahedral (O). Generally, smectite (Hectorite, saponite, and montmorillonite) type layered silicates are employed for the synthesis of nanocomposites [6, 20, 28].

2. **Carbon Nanotube-Reinforced Composites** – In the year 1960, Roger Bacon discovered that micrometer-sized carbon tubes are akin to multi-walled carbon nanotubes in terms of structure; however, they differ in dimensions. The carbon nanotubes were first discovered by Sumio Iijima of NEC Corporation of Japan in the year 1991. It was noted that multi-walled nanotubes were the first nanotubes, and they include more than two concentric cylindrical shells of graphene sheets. Like graphite (0.34 nm), the graphene sheets are arranged in such a manner that they surround a central hollow core with interlayer partition. In contrast, single-walled nanotubes are comprised of single graphene cylinders with a restricted size distribution (1–2 nm) [56, 57].

3. **Nano-Fiber-Reinforced Composites** – Carbon nano-fibers are described as a rare kind of vapor-grown fibers and help in restoring the physical properties between the usual carbon fibers (5–10 μm) and carbon nanotubes (1–10 μm) [21, 58].

4. **Inorganic particle-reinforced composites** – The diameter of nano particle is less than 100nm. Nanometer –sized particles are prepared by many organic and inorganic particles and provide better features to composite materials. Polymer/inorganic nano composites are prepared by particles such as metal oxides, metals and non-metals. Nano particles are selected on the basis of thermal, electrical and mechanical properties of nano composites.

6.6 MECHANICAL PROPERTIES OF NANOCOMPOSITES

The mechanical properties deal with Young's modulus, stress at break, and strain at break of all nanocomposites and new polymers reported by an author. The mechanical properties of the nanocomposites vary depending on the quantity of clay; that is, the mechanical properties increase when the clay is less and vice versa. Other reports state that when nanoparticles are added to the polymer matrix, an effect is seen in the properties of materials such as hardness and scratch resistance [28, 56, 59]. The enhancement of mechanical properties such as stiffness and strength can be modified through reinforcement mechanisms. Proper distribution and orientation of clay are found to be beneficial for enhancing the stiffness of the polymer matrix [56].

6.7 SYNTHESIS METHODS

To synthesize nanocomposites, there are diverse processes that yield high-quality nanocomposites. The basic aspect of these synthesis methods is their ease, flexibility, or diversity [1, 6, 20, 28, 34]. The strategy depends on many parameters such as structure, reactivity of the species, physical properties of the constituent materials, and so forth. The synthesis methods include electrospinning, centrifugal infiltration process, high-energy ball milling (HEBM), liquid phase infiltration process, melt intercalation process, grafting melt intercalation process, and solution intercalation process [40, 41, 56]. Other methods include dry mixing/thermal pressing, solution blending, emulsion mixing, *in situ* polymerization, and lamination stacking [59].

6.7.1 *IN SITU POLYMERIZATION*

In this method, nanocomposite coatings are created with the aid of organic matrices (conducting polymer) or other monomers, cross-linkers, and templates with initiators [60]. Metals or metal oxides are employed as nanofillers. The polymerization process occurs using electrodeposition, an oxidizing agent, or photons (photo-polymerized). Furthermore, the template molecules form a complex with functional monomers, which are polymerized to form a porous polymer matrix. Diverse weak interactions, namely hydrogen bonds, dipole-dipole interactions, and electrostatic interactions, are observed in addition to covalent bonds between the template and the functional monomers. These interactions help in holding a template molecule in the polymer matrix. After the removal of the template by disrupting the interaction, a molecular memory of the template (target analyte) remains, existing with cavities that are similar in size, shape, and position to different groups.

6.7.2 MELT-BLENDING

This method is the desired method to prepare diverse polymer hybrids with inorganic nanoparticles. They are inexpensive and eco-friendly, with one benefit being that there is no need for a solvent. In the molten polymer matrix, the graphene can be directly mixed. Melt blending is the method in which the polymer is melted to form a viscous liquid. At high temperatures, the nanofillers are added to the polymer matrix with the help of a high shear mixer. The polymer matrix is heated to the point of glass transition temperature, after which the fillers are added and mixed consistently. The extent of intercalation depends on many factors, such as mixing speeds and times, temperature, compatibility of the polymer matrix and the fillers, the fillers' interlayer forces, and filler surface preparation. Melt blending is suitable for producing composites; however, it is ineffective in diffusing nanofillers compared to solution blending [41].

6.7.3 TEMPLATE SYNTHESIS

This method includes the preparation of inorganic material in the presence of a polymer matrix, further guiding it towards the path of nucleation and growth of the inorganic host crystals and trapping through the layers.

6.8 CHARACTERIZATION OF NANO COMPOSITES

Characterization is required to study and determine the structure of nanocomposites [3, 20, 28, 40, 49]. It also briefs us about the diffusion of nanoparticles in the polymer matrix, the connection between the nanofillers' surface and polymer chains, and the effects on the final properties of nanocomposites. To acquire detailed information about the specimen, more than one characterization method should be performed [56, 59].

6.8.1 SCANNING ELECTRON MICROSCOPY (SEM)

SEM is employed to investigate the surface morphology, roughness, and homogeneity of the dispersion of nanomaterials in the polymer matrix. It is considered the most conventional method due to its simplicity in preparing the samples and in understanding the images [61]. It also helps us to anticipate the specimen in a broader way. In one of the studies, it was revealed that local strain in a testing sample can be calculated by using the digital image correlation (DIC) of SEM images, which were taken during the *in situ* deformation experiments. Along with the macro-scale testing, the DIC method is reformed to assist micro and nanoscale testing by switching the method from optical microscopy to SEM [61, 62].

6.8.2 INFRARED SPECTROSCOPY (IR)

In this technique, we can study the numerous types of interatomic bond vibrations in organic molecules, polymers, composites, and so forth. Near-IR radiation, also identified as the visible range, holds the ability to penetrate within the samples, allowing for the analysis of larger samples at this range. It has enormous applications in fields like rapid grain analysis, medical diagnosis, biotechnology, genomic analysis, interatomic research, inline textile monitoring, food analysis, chemical imaging/hyperspectral imaging, plastics, textiles, insect detection, and forensic and crime detection [8, 16]. Polymer nano composites for instance montmorillonite can be characterized by altering the Si-O clay band. It affected its role of processing, intercalation and exfoliation from the range of 1350–750cm^{-1}. According to an author, polymer composites were treated with a compatibilizing agent; the interaction between the agent and the Si-O dipoles of the nanoclays can also be comparatively accountable for the observed results [20, 34].

6.9 APPLICATION OF POLYMER BASED NANO COMPOSITES IN CLINICAL DIAGNOSIS

This particular section will deal with clinical diagnosis via nanocomposites [63]. It will discuss the diverse aspects of carbon-based nanocomposites, gold and silver nanocomposites, and other nanocomposites [1, 42–44]. Nanotechnology has been employed in the field of medicine for a long time [16]. It shows diverse features, which is why it is utilized in medical imaging. It is divided into four areas: targeted pharmaceutics, tissue engineering (molecular engineering and biosensors), biosensors, and diagnosis [9–13, 64, 65]. Polymer nanocomposites have various applications in different domains, imparting advantages like improved features, reduction of solid waste, and increased potential, and so forth [66, 67]. Gold nanoparticles utilized in biomedicine comprise polymeric nanoparticles, metal, and semiconductor nanoparticles [43, 44]. An example of the first composite nanoparticle is the composite of gold nanoparticles with polyaminoamide dendrimer (PAMAM). A few examples of polymer filler nanocomposites in biomedical sciences are bone fracture, joint replacement, dental applications, and so forth [68].

6.9.1 CANCER TREATMENT

Some cells that proliferate rapidly and are unable to be controlled lead to a certain group of diseases called cancer. In the adult body, the process of cell division happens for two reasons: to replace damaged cells or to repair injuries. DNA in a normal cell can be repaired or it can die, but this is not the case in cancerous cells; they tend to multiply and spread to other parts of the body, forming tumors, and this process is called metastasis [37]. Nanomaterials for cancer diagnosis include liposomes, polymeric nanoparticles (nanospheres and nanocapsules), solid lipid particles, nanocrystals, and polymer therapeutics such as dendrimers, fullerenes, and inorganic nanoparticles (e.g., gold and magnetic nanoparticles) [38, 39]. Recent approaches to diagnose cancer include surgery, CT, and radiotherapy [69].

Nanoparticles can be employed for binary imaging of cancer. A combination of quantum dots and magnetic iron oxide nanoparticles is used to fabricate a single nanoparticle probe, which will be beneficial for diagnosing images of tumors and molecules involved in cancer. Silica nanoparticles, nearly 30 nm in size, are loaded with rhodamine and iron oxide nanoparticles (9 nm), which are water-soluble in nature. The best outcomes can be seen in MRI and fluorescent imaging when both elements are combined rather than using single elements. Gold nanoparticles are immensely useful in detecting cancer and also in disrupting it.

Specifically, gold nanoparticles are coupled to anti-epidermal growth factor receptor monoclonal antibodies. They homogeneously bind to the surface of the cancer cell with 100% affinity. It is observed that specific and homogeneous binding produces a sharper SPR absorption band with a red shift maximum when added to a non-cancerous cell. Rapidly growing cancer cells can be detected and measured by gold nanoparticles depending on electro-catalytic methods. For brain cancer or tumors, nanomaterials such as gold NPs, liposomes, dendrimers, carbon nanotubes, and micelles can be employed to treat it [38].

6.9.2 ALZHEIMER'S DISEASE

This disease can be managed by nano constructs. They provide a medium to transport medication or other therapeutic or neuroprotective molecules accurately to the brain [38]. They can be modified directly to help in the removal of pathogenic factors, such as the accumulation of proteins in oligomers and fibrils. More specifically, it is the accumulation of amyloid protein in the brain and the production of extracellular amyloid plaques that lead to Alzheimer's disease. Selenium in nano-size can help to treat this disease. It has been observed that the small size of selenium nanoparticles, ranging between 5–15 nm, can reduce the production of amyloid β by lowering the production of reactive oxygen species (ROS). Gold nanoparticles can also aid in diagnosing this disease [43, 44]. They demonstrate powerful features and hold the potential to cross the blood-brain barrier by associating with different ligands or by adjusting their sizes accordingly. The characterization of gold nanoparticles was performed via dynamic light scattering, which provides details about them. The results showed that if the gold nanoparticles were smaller in size, it would be easier to prevent the accumulation of β-peptides into oligomers, thereby escaping the nucleation of fibrils.

6.9.3 ORTHOPEDIC INFECTIONS AND WOUND DRESSING

Infection is the most serious issue in the field of orthopedics, which can cause slow healing, failure in implantation, and the need for repeat surgery. The origin of infection is bacterial biofilms that need to be treated. Thus, to remove this barrier, an anti-biofilm was prepared with nanoparticles. Nanophase silver is the best material in orthopedics and is employed to treat wound care. Antimicrobial nanophase silver is determined to be effective in inhibiting and curing infections rather than ordinary dressings [1, 42]. A freeze-drying approach is employed to prepare a biodegradable and biocompatible silk fibroin/chitin nanocomposite scaffold by adding silver nanoparticles. The permeability level is reduced when the amount of silver nanoparticles is increased in the nanocomposites, resulting in outstanding outcomes for wound dressing purposes [70]. An increase in the amount of silver enhances the tensile strength of the newly synthesized nanocomposites.

6.9.4 DRUG DELIVERY AND PROTEIN DELIVERY

Several polymeric nanostructured materials have been utilized in the past for controlling the delivery of different kinds of bioactive molecules, comprising low molecular weight drugs and peptides/proteins. These materials have many advantages [71–73]. Polymer nanotube composites have two benefits for the purpose of drug delivery. Firstly, the polymer provides biocompatibility and biodegradability. Secondly, the carbon nanotubes provide stability, cellular uptake, and magnetic and electromagnetic features. Carbon nanotubes are especially used in DDS, such as in cancer therapies; however, cytotoxicity is a barrier related to them. One of the authors synthesized chitosan carbon nanotubes through the process of chemical oxidation, which can be applied for biomedical purposes. Another author synthesized chitosan-related graphene oxide (GO), which acts as a nanocarrier for drug and gene delivery. In addition to biocompatibility, natural polymers encapsulated in graphene help in depleting the adverse effects of the sample [74]. The oral route is considered to be the safest and most common method for drug delivery. Employing nanoparticles in drug delivery provides benefits, and because of these benefits, they reduce toxic side effects and enhance the function of drugs; thus, they are broadly utilized in drug formulations.

6.9.5 TISSUE ENGINEERING AND BONE GRAFTING

In tissue engineering, additive manufacturing (AM) is utilized to modify personalized scaffolds or artificial tissues and organs for transplants, DDS, probes and tools to analyze specific medical factors, orthoses, prostheses, implants, anatomical models, and medical instruments for diagnostics and surgery [75]. Some of the features required for tissue engineering are biocompatibility and biodegradability for *in vivo* applications, extremely permeable structures for cellular migration and multiplication, and good mechanical strength and elasticity, and so forth. Supramolecular polymer nanocomposites are outstanding materials for tissue engineering as they show the potential to mix biodegradable polymers with different nanofillers [50]. Graphene-based nanomaterials possess features such as high elasticity, flexibility, and adaptability to flat or irregularly shaped surfaces, and can be a part of proliferation, adhesion, and differentiation [53–57]. One report stated that using graphene with chitosan poly(vinyl alcohol) for total skin cure took 10 days. Natural polymers or biodegradable-based polymeric composites are helpful in forming scaffolds for tendons and ligaments. Carbon nanotubes are also employed for the purpose of tissue engineering and regenerative medicine. The procedure for this approach is that the formation of new tissues will occur when the cell is enclosed with the desired biological components. Some of the uses of carbon nanotubes include enhancing the mechanoelectrical features of the scaffolds, impacting the micro-ambiance of the cell, and empowering the chemical reactions occurring in the cell. In bone grafting, nanocomposites are regarded as crucial, utilizing different nanoscale bone graft materials in association with various factors [76].

6.10 CONCLUSION

Polymer-based nanocomposites are trending materials due to their great features and their role in the industrial and medical domains. Gold and silver nanoparticles give tough competition to each other because of their excellent features, and both of them are equally devoted to numerous fields. Graphene-based polymer nanocomposites are also favorable in many fields, and they too possess great features. Altogether, we can use the nanocomposite as per the needs of society and ease the complications. Nanotechnology is a trend and can be applied to interdisciplinary as well as multidisciplinary fields. Since nanotechnology is the study of nanoscale objects, it raises opportunities in many regions by tailoring the size of the material and utilizing it for further use. This technology is not new; it has been practiced for a very long time, and with the coming technologies, we can customize it more and more for enhanced purposes.

KEYWORDS

- **additive manufacturing**
- **carbon nanotubes**
- **clinical diagnosis**
- **medicine**
- **nano materials**
- **polymer nano composites**
- **silver nanoparticles**
- **supramolecular polymer nanocomposites**
- **tissue engineering**

REFERENCES

1. Sadasivuni, K. K., Rattan, S., Waseem, S., Bramhe, S. K., Kondawar, S. B., Ghosh, S., Das, A. P., Chakraborty, P. K., Adhikari, J., Saha, P., & Mazumdar, P. (n.d.). Silver nanoparticles and its polymer nanocomposites—synthesis, optimization, biomedical usage, and its various applications. In *Polymer Nanocomposites in Biomedical Engineering. Lecture Notes in Bioengineering*. https://doi.org/10.1007/978-3-030-04741-2_11 (accessed on 4th July 2025).
2. Suryanarayana, C., & Koch, C. C. (2000). Nanocrystalline materials—current research and future directions. *Hyperfine Interactions*, *130*, 5–44. http://dx.doi.org/10.1023/A:1011026900989 (accessed on 4th July 2025).
3. Vinyas, M., Athul, S. J., Harursampath, D., Loja, M. A. R., & Nguyen, T. T. (2019). A comprehensive review on analysis of nanocomposites: From manufacturing to properties characterization. *Materials Research Express*. https://doi.org/10.1088/2053-1591/ab3175 (accessed on 4th July 2025).
4. Karak, N. (2019). Fundamentals of nanomaterials and polymer nanocomposites. In *Nanomaterials and Polymer Nanocomposites* (Ch. 1, pp. 1–45). https://doi.org/10.1016/B978-0-12-814615-6.00001-1 (accessed on 4th July 2025).
5. Mikličanin, E. O., Badnjević, A., Kazlagić, A., & Hajlovac, M. (2019). Nanocomposites: A brief review. *Health and Technology*. https://doi.org/10.1007/s12553-019-00380-x (accessed on 4th July 2025).
6. Rane, A. V., Kanny, K., Abitha, V. K., & Thomas, S. (2018). Methods for synthesis of nanoparticles and fabrication of nanocomposites. In *Synthesis of inorganic nanomaterials* (pp. 121–139). https://doi.org/10.1016/B978-0-08-101975-7.00005-1 (accessed on 4th July 2025).

7. Sen, M. (2000). Nanocomposite materials. In *Nanotechnology and the Environment* (pp. 1–12). http://dx.doi.org/10.5772/intechopen.93047 (accessed on 4th July 2025).
8. Mousavi, S. M., Low, F. W., Hashemi, S. A., Lai, C. W., Ghasemi, Y., & Soroshnia, S. (2020). Development of graphene-based nanocomposites towards medical and biological applications. *Artificial Cells, Nanomedicine, and Biotechnology: An International Journal*, *48*, 1189–1205. https://doi.org/10.1080/21691401.2020.1817052 (accessed on 4th July 2025).
9. Jackson, C., Patani, B. O., & Ekpa, D. E. (2017). Nanotechnology in diagnosis: A review. *Advances in Nanoparticles*, *6*, 93–102. https://doi.org/10.4236/anp.2017.63008 (accessed on 4th July 2025).
10. Shurygina, I. A., & Shurygin, M. G. (2021). Selenium nanocomposites in diagnosis, drug delivery, and treatment. In *Nanobiotechnology in Diagnosis, drug delivery, and treatment* (pp. 25–45). https://doi.org/10.1002/9781119671732.ch2 (accessed on 4th July 2025).
11. Bilal, M., Barani, M., Sabir, F., Rahdar, A., & Kyzas, G. Z. (2020). Nanomaterials for the treatment and diagnosis of Alzheimer's disease: An overview. *NanoImpact*, *20*. https://doi.org/10.1016/j.impact.2020.100251 (accessed on 4th July 2025).
12. Jain, K. K. (2005). Nanotechnology in clinical laboratory diagnostics. *Clinica Chimica Acta*, *358*, 37–54. https://doi.org/10.1016/j.cccn.2005.03.014 (accessed on 4th July 2025).
13. Wang, J., Sui, L., Huang, J., Miao, L., Nie, Y., Wang, K., Yang, Z., Huang, Q., Gong, X., Nan, Y., & Ai, K. (2021). *MoS_2*-based nanocomposites for diagnosis and therapy. *Bioactive Materials*, *6*, 4209–4242. https://doi.org/10.1016/j.bioactmat.2021.04.021 (accessed on 4th July 2025).
14. Jain, K. K. (2007). Applications of nanobiotechnology in clinical diagnostics. *Clinical Chemistry*, *53*, 2002–2009. https://doi.org/10.1373/clinchem.2007.090795 (accessed on 4th July 2025).
15. Escoto, J. L. V., & Huang, Y. T. (2011). Inorganic-organic hybrid nanomaterials for therapeutic and diagnostic imaging applications. *International Journal of Molecular Sciences*, *12*, 3888–3927. https://doi.org/10.3390/ijms12063888 (accessed on 4th July 2025).
16. Orcid, B. P., Alexiou, C., Alvarez, R. A., Alves, F., Ashraf, S., Balogh, L. P., Bestetti, A., Brendel, C., Bosi, S., Cheng, Z., Cui, D., Dullin, C., Feli, N., George, M., Grünweller, A., Hartmann, R. K., Hunziker, P., Kataoka, K., Krug, H. F., & Zhang, X. E. (2017). Diverse applications of nanomedicine. *ACS Nano*, *11*, 2313–2381. https:///doi.org/10.1021/acsnano.6b06040 (accessed on 4th July 2025).
17. Laroui, H., Rakhya, P., Xiao, B., Viennois, E., & Merlin, D. (2013). Nanotechnology in diagnostics and therapeutics for gastrointestinal disorders. *Digestive and Liver Disease*, *45*, 995–1002. https://doi.org/10.1016/j.dld.2013.03.019 (accessed on 4th July 2025).
18. Hulla, J. E., Sahu, S. C., & Hayes, A. W. (2015). Nanotechnology: History and future. *Human and Experimental Toxicology*, *34*, 1318–1321. https://doi.org/10.1177/0960327115603588 (accessed on 4th July 2025).
19. Leon, L., Chung, E. J., & Rinaldi, C. (2020). A brief history of nanotechnology and introduction to nanoparticles for biomedical applications. In *Nanoparticles for Biomedical Applications* (pp. 1–4). https://doi.org/10.1016/B978-0-12-816662-8.00001-1 (accessed on 4th July 2025).

20. Ealias, A. M., & Saravanakumar, M. P. (2017). A review on the classification, characterization, synthesis of nanoparticles and their application. *Materials Science and Engineering*, *263*, 032019. https://doi.org/10.1088/1757-899X/263/3/032019 (accessed on 4th July 2025).
21. Tjong, S. C. (2012). Polymer nanocomposites for biomedical applications. In *Polymer Composites with Carbonaceous Nanofillers* (pp. 285–329). https://doi.org/10.1002/9783527648726.ch7 (accessed on 4th July 2025).
22. Kurahatti, R. V., Surendranathan, A. O., Kori, S. A., Singh, N., Kumar, A. V. R., & Srivastava, S. (2010). Defence applications of polymer nanocomposites. *Defence Science Journal*, *60*, 551–563. https://doi.org/10.14429/dsj.60.578 (accessed on 4th July 2025).
23. Kumar, S., Sarita, Nehra, M., Dilbaghi, N., Tankeshwar, K., & Kim, K. H. (2018). Recent advances and remaining challenges for polymeric nanocomposites in healthcare applications. *Progress in Polymer Science*, *1–38*. https://doi.org/10.1016/j.progpolymsci.2018.03.001 (accessed on 4th July 2025).
24. Emmanuel, A., & Aziz, S. (2014). *Polymer Nanocomposites*. Kurdistan Regional Government – Iraq, Ministry of Higher Education & Scientific Research, University of Sulaimani. www.ijriit.com (accessed on 4th July 2025).
25. Zaferani, S. H. (2018). Polymer-based nanocomposites for energy and environmental applications. In *Introduction of Polymer–Based Nanocomposites* (Ch. 1, pp. 1–25). Elsevier. https://doi.org/10.1016/B978-0-08-102262-7.00001-5 (accessed on 4th July 2025).
26. Silvestre, J., Silvestre, N., & De Brito, J. (2016). Polymer nanocomposites for structural applications: Recent trends and new perspectives. *Mechanics of Advanced Materials and Structures*, *23*, 1263–1277. https://doi.org/10.1080/15376494.2015.1068406 (accessed on 4th July 2025).
27. Armstrong, G. (2015). An introduction to polymer nanocomposites. *European Journal of Physics*, *36*, 1–39. http://dx.doi.org/10.1088/0143-0807/36/6/063001 (accessed on 4th July 2025).
28. Puggal, S., Dhall, N., Singh, N., & Singh, M. (2016). A review on polymer nanocomposites: Synthesis, characterization and mechanical properties. *Science and Technology India Journal*, *9*. https://doi.org/10.17485/ijst/2016/v9i4/81100 (accessed on 4th July 2025).
29. Fu, S., Sun, Z., Huang, P., Li, Y., & Hu, N. (2019). Some basic aspects of polymer nanocomposites: A critical review. *Nano Materials Science*, *1*, 2–30. https://doi.org/10.1016/j.nanoms.2019.02.006 (accessed on 4th July 2025).
30. Chen, X., Zhao, Y., Li, L., Wang, Y., Wang, J., Xiong, J., Du, S., Zhang, P., Shi, X., & Yu, J. (2020). MXene/polymer nanocomposites: Preparation, properties, and applications. *Polymer Reviews*. https://doi.org/10.1080/15583724.2020.1729179 (accessed on 4th July 2025).
31. Müller, K., Bugnicourt, E., Latorre, M., Jorda, M., Sanz, Y. E., Lagaron, J. M., Miesbauer, O., Bianchin, A., Hankin, S., Bölz, U., Pérez, G., Jesdinszki, M., Lindner, M., Scheuerer, Z., Castelló, S., & Schmid, M. (2017). Review on the processing and properties of polymer nanocomposites and nanocoating's and their applications in the packaging, automotive and solar energy fields. *Nanomaterials*, *7*, 74. https://doi.org/10.3390/nano7040074 (accessed on 4th July 2025).

32. Anbusagar, N. R. R., Palanikumar, K., & Ponshanmugakumar, A. (2018). Preparation and properties of nano-polymer advanced composite: A review. In *Introduction of Polymer–Based Nanocomposites* (pp. 27–73). https://doi.org/10.1016/B978-0-08-102262-7.00002-7 (accessed on 4th July 2025).
33. Wang, X., Xing, W., Feng, X., Song, L., & Hu, Y. (2017). Polymer nanocomposites: Preparation, properties and application. *Polymer Reviews*, *57*, 440–466. https://doi.org/10.1080/15583724.2017.1309662 (accessed on 4th July 2025).
34. Camargo, P. H. C., Satyanarayan, K. G., & Wypych, F. (2009). Nanocomposites: Synthesis, structure, properties and new application opportunities. *Materials Research*, *12*, 1–39. https://doi.org/10.1590/S1516-14392009000100002 (accessed on 4th July 2025).
35. Han, J., Zhao, D., Li, D., Wang, X., Jin, Z., & Zhao, K. (2018). Polymer-based nanomaterials and applications for vaccines and drugs. *Polymers*, *10*, 1–31. https://doi.org/10.3390/polym10010031 (accessed on 4th July 2025).
36. Ali, A., & Ahmed, S. (2018). A review on chitosan and its nanocomposites in drug delivery. *International Journal of Biological Macromolecules*, *109*, 273–286. https://doi.org/10.1016/j.ijbiomac.2017.12.078 (accessed on 4th July 2025).
37. Poonia, M., Ramalingam, K., Goyal, S., & Sidhu, S. K. (2017). Nanotechnology in oral cancer: A comprehensive review. *Journal of Oral and Maxillofacial Pathology*, *21*, 407–414. https://doi.org/10.4103/jomfp.JOMFP_29_17 (accessed on 4th July 2025).
38. Mukhtar, M., Bilal, M., Rahdar, A., Barani, M., Arshad, R., Behl, T., Brisc, C., Banica, F., & Bunga, S. (2020). Nanomaterials for diagnosis and treatment of brain cancer: Recent updates. *Chemosensory*, *8*, 117. https://doi.org/10.3390/chemosensors8040117 (accessed on 4th July 2025).
39. Dhas, N., Kudarha, R., Garkal, A., Ghate, V., Sharma, S., Panzade, P., Khot, S., Chaudhari, P., Singh, A., Paryani, M., Lewis, S., Garg, N., Singh, N., Bangar, P., & Mehta, T. (2020). Molybdenum-based hetero-nanocomposites for cancer therapy, diagnosis and biosensing application: Current advancement and future breakthroughs. *Journal of Controlled Release*. https://doi.org/10.1016/j.jconrel.2020.12.015 (accessed on 4th July 2025).
40. Masoud, E. M., Liu, L., & Peng, B. (2020). Synthesis, characterization, and applications of polymer nanocomposites. *Nanomaterials*, *2020*, 1, 2. https://doi.org/10.1155/2020/5439136 (accessed on 4th July 2025).
41. Hanemann, T., & Szabó, D. V. (2010). Polymer-nanoparticle composites: From synthesis to modern applications. *Materials*, *3*, 3468–3517. https://doi.org/10.3390/ma3063468 (accessed on 4th July 2025).
42. Umana, S., Baudrit, V., & Roberto, J. (2015). Silver nanotechnology on medicine. *Journal of Chemistry and Biochemistry*, *3*, 21–33. https://doi.org/10.15640/jcb.v3n1a2 (accessed on 4th July 2025).
43. Dykman, L. A., & Khlebtsov, N. G. (2016). Biomedical applications of multifunctional gold-based nanocomposites. *Biochemistry (Moscow)*, *81*, 1771–1789. https://doi.org/10.1134/S0006297916130125 (accessed on 4th July 2025).
44. Chandra, P., Singh, J., Singh, A., Srivastava, A., Goyal, R. N., & Shim, Y. B. (2013). Gold nanoparticles and nanocomposites in clinical diagnostics using electrochemical

methods. *Nanoparticles*, *2013*, 1–12. https://doi.org/10.1155/2013/535901 (accessed on 4th July 2025).
45. Bopche, Y. S., & Bisen, S. R. (2015). Review on polymer nanotechnology: Nanocomposite. *International Journal of Researches in Biosciences, Agriculture and Technology*, *2*, 378–382.
46. Shameem, M. M., Sasikanth, S. M., Annamalai, R., & Raman, R. G. (2021). A brief review on polymer nanocomposites and its applications. *Materials Today: Proceedings*, *45*, 2536–2539. https://doi.org/10.1016/j.matpr.2020.11.254 (accessed on 4th July 2025).
47. Jeevanandam, J., Barhoum, A., Chan, Y. S., Dufresne, A., & Danquah, M. K. (2018). Review on nanoparticles and nanostructured materials: History, sources, toxicity and regulations. *Beilstein Journal of Nanotechnology*, *9*, 1050–1074. https://doi.org/10.3762/bjnano.9.98 (accessed on 4th July 2025).
48. Thostenson, E. T., Li, C., & Chou, T. W. (2005). Nanocomposites in context. *Composites Science and Technology*, *65*, 491–516. https://doi.org/10.1016/j.compscitech.2004.11.003 (accessed on 4th July 2025).
49. Pandey, P. P. (2020). Preparation and characterization of polymer nanocomposites. *Soft Nanoscience Letters*, *10*, 1–15. https://doi.org/10.4236/snl.2020.101001 (accessed on 4th July 2025).
50. Li, X., Xu, W., X., Y., Yuan, J., Ji, Y., Chu, S., Liu, J., & Luo, Q. (2021). Supramolecular polymer nanocomposites for biomedical applications. *Polymers*, *13*, 1–17. https://doi.org/10.3390/polym13040513 (accessed on 4th July 2025).
51. Tang, Z., He, C., Tian, H., Ding, J., Hsiao, B. S., Chu, B., & Chen, X. (2016). Polymeric nanostructured materials for biomedical applications. *Progress in Polymer Science*, *60*, 86–128. https://doi.org/10.1016/j.progpolymsci.2016.05.005 (accessed on 4th July 2025).
52. Pandya, S. (n.d.). Nanocomposites and its application—review. https://doi.org/10.13140/RG.2.1.2798.9840 (accessed on 4th July 2025).
53. Silva, M., Pinho, I. S., Covas, J. A., Alves, N. M., & Paiva, M. C. (2021). 3D printing of graphene-based polymeric nanocomposites for biomedical applications: Review. *Functional Composite Materials*, *2*, 1–21. https://doi.org/10.1186/s42252-021-00020-6 (accessed on 4th July 2025).
54. Bertana, V., Catania, F., Cocuzza, M., Ferrero, S., Scaltrito, L., & Pirri, C. F. (2020). Medical and biomedical applications of 3D and 4D printed polymer nanocomposites. In *Processes, Applications, and Challenges* (pp. 325–366). https://doi.org/10.1016/B978-0-12-816805-9.00011-9 (accessed on 4th July 2025).
55. Sachinjith, K. R., & Krishna, K. R. S. (2018). A review on types of nanocomposites and their applications. *Advanced Research International Journal: Ideas and Innovations in Technology*, *4*, 235–236. www.ijriit.com (accessed on 4th July 2025).
56. Ibrahim, A., Klopocinska, A., Horvat, K., & Hamid, Z. A. (2021). Graphene-based nanocomposites: Synthesis, mechanical properties and characterizations. *Polymers*, *13*, 2869. https://doi.org/10.3390/polym13172869 (accessed on 4th July 2025).
57. Silva, M., Alves, N. M., & Paiva, M. C. (2017). Graphene-polymer nanocomposites for biomedical applications. *Polymers for Advanced Technologies*, *29*, 687–700. https://doi.org/10.1002/pat.4164 (accessed on 4th July 2025).

58. Raphey, V. R., Henna, T. K., Nivitha, K. P., Mufeedha, P., Sabu, C., & Pramod, K. (2019). Advanced biomedical applications of carbon nanotube. *Materials Science and Engineering: C, 100*, 616–630. https://doi.org/10.1016/j.msec.2019.03.043 (accessed on 4th July 2025).
59. Roy, S., Ryan, J., Webster, S., & Nepal, D. (2017). A review of *in-situ* mechanical characterization of polymer nanocomposites: Prospect and challenges. *Applied Mechanics Reviews, 69*. https://doi.org/10.1115/1.4038257 (accessed on 4th July 2025).
60. Prasad, B., Panwar, V., Chaturvedi, M., Rathi, V., Gill, F. S., Sharma, K., & Patil, P. P. (2018). Development of conductive nanocomposite for sensing application. *Engineering and Technology International Journal, 7*, 1025–1029. http://dx.doi.org/10.14419/ijet.v7i3.12.17625 (accessed on 4th July 2025).
61. Bokobza, L. (2018). Spectroscopic techniques for the characterization of polymer nanocomposites: A review. *Polymers, 10*, 7. https://doi.org/10.3390/polym10010007 (accessed on 4th July 2025).
62. Ponnamma, D., Rouxel, D., & Thomas, S. (2016). Spectroscopy—Introducing the advantages and application areas in polymer nanocomposites. In *Spectroscopy of Polymer Nanocomposites*. http://dx.doi.org/10.1016/B978-0-323-40183-8.00001-X (accessed on 4th July 2025).
63. N-Tri, P., Nguyen, T. A., Carriere, P., & Xuan, C. N. (2018). Nanocomposite coatings: Preparation, characterization, properties, and applications. *Corrosion Hindawi International Journal*. https://doi.org/10.1155/2018/4749501 (accessed on 4th July 2025).
64. Silva, M., Ferreira, F. N., Alves, N. M., & Paiva, M. C. (2020). Biodegradable polymer nanocomposites for ligament/tendon tissue engineering. *Journal of Nanobiotechnology*, 1–33. https://doi.org/10.1186/s12951-019-0556-1 (accessed on 4th July 2025).
65. Lam, C. Y. K., Yin, Q. Z. B., Huang, Y., Wang, H., Yang, M., & Wong, S. H. D. (2021). Recent advances in two-dimensional transition metal dichalcogenide nanocomposites biosensors for virus detection before and during COVID-19 outbreak. *Journal of Composites Science, 5*, 190. https://doi.org/10.3390/jcs5070190 (accessed on 4th July 2025).
66. Ma, Y., Xu, S., Wang, S., & Wang, L. (2015). Luminescent molecularly-imprinted polymer nanocomposites for sensitive detection. *Trends in Analytical Chemistry, 67*, 209–216. http://dx.doi.org/10.1016/j.trac.2015.01.012 (accessed on 4th July 2025).
67. Nayak, R. K., Mahato, K. K., & Ray, B. C. (2020). Hydrothermal behavior of fiber and nanomaterial-reinforced polymer composites. https://doi.org/10.1201/9780429287824 (accessed on 4th July 2025).
68. Murugan, R., & Ramakrishna, S. (2005). Development of nanocomposites for bone grafting. *Composites Science and Technology, 65*, 2385–2406. https://doi.org/10.1016/j.compscitech.2005.07.022 (accessed on 4th July 2025).
69. Clair, B. S. (2016). Nanotechnology and predicting the future (review of the current state of nanotechnology and making future predictions with a discussion of forecasting methods). *The Amateur Academic, 1*. https://www.researchgate.net/publication/311753193 (accessed on 4th July 2025).

70. Gobi, R., Ravichandiran, P., Babu, R. S., & Yoo, D. J. (2021). Biopolymer and synthetic polymer-based nanocomposites in wound dressing applications: A review. *Polymers*, *13*, 1–23. https://doi.org/10.3390/polym13121962 (accessed on 4th July 2025).
71. Gupta, P. D., & Sood, P. P. (2017). Fast and effective role of nanotechnology in health care system: A review. *Cell and Tissue Research Journal*, *17*, 6217–6221.
72. Smith, W. R., Hudson, P. W., Ponce, B. A., & Manoharan, S. R. R. (2018). Nanotechnology in orthopedics: A clinically oriented review. *BMC Musculoskeletal Disorders*, *19*, 1–12. https://doi.org/10.1186/s12891-018-1990-1 (accessed on 4th July 2025).
73. Nikaeen, G., Abbaszadeh, S., & Yousefinejad, S. (2020). Application of nanomaterials in treatment, anti-infection and detection of coronaviruses. *Nanomedicine (London)*, *15*, 1501–1512. https://doi.org/10.2217/nnm-2020-0117 (accessed on 4th July 2025).
74. Rao, G. S. S., Mathur, A. B., & Jasra, R. (2017). Polyolefin/graphene nanocomposites: A review. *RSC Advances*, *7*, 23615–23632. https://doi.org/10.1039/C6RA28392F (accessed on 4th July 2025).
75. Zhao, H., Lin, Z. Y., Yildirimer, L., Dhinakar, A., Zhao, X., & Wu, J. (2016). Polymer-based nanoparticles for protein delivery: Design, strategies and applications. *Materials Chemistry B*, *4*, 4060–4071. https://doi.org/10.1039/C6TB00308G (accessed on 4th July 2025).
76. Farhoodi, M. (2015). Nanocomposite materials for food packaging applications: Characterization and safety evaluation. *Food Engineering Reviews*, *8*, 35–51. https://doi.org/10.1007/s12393-015-9114-2 (accessed on 4th July 2025).

CHAPTER 7

Recent Advancements in Cancer Therapy by Using Polymers and Their Composites

APARAJITA BANERJEE

Department of Zoology, Changu Kana Arts, Commerce and Science College, New Panvel, Raigad, Maharashtra, India

ABSTRACT

Polymers, both synthetic and biodegradable, their hybrids, as well as nanocomposites, have been used in different fields of medicine. In recent years, their use in cancer therapy has also gained much attention. The application of polymers in the form of micelles, polymerosomes, liposomes, hydrogels, and so forth, has been experimented with for both cancer diagnosis and treatment. For diagnosis, polymer-based probes are designed to improve the optical resolution of imaging techniques. However, more research is required for the mass-scale application of different polymers in cancer diagnosis. Relatively, substantial work has been done on the use of polymers in cancer treatment. An array of polymers has been successfully demonstrated to act as efficient drug carrier systems. These polymers and their composites can be used in the delivery of a single drug as well as the co-delivery of multiple drugs or the co-delivery of drugs and other therapeutic agents or even genes of interest. Such polymer applications are known to lower the side effects of conventional drug delivery platforms. Hence, significant replacement of conventional drug delivery systems (DDS) by polymers is anticipated in the future.

Polymer Applications in Medicine: Revolutionizing Treatment and Therapeutics.
Mohd. Imran Ahamed, Faheem Ahmad, and Ishaat M. Khan (Eds.)

DOI: 10.1201/9781779640871-7

7.1 INTRODUCTION

The uncontrolled division of cells leads to a fatal manifestation called cancer. Although cancer has been taking lives since time unknown, its scary existence has actually gained prominence since the Second World War, owing to the profound developments in imaging tools and other diagnostic techniques, genetics, and molecular biology. In fact, on a global scale, millions of people are currently diagnosed with cancer every year, and alarmingly, more than 50% cannot be cured. A worldwide estimation has revealed that non-communicable diseases (NCDs) account for 71% of global deaths, while in India, NCDs cause 63% of total deaths, and cancer is one of the key causes (9%) [1].

Yearly, a considerable fund for biological research is allotted to cancer research; still, cancer is a very complicated entity driven by the fact that it is not a single disease but a group of diseases with a common attribute, that is, uncontrolled cell division. Current therapy pertaining to cancer involves diagnosis followed by suitable treatment. For successful cancer treatment, the diagnosis needs to be early and accurate. The conventional diagnostic tools comprise histological and pathological assessments of tissue samples. However, such diagnostic techniques are strongly dependent on the skills and expertise of the technician and are very much open to experimental errors. Furthermore, to diagnose and determine the stage of cancer, six imaging modalities are available to clinicians, including X-ray, CT, sonograms, MRI, single-photon emission CT, PET, and optical imaging [2]. However, for efficient screening of smaller cancers, the sensitivity and resolution of these techniques need further improvement.

Conventional treatment of cancer usually includes CT, radiotherapy, and surgery [2]. Unconventional therapies like hyperthermia, targeted therapy, immuno- or phototherapy, and stem cell transplants are also available; however, these complementary therapies are still in the experimental phase of research [2]. The conventional CT drugs have poor solubility, tend to degrade and get cleared from the body soon, and also have poor ability to cross biological barriers [2]. Optimizing a suitable drug delivery system is very important in cancer treatment. Polymers can prove very beneficial for the same, owing to their superior pharmacokinetic properties, and can better control the location, dose, and time of drug delivery [3].

Polymers are products of the sequential connection of repeating units called monomers. The physical and chemical properties of polymers, such as size, hydrophilicity, flexibility, and charge density, are determined by the monomers [4]. According to the type and connection between monomers, the polymers are classified into groups; homopolymers are polymers that comprise the same monomers, while heteropolymers are composed of different monomers. Copolymers are polymers in which more than two monomers are used [4]. Polymers, both synthetic and natural, and their composites can add lucrative benefits to cancer therapy. When two or more different components are mixed together, the amalgam is called a composite [3]. When composites of polymers are formed, the additive can improve the properties of the individual polymers, such as physical strength, base characteristics, and compatibility with biological counterparts. This can bring overall enrichment in their physical properties and biological activity [5]. Polymer-based composites are commonly used in space research, military purposes, automobile engineering, and sports applications, and are currently gaining importance in biomedicine as well. Polymers and their composites in different forms, such as polymersomes, dendrimers, micelles, hydrogels, microcapsules, and liposomes, have important potential in cancer diagnosis and treatment [2]. The water-soluble polymers and their composites can effectively maintain a balance between decreased renal clearance and enhanced permeation and retention (EPR) effect by tumor cells [4]. This balance is attributed to the molecular architecture of the polymers, which includes their molecular weight, molecular conformation, chain flexibility, and branching. The general architecture is such that the hydrodynamic diameter of the polymer is comparable to the pore size of the walls of the kidney; in contrast, its size is smaller than the openings in blood vessels that traverse tumors, thereby easing the traversing of these molecules from blood to tumors [4]. In the current review, various aspects of cancer therapy with respect to the use of polymers are discussed. A brief discussion on the role of polymers in cancer diagnosis is covered, followed by their role as a drug delivery system and in additional therapy.

7.2 POLYMER IN CANCER DIAGNOSIS

One of the most important requirements of effective cancer treatment is early and accurate detection. However, due to the lack of definite symptoms, early diagnosis often becomes very challenging. Especially for small cancers, diagnosis is usually tricky. Hence, a highly sensitive diagnostic technique is the need of the hour. Molecular imaging is one such technique that can give an actual peek into the biological processes taking place in a particular site of the body. However, such imaging techniques are largely dependent on suitable optical contrast molecules that can highly enhance the resolution of the image, thereby enhancing the sensitivity of the technique. A number of small molecule optical agents, like indocyanine green, are currently being approved by the US Food and Drug Administration (FDA) for the same [6]; however, some negative artifacts, like lower miscibility in water, quenching, and fast clearance from the body, restrict their application on a mass level [7]. One very efficient method to overcome these limitations is the application of polymers. The polymer can be attached to the optical probe either by conjugation or by encapsulation. The inherent characteristics of the polymer determine the nature of the bond between the polymer and the probe. In the first case, when a hydrophilic polymer is used, covalent bonds help in forming a polymer-probe conjugate. If an amphiphilic polymer is used, nano-precipitation occurs, forming a polymer-based nanosize optical probe. In the third case, self-assembly between probe-polymer units is promoted to form an encapsulated complex. The conjugation or encapsulation of the polymer builds a hydrophilic layer around the probe, which vividly enhances its water solubility. Furthermore, it decreases the chances of proteins binding to the probe *in vivo*, thereby extending blood circulation time and reducing renal clearance. In this respect, a number of polymers, both hydrophilic and amphiphilic, have been permitted by the FDA for clinical use. Polyethylene glycol (PEG), a polymer formed by the condensation of ethylene glycol, "generally recognized as safe," can be linked to small molecules or macrostructures, such as a drug, therapeutic protein, or optical agents [7].

Polymer-probe conjugates can thus be developed as a much more sensitive and specific technique for cancer diagnosis. Even more promising is the development of 'inducible' or 'activatable' optical probes, which get activated or emit a strong signal in only certain biomolecular environments. This specific biomolecular environment can be the tumor microenvironment (TME), which exhibits an abnormal physiological environment, like a weakly acidic environment, hypoxia, an increase in reactive oxygen and reactive nitrogen species, and overexpression of certain tumor-specific enzymes. Such modifications in polymer-probe conjugates can provide a high signal-to-background ratio for cancer diagnosis. However, despite imposing many positive attributes, the long-term safety of these polymer-based optical probes requires further research. Currently, many serum-based techniques are under study owing to their potential sensitivity, specificity, and cost-effectiveness. These techniques rely on serum-based cancer-specific biomarkers. Liu et al. [8] reported a polymer-based sensor that can rapidly detect changes in serum protein levels in cancerous tissue. The authors have combined the benefits endowed by polymer chemistry with radiometric fluorescent dyes for the diagnosis of early-stage and metastatic cancer with a high level of accuracy. Another serum-based technique was developed by Liu et al. [8], wherein a carbon-based polymer dots (CPDs) sensor was constructed, which could identify breast cancer cells based on changes in peripheral blood cells. While this field of research can provide a promising approach for developing accurate diagnostic tools, challenges still remain to make these techniques clinically applicable at a large scale.

7.3 POLYMER IN CANCER TREATMENT

The conventional treatment of cancer includes surgery, radiotherapy, CT, immunotherapy, and hormonal therapy. Although surgery and radiotherapy can lead to the most effective cure of localized tumors or non-metastatic cancer, metastatic cancers require the use of specific drugs (chemotherapy, hormonal, and biological therapies) as these therapies cause effective distribution of the drugs into different organs of the body via the bloodstream [9]. An effective drug delivery system forms one of the most important requisites of cancer treatment. A drug delivery system includes the carriers that can bind to the therapeutic agent efficiently and deliver them to the site of action [5]. An efficient drug delivery system is the key to effective cancer treatment. The most popular DDS include synthetic polymers, biopolymers, and polymer nanocomposites [9]. Nanocomposites have distinctive design capacity, are environmentally friendly, can be mass-produced, and are cost-effective, which makes their use very promising [9]. Another very important drawback associated with cancer therapeutic agents is the development of multidrug resistance (MDR), which significantly reduces their anticancer effect [10]. Therefore, polymer-based co-delivery systems are very effective, as they can simultaneously deliver two or more different chemotherapeutic agents to the same tumor site, which are known to demonstrate considerable MDR reversal compared to single-drug-loaded systems. Particularly, co-delivery systems for chemotherapeutic agents and genes have demonstrated promising solutions to MDR driven by gene therapy [10].

7.3.1 SYNTHETIC POLYMERS AS NANOCOMPOSITES IN CANCER THERAPY

Nanotechnology in the current century has gained increased limelight for its role in the effective diagnosis and treatment of many cancer tissues. Nanocomposites in the form of nanocarriers can act as effective DDS; these carriers can lower the side effects of conventional DDS and thereby enhance the therapeutic quality of the anticancer drug. Furthermore, the nanocarriers are known to increase target-specific accumulation of drugs. The nanocarriers can even act as smart carriers by controlling the release and accumulation of drugs at specific sites, lowering the damage to non-cancerous tissues and organs, and reducing the ill effects caused by conventional anticancer drugs [9]. A number of synthetic polymers have shown promising results as nanocarriers.

Polyester/ether urethanes (PURs) are one such polymer that can be modified to create a suitable hydrophilic/hydrophobic balance, thus promoting targeted drug delivery [9]. Nanocarriers of different polymers like Poly(cyclotriphosphazene-co-dopamine), poly(lactic acid), PEG, poly(vinyl pyrrolidone-co-vinyl acetate) copolymer, poly(acrylic acid) (PAA), and poly(vinyl alcohol) (PVA)-co-albumin copolymer, polyurethane (PU), and poly(l-lactide-co-glycolic acid) are being used to deliver drugs like acriflavine, Sorafenib, DOX, and Docetaxel (DTXL) [11–14]. Smart or intelligent nanocomposites have also been designed using various polymeric combinations. A thermoresponsive nanocomposite using oligoethylene glycol methyl methacrylate, diethylene glycol methyl methacrylate, and 2-aminoethyl methacrylate was designed for the delivery of DOX [15]. A pH-receptive nanocomposite has been designed by [16], using nanoparticles of silica (nSi) and PEG-co-poly(vinyl pyridine) (PEG-co-PVP) for the delivery of DOX. Furthermore, Pourjavadi et al., [16] designed a novel nanocomposite processing both pH and temperature responsiveness with a combination of nSi, 1-β-cyclodextrin, and poly(N-isopropyl acrylamide).

Besides acting as an effective drug delivery system, nanocomposites have also been demonstrated to be successfully used in alternative therapies for cancer. A novel nanoparticle system was constructed by Su et al. [17], from PEG and bis-pyrene, that could generate reactive oxygen species under UV irradiation in cancer cells, causing their apoptosis. In another study, polyaminoamide dendrimers were used for the successful encapsulation of DOX [18]. These nanocomposites could bring about effective deformation in cancer cells without the need for any additional stimuli for cancer therapy. Different synthetic polymers and their effects as DDS are tabulated in Table 7.1.

TABLE 7.1 Synthetic Polymer Nanocomposites as Drug Delivery System

Carrier	Drug	Effect	References
Polyester/ether urethanes	Various	Targeted delivery system	[13]
Poly(cyclotriphosphazene-co-dopamine)	Acriflavine	Sustained release of drug for upto 7 days	[14]
(PLA-PEG-PLL-DTPA) PEG-PLGA/PLGA	Sorafenib	Enhanced drug entrapment efficiency	[12]
Polyurethane (PU)	DOX	Enhanced inhibition effect on the proliferation of breast cancer cell line (MCF-7)	[11]
Heparin-biotin/heparin/ $CaCO_3$/Ca phosphate	DOX	pH sensitivity and tumor-targeting property	[19]
PLGA+P3HB	Docetaxel (DTXL)	Delivery and controlled release of hydrophobic therapeutic molecules.	[20]
Diethylene glycol methyl methacrylate, oligoethylene glycol methyl methacrylate, and 2-aminoethyl methacrylate	DOX	pH sensitivity	[15]
PEG-co-poly (vinyl pyridine)	DOX	Optimum particle size and high colloidal stability	[16]
Methacrylic acid (MMA) and a mesoporous nanostructured silica	Naproxen	Enhanced drug entrapment efficiency	[21]
PEG and bis-pyrene		Increase in reactive oxygen level concentration UV irradiation in cancer cells, causing apoptosis.	[17]
Polyaminoamide dendrimers	DOX	Effective deformation of cancer cells without external additional stimuli	[18]
Poly(vinyl pirrolidone) and poly(ethylene adipate)	Artenisimin (ART)	Decreased prostatic cancer cell viability	[22]

7.3.2 BIOPOLYMER AS NANOCOMPOSITES IN CANCER THERAPY

Synthetic polymers, although widely used, have major environmental concerns due to being non-degradable in nature. Therefore, biodegradable polymers or biopolymers are gaining limelight in the field of medicine and healthcare. These polymers can completely degrade in nature by the action of microorganisms [23]. The nanocomposites of biopolymers are even more desirable as antimicrobial agents, drug carriers, sensors, in the diagnosis of diseases, tissue engineering, wound healing, and also in cancer therapy [9]. In cancer therapy, biopolymers have been efficiently demonstrated to work as DDS. Such DDS, along with the conjugated drug, can easily penetrate through cells, and through specific modifications, these nanoparticles can show tissue-specific responsiveness, thereby acting as smart polymers.

An array of different biopolymers has been experimented with for designing various DDS for cancer therapy. A polymer widely used in cancer therapy is chitosan (CS). CS is a linear cationic biopolymer comprising repeating units of glucosamines. CS can be easily prepared, can encapsulate various hydrophilic drugs, has low toxicity, and is inexpensive. CS-based nanoparticles were constructed by Gupta et al. [24], using the water-in-oil (W/O) nanoemulsion technique with the drug PTX. This combination was found to render a positive effect in treating breast cancer cells. Further, CS-based nanoparticles loaded with the anticancer drug Alphastatin were found to possess enhanced antiangiogenic effects both *in vitro* and *in vivo* [24]. In another study, Csikós et al. [26] constructed nanocomposites from poly-g-glutamic acid (PGA), chitosan, and folic acid for delivering DOX. The addition of folic acid adds tissue specificity to the drug delivery system since cancer cells have additional receptors for folic acid. This nanocomposite has shown better specificity towards nasopharyngeal epithelium. Chitosan-based composites bound to hydroxyapatite (HAP) and a sugar-based polymer embedded on a Cloisite 30B clay surface (CS/HAP/clay-g), as well as another one comprising CS/HAP pristine Cloisite 30B (CS/HAP/clay-g), have been constructed by Amin et al. [27] for drug delivery. In general, the therapeutic application of CS-based nanocomposites has lately been the topic of research for various types of cancers, such as lung, bladder, pancreas, breast, colon, and prostate cancer [9].

Another popularly studied biopolymer is Poly(lactic-co-glicolic acid) (PLGA), approved by the FDA [28]. Being biocompatible with the human body, it has been demonstrated to be a promising carrier for drugs, proteins, and other molecules such as DNA, RNA, and peptides. Geng et al. [29] studied the effect of PLGA-enclosed cisplatin on a human hepatoma cell line. Folic acid-conjugated nanocomposites of chitosan and PLGA as nanocarriers for carboplatin were constructed by Profirio & Pessine [30].

Curcumin, a popular anticancer molecule, is often recommended as a part of cancer therapy. However, its use is restricted owing to its low solubility and hence requires an efficient drug delivery system [9]. An effective drug delivery system for curcumin has been designed by Raveendran et al. [31] using block copolymers of poly (alkyl-2-oxazoline), which are amphiphilic in nature. Another efficient and safe delivery carrier for curcumin was developed by Lachowicz et al. [32] as bioconjugated micelles of alginate and curcumin. This bioconjugate (0.7 mg/ml) drops the viability of cancer cells by about 80% and was also effectively taken up by cells within an hour of administration. Thiolated starch-coated nano-iron oxide particles loaded with curcumin also revealed enhanced anticancer effects [33]. A potential application of methoxy-PEG-b-poly (δ-valerolactone) (mPEG-b-PVL) copolymer as a vehicle for curcumin delivery has also been achieved by Song et al. [34]. Methoxy-PEG-b-PLA diblock copolymers have also shown promising results against breast cancer cells [34].

Various other biopolymers have also exhibited fruitful results as efficient DDS. A nanocomposite with biodegradable properties constructed of starch and cellulose acetate-co-acrylate laden with DOX was found to possess growth inhibition capacity against liver and colon cancer cell lines [35]. Plaxitel-laden microspheres with fluorescent properties were designed from PLA and PEG with grafted fluorescein [36]. This complex was found to have anticancer potency against the colorectal cancer cell line Caco-2. In a study on hepatocancer cell lines, dextran-layered goldmag nAu/Fe_3O_4 particles were used as a potential delivery system for DOX. The application of biopolymers has also been helpful in adjuvating the effect of alternative therapy with conventional CT. Poly-γ-glutamic acid-g-poly(lactic-co-glycolic acid) nanocarriers were designed for the delivery of DOX and indocyanine green (ICG). This complex could facilitate the rapid release of DOX along with photoinduced hyperthermia, which was successful in suppressing the proliferation of cancer even at low doses. This study presented a wonderful possibility of enhancing the efficiency of chemo-photothermal cancer therapy by the application of biopolymers. Table 7.2 tabulates various biopolymeric DDS used in cancer treatment.

TABLE 7.2 Biopolymer Nanocomposites as Drug Delivery System

Carrier	Drug	Effect	References
Chitosan	PTX	Demonstrates cytotoxicity on breast cancer cell	[24]
Chitosan	Alphastatin	Antiangiogenic effect on lung carcinoma	[25]
Poly-g- glutamic acid (PGA), chitosan and folic acid	DOX	Enhanced specificity towards nasopharyngeal epithelium	[26]
Chitosan, hydroxy apatite (HAP), Cloisite 30B clay	-	Cytotoxicity against breast carcinoma cell line (Hep G-2) and a normal human skin fibroblast cell line (BJ-I)	[27]
Poly lactic-co-Glycolic Acid (PLGA), maleimide, TP13	Cisplatin	Antineoplastic	[29]
PLGA, chitosan	Cisplatin	Specificity along with cytotoxicity.	[37]
Chitosan, PLGA, folic acid	Carboplatin	Enhanced cellular uptake	[30]
Poly (alckyl-2-oxazoline).	Curcumin	Enhanced solubility	[31]
Alginate and curcumin	Curcumin	Enhanced cytotoxicity and cellular uptake	[32]
Thiolated starch-coated nano-iron oxide particles	Curcumin	Enhanced anticancer effect	[33]
Metoxy-PEG-b-poly (δ-valerolactone)	Curcumin	Increased solubility of curcumin and improved pharmacokinetic properties	[34]
Metoxy-PEG-b-PLA	Curcumin	Decreased breast cancer cells viability	[34]
Starch, cellulose acetate-co-acrylate	DOX	Enhanced growth inhibition potency against colon and liver cancer cell lines	[35]
PLA, PEG, fluorescein	Plaxitel	Anticancer activity against the colorectal cancer cell line.	[36]
Poly-γ-glutamic acid-g-poly(lactic-co-glycolic acid)	DOX and Indocianine green	Rapid release of DOX and photoinduced hyperthermia	[38]

7.3.3 POLYMER AS LIPOSOMES IN CANCER THERAPY

Liposomes are lipid-based nanoparticles that can associate with a large number of cancer drug molecules. When amphiphilic polymers self-assemble into polymeric vesicles, the structure is called a polymersome.

The first polymersome was designed by Langer and co-workers in 1976 from PVA for the restricted release of peptides and other biomolecules [39]. The hydrophilic core of the polymersome can encapsulate hydrophilic drugs with high encapsulation efficiency. The polymerosomes have been reported to effectively deliver drugs like DOX, 5-FU, and Leucovorin. A very commonly studied polymersome is that prepared from PEG. Such (PEG)ylated polymerosomes can passively accumulate in tumorous cells by the enhanced permeability and retention (EPR) effect [40–42]. Cisplatin and carboplatin-loaded (PEG)ylated polymerosomes have been demonstrated to be successful in treating lung cancer and liver cancer, respectively [43, 44]. The polymerosomes can be modified according to the target cell; for instance, specific antibodies or specific receptor ligands can be bound to the surface of the liposomes, which in turn can increase the binding of the liposomes to the target cells. Polymer-based liposomes thus provide improved biodistribution and tumor accumulation for the attached therapeutics. However, to achieve the maximum EPR effect, the physical and chemical properties of polymerosomes, such as their size, charge, and polarity, must be precisely regulated [45, 46]. For example, the size of PEGylated liposomes needs to be less than 500 nm, as a larger diameter can lead to removal by opsonization in the blood.

The polymerosomes are also ideal as co-delivery systems. The polymerosomes can deliver drugs with different solubilities together, which is otherwise difficult to achieve. One such example is the co-delivery of the drug PTX (hydrophobic in nature) and DOX·HCl (hydrophilic in nature) by liposomes constructed from the pH-responsive degradable copolymers poly(2,4,6-trimethoxy benzylidene pentaerythritol carbonate) (PEG-PTMBPEC) and PEG-PLA [47, 48]. Besides co-delivering two different chemotherapeutic drugs, polymerosomes have also been demonstrated to co-deliver a chemotherapeutic drug and gene together; such a combination can effectively help in MDR reversal. In one such system developed by Ding et al. [49], an amphiphilic polypeptide polymersome was formed into a cationic vesicle by dissolving it in phosphate buffer solution. The hydrophilic core could bind to the chemotherapeutic drug DOX-HCl, while the polypeptide could bind to DNA, indicating its use as a carrier for the delivery of genes. In another research conducted by Kim et al. [50], the synergistic effect of gene and drug administration was studied. In this chapter, polymerosomes constructed of methoxy-poly(ethylene glycol)-block-poly(D, L-lactic acid) (mPEG-b-PLA) block polymers were used for the co-delivery of Bcl-xL siRNA and doxorubicin [50]. Such polymerosomes demonstrated better inhibition of the proliferation of MKN-45 and MKN-28 human gastric cancer cell lines compared to the sole delivery of only gene or drug-loaded polymerosomes. The authors thus indicate the potential use of polymerosomes as efficient nanocarriers for combined cancer therapy. Table 7.3 enlists different polymerosomes used in cancer treatment.

TABLE 7.3 Polymersomes as Drug Delivery System

Carrier	Drug	Effect	References
Polyethylene glycol	Cis-platin	Cytotoxicity against lung cancer	[43]
Polyethylene glycol	carboplatin	Cytotoxicity against liver cancer	[44]
PEG-PTMBPEC)	DOX and PTX	Co-delivery of drugs	[48]
PEG-PLA	DOX and PTX	Co-delivery of drugs	[47]
Polypeptide polymersome	DOX-HCL and gene of interest	Codelivery of drug and gene	[49]
mPEG-*b*-PLA	Bcl-xL siRNA and doxorubicin	Codelivery of drug and gene	[50]

7.3.4 POLYMER AS MICELLES IN CANCER THERAPY

Micelles are two-layered structures formed of an outer hydrophilic shell and an inner hydrophobic core. The addition of polymers to micelles decreases their critical micelle concentration (CMC) and increases their stability upon dilution [51, 52]. The use of polymeric micelles as drug carriers was first proposed by Bader and co-workers in 1984 [53]. Since then, the effect of a number of chemotherapeutic drugs loaded onto different polymeric micelles has been studied for different cancer types. DOX-laden micelles constructed of PEG–PLA–PEG triblock copolymer damaged more tumor cells than free DOX. Polymeric micelles constructed of hydrophobic polyethyleneimine and cis-1,2-cyclohexanedicarboxylic anhydride loaded with chemotherapeutic drugs Candesartan and Paclitaxel (PTX) have been used in treating cervical cancer [54]. A diblock copolymer micelle constructed of PEG-poly (DL-lactide) has been demonstrated to be an effective carrier for the delivery of DTX to cervical cancer cells. In another study involving PEGylated micelles (a mixture of PEG, dimethyl thioketal (DMTK), SS, and PLA (PEG–DMTK–SS–PLA)), efficient drug delivery on various cancer cells like cervix, lung, gastric, and colon was successfully demonstrated.

Smart and multifunctional micelles with additional properties have been prepared with several modifications. Biodegradable micelles developed from polycaprolactone–disulfide bond–photoluminescent polymer (PCL–SS–BPLP) and biotin PEG-cypate demonstrated promising drug delivery along with photothermal/photodynamic effects, which present an excellent example of chemo/PTT/PDT combination therapy [25]. Another work on smart micelles involved micelles prepared from PAA, poly(methacrylic acid), and poly(N, N-dimethylaminoethyl methacrylamide); these micelles are pH-responsive [55]. Several studies have also been conducted on temperature-responsive, light-responsive, and multiresponsive polymer micelles [55]. Different micelle carriers used for drug delivery are listed in Table 7.4.

TABLE 7.4 Polymeric Micelles as Drug Delivery System

Carrier	Drug	Effect	References
PEG–PLA–PEG	DOX	Increased cell killing	[11]
Polyethyleneimine and cis 1,2-cyclohexandycarboxylic anhydride	Candesartan and Paclitaxel (PTX)	Co-delivery of drugs	[54]
PEG-poly(DL-lactide)	DTX	Effective delivery to cervical cancer cells	[3]
Polycaprolactone–disulfide bond–biodegradable photoluminescent polymer (PCL–SS–BPLP) and biotin PEG-cypate	Various	Combined chemo and phototherapy	[25]
PAA, poly(methacrylic acid), and poly(N, N dimethyl aminoethyl methacrylamide).	DOX-HCL and gene of interest	pH-responsiveness	[55]

7.4 CONCLUSION

A quarter of the adult population worldwide is estimated to succumb to cancer sooner or later. Researchers and doctors are therefore always at the forefront of developing strategies to combat this deadly disease.

Early and accurate detection can lay the path for successful treatment of this disease. However, the lack of specific symptoms and the rapid development of cancer in the human body make both diagnosis and treatment difficult. Polymers, both synthetic and biodegradable, in different forms like polymersomes, micelles, dendrimers, hydrogels, and so forth, are known to aid in cancer therapy. Although more research is required in the use of polymers in cancer diagnostics, substantial work has been done on the application of polymers in cancer treatment. Being more prone to easy modifications, tailor-made smart polymers can be designed for cancer therapy. The current review presents a concise discussion on recent advancements in cancer therapy using polymers and their composites. The trends in this field, as discussed here, suggest a substantial replacement of conventional DDS by polymers in the future.

KEYWORDS

- **biodegradable micelles**
- **biopolymer nanocomposites**
- **carbon-based polymer dots**
- **curcumin**
- **drug delivery system**
- **immunotherapy**
- **liposomes**
- **radiotherapy**
- **synthetic polymers**

REFERENCES

1. Mathur, P., Sathishkumar, K., Chaturvedi, M., Das, P., Sudarshan, K. L., Santhappan, S., & ICMR-NCDIR-NCRP Investigator Group. (2020). Cancer statistics, report from national cancer registry programmed, India. *JCO Global Oncology, 6*, 1063–1075.
2. Luk, B. T., & Zhang, L. (2014). Current advances in polymer-based nanotheranostics for cancer treatment and diagnosis. *ACS Applied Materials & Interfaces, 6*(24), 21859–21873.

3. Srivastava, A., Yadav, T., Sharma, S., Nayak, A., Kumari, A. A., & Mishra, N. (2015). Polymers in drug delivery. *Journal of Biosciences and Medicines, 4*(1), 69–84.
4. Fox, M. E., Szoka, F. C., & Fréchet, J. M. (2009). Soluble polymer carriers for the treatment of cancer: The importance of molecular architecture. *Accounts of Chemical Research, 42*(8), 1141–1151.
5. Huang, H. M. (2020). Medical application of polymer-based composites. *Medical Application of Polymer-Based Composites*, 1–2.
6. Kosaka, N., Mitsunaga, M., Longmire, M. R., Choyke, P. L., & Kobayashi, H. (2011). Near infrared fluorescence-guided real-time endoscopic detection of peritoneal ovarian cancer nodules using intravenously injected indocyanine green. *International Journal of Cancer, 129*(7), 1671–1677.
7. WIREs Authors. (2019). Polymers are improving our ability to diagnose cancer. *Advanced Science News.* https://www.advancedsciencenews.com/polymers-are-improving-our-ability-to-diagnose-cancer/ (accessed on 4th July 2025).
8. Liu, M. X., Chen, S., Ding, N., Yu, Y. L., & Wang, J. H. (2020). A carbon-based polymer dot sensor for breast cancer detection using peripheral blood immunocytes. *Chemical Communications, 56*(20), 3050–3053.
9. Feldman, D. (2019). Polymers and polymer nanocomposites for cancer therapy. *Applied Sciences, 9*(18), 3899.
10. Lee, H. J., Ponta, A., & Bae, Y. (2010). Polymer nano assemblies for cancer treatment and imaging. *Therapeutic Delivery, 1*(6), 803–817.
11. Huang, D., Zhou, Y., Xiang, Y., Shu, M., Chen, H., Yang, B., & Liao, X. (2018). Polyurethane/doxorubicin nanoparticles based on electrostatic interactions as pH-sensitive drug delivery carriers. *Polymer International, 67*(9), 1186–1193.
12. Khan, M. A., Raza, A., Ovais, M., Sohail, M. F., & Ali, S. (2018). Current state and prospects of nano-delivery systems for sorafenib. *International Journal of Polymeric Materials and Polymeric Biomaterials, 67*(18), 1105–1115.
13. Mattu, C., Silvestri, A., Wang, T. R., Boffito, M., Ranzato, E., Cassino, C., & Ciardelli, G. (2016). Surface-functionalized polyurethane nanoparticles for targeted cancer therapy. *Polymer International, 65*(7), 770–779.
14. Mehmood, S., Wang, L., Yu, H., Haq, F., Amin, B. U., Uddin, M. A., & Ni, Z. (2020). Preparation of poly (cyclotriphosphazene-co-piperazine) nanospheres and their drug release behavior. *International Journal of Polymeric Materials and Polymeric Biomaterials, 71*(2), 1–9.
15. Lipowska-Kur, D., Szweda, R., Trzebicka, B., & Dworak, A. (2018). Preparation and characterization of doxorubicin nanocarriers based on thermoresponsive oligo (ethylene glycol) methyl ether methacrylate polymer-drug conjugates. *European Polymer Journal, 109*, 391–401.
16. Pourjavadi, A., Tehrani, Z. M., & Bennett, C. (2015). PEG-co-polyvinyl pyridine coated magnetic mesoporous silica nanoparticles for pH-responsive controlled release of doxorubicin. *International Journal of Polymeric Materials and Polymeric Biomaterials, 64*(11), 570–577.
17. Su, T., Cheng, F., Lin, S., Xiao, T., Zhu, Y., Cao, J., & He, B. (2018). Reduction-induced decomposition and self-aggregation strategy to induce reactive oxygen species generation for cancer therapy. *ACS Applied Bio Materials, 1*(4), 954–960.

18. Yuan, S., Wu, M., Han, L., Song, Y., Yuan, S., Zhang, Y., & Qi, X. (2018). Surface partially neutralized dendritic polymer demonstrating proton-triggered self-assembled aggregation for tumor therapy. *European Polymer Journal, 103*, 59–67.
19. Liang, P., Wang, C. Q., Chen, H., Zhuo, R. X., & Cheng, S. X. (2015). Multi-functional heparin–biotin/heparin/calcium carbonate/calcium phosphate nanoparticles for targeted co-delivery of gene and drug. *Polymer International, 64*(5), 647–653.
20. Di Mascolo, D., Basnett, P., Palange, A. L., Francardi, M., Roy, I., & Decuzzi, P. (2016). Tuning core hydrophobicity of spherical polymeric Nano constructs for docetaxel delivery. *Polymer International, 65*(7), 741–746.
21. Rafi, A. A., Fakheri, F., & Mahkam, M. (2016). Synthesis and preparation of new pH-sensitive nanocomposite and nano capsule based on "MCM-41/poly methacrylic acid" as drug carriers. *Polymer Bulletin, 73*, 2649–2659.
22. Bonadies, I., Maglione, L., Ambrogi, V., Paccez, J. D., Zerbini, L. F., e Silva, L. F. R., & Carfagna, C. (2017). Electrospun core/shell nanofibers as designed devices for efficient Artemisinin delivery. *European Polymer Journal, 89*, 211–220.
23. Van de Velde, K., & Kiekens, P. (2002). Biopolymers: Overview of several properties and consequences on their applications. *Polymer Testing, 21*(4), 433–442.
24. Gupta, U., Sharma, S., Khan, I., Gothwal, A., Sharma, A. K., Singh, Y., & Kumar, V. (2017). Enhanced apoptotic and anticancer potential of paclitaxel loaded biodegradable nanoparticles based on chitosan. *International Journal of Biological Macromolecules, 98*, 810–819.
25. Zhang, L., & Hu, Y. (2019). Alphastatin-loaded chitosan nanoparticle preparation and its antiangiogenic effect on lung carcinoma. *International Journal of Polymer Science*, 1–9.
26. Csikós, Z., Kerekes, K., Fazekas, E., Kun, S., & Borbély, J. (2017). Biopolymer based nano system for doxorubicin targeted delivery. *American Journal of Cancer Research, 7*(3), 715.
27. Amin, A., Kandil, H., Awad, H. M., & Ismail, M. N. (2015). Preparation and characterization of chitosan–hydroxyapatite–glycopolymer/Cloisite 30 B nanocomposite for biomedical applications. *Polymer Bulletin, 72*, 1497–1513.
28. López-Mendoza, C. M., Terán-Figueroa, Y., & Alcántara-Quintana, L. E. (2020). Use of biopolymers as carriers for cancer treatment. *Journal of Bioengineering and Biomedicine Research, 4*, 6–22.
29. Geng, X., Ye, H., Feng, Z., Lao, X., Zhang, L., Huang, J., & Wu, Z. R. (2012). Synthesis and characterization of cisplatin-loaded, EGFR-targeted biopolymer and *in vitro* evaluation for targeted delivery. *Journal of Biomedical Materials Research Part A, 100*(10), 2839–2848.
30. De Moraes Profirio, D., & Pessine, F. B. T. (2018). Formulation of functionalized PLGA nanoparticles with folic acid-conjugated chitosan for carboplatin encapsulation. *European Polymer Journal, 108*, 311–321.
31. Raveendran, R., Mullen, K. M., Wellard, R. M., Sharma, C. P., Hoogenboom, R., & Dargaville, T. R. (2017). Poly (2-oxazoline) block copolymer nanoparticles for curcumin loading and delivery to cancer cells. *European Polymer Journal, 93*, 682–694.
32. Lachowicz, D., Karabasz, A., Bzowska, M., Szuwarzyński, M., Karewicz, A., & Nowakowska, M. (2019). Blood-compatible, stable micelles of sodium

alginate–Curcumin bioconjugate for anti-cancer applications. *European Polymer Journal, 113*, 208–219.

33. Saikia, C., Das, M. K., Ramteke, A., & Maji, T. K. (2017). Controlled release of curcumin from thiolated starch-coated iron oxide magnetic nanoparticles: An *in vitro* evaluation. *International Journal of Polymeric Materials and Polymeric Biomaterials, 66*, 349–358.
34. Song, Z., Zhu, W., Yang, F., Liu, N., & Feng, R. (2015). Preparation, characterization, *in vitro* release, and pharmacokinetic studies of curcumin-loaded mPEG–PVL nanoparticles. *Polymer Bulletin, 72*(1), 75–91.
35. Helaly, F. M., El Nashar, D. E., Khalaf, A. I., Abdelhamid, H. F., Wietrzyk, J., Psurski, M., & Soliman, A. (2017). Slow-release nano polymeric biodegradable composites holding doxorubicin and evaluation its antiproliferative potency on cancer. *Polymer Composites, 38*, E34–E41.
36. Icart, L. P., Santos, E. R. F., Aguero, L., Andrade, L. R., de Souza, C. Z., d'Avila, L. A., Zaldivar, D., & Dias, M. L. (2018). Paclitaxel-loaded PLA/PEG/fluorescein anticancer agent prepared by Ugi reaction. *International Journal of Polymeric Materials and Polymeric Biomaterials, 67*(13), 776–782.
37. Mansur, A. A., Caires, A. J., Carvalho, S. M., Capanema, N. S., Carvalho, I. C., & Mansur, H. S. (2019). Dual-functional supramolecular nanohybrids of quantum dot/ biopolymer/chemotherapeutic drug for bioimaging and killing brain cancer cells *in vitro*. *Colloids and Surfaces B: Bio Interfaces, 184*, 110507.
38. Hou, K. T., Liu, T. I., Chiu, H. C., & Chiang, W. H. (2019). DOX/ICG-carrying γ-PGA-g-PLGA-based polymeric nano assemblies for acid-triggered rapid DOX release combined with NIR-activated photothermal effect. *European Polymer Journal, 110*, 283–292.
39. Li, N., Zhao, L., Qi, L., Li, Z., & Luan, Y. (2016). Polymer assembly: Promising carriers as co-delivery systems for cancer therapy. *Progress in Polymer Science, 58*(6), 1–26.
40. Fang, J., Nakamura, H., & Maeda, H. (2011). The EPR effect: Unique features of tumor blood vessels for drug delivery, factors involved, and limitations and augmentation of the effect. *Advanced Drug Delivery Reviews, 63*(3), 136–151.
41. Maruyama, K. (2011). Intracellular targeting delivery of liposomal drugs to solid tumors based on EPR effects. *Advanced Drug Delivery Reviews, 63*(3), 161–169.
42. Ozcelikkale, A., Ghosh, S., & Han, B. (2013). Multifaceted transport characteristics of nanomedicine: Needs for characterization in dynamic environment. *Molecular Pharmaceutics, 10*(6), 2111–2126.
43. Foroud, N., Ardjmand, M., Heidarinasab, A., & Akbarzadeh, A. (2018). Delivery of cisplatin by folic acid-targeted liposomal nanoparticles into liver cancer cell line. *International Journal of Polymeric Materials and Polymeric Biomaterials, 67*(14), 865–872.
44. Poy, D., Ebrahimi Shahemabadi, H., Akbarzadeh, A., Moradi-Sardareh, H., & Ebrahimifar, M. (2018). Carboplatin liposomal nanoparticles: Preparation, characterization, and cytotoxicity effects on lung cancer *in vitro* environment. *International Journal of Polymeric Materials and Polymeric Biomaterials, 67*(4), 367–370.

45. Maeda, H. (2015). Toward a full understanding of the EPR effect in primary and metastatic tumors as well as issues related to its heterogeneity. *Advanced Drug Delivery Reviews, 91*, 3–6.
46. Ojha, T., Pathak, V., Shi, Y., Hennink, W. E., Moonen, C. T., Storm, G., & Lammers, T. (2017). Pharmacological and physical vessel modulation strategies to improve EPR-mediated drug targeting to tumors. *Advanced Drug Delivery Reviews, 119*, 44–60.
47. Ahmed, F., Pakunlu, R. I., Brannan, A., Bates, F., Minko, T., & Discher, D. E. (2006). Biodegradable polymerases loaded with both paclitaxel and doxorubicin permeate and shrink tumors, inducing apoptosis in proportion to accumulated drug. *Journal of Controlled Release, 116*(2), 150–158.
48. Chen, W., Meng, F., Cheng, R., & Zhong, Z. (2010). pH-sensitive degradable polymerases for triggered release of anticancer drugs: A comparative study with micelles. *Journal of Controlled Release, 142*(1), 40–46.
49. Ding, J., Xiao, C., Zhuang, X., He, C., & Chen, X. (2012). Direct formation of cationic polypeptide vesicle as potential carrier for drug and gene. *Materials Letters, 73*, 17–20.
50. Kim, H. O., Kim, E., An, Y., Choi, J., Jang, E., Choi, E. B., & Haam, S. (2013). A biodegradable polymer some containing Bcl-xL siRNA and doxorubicin as a dual delivery vehicle for a synergistic anticancer effect. *Macromolecular Bioscience, 13*(6), 745–754.
51. Kang, L., Gao, Z., Huang, W., Jin, M., & Wang, Q. (2015). Nanocarrier-mediated co-delivery of chemotherapeutic drugs and gene agents for cancer treatment. *Acta Pharmaceutica Sinica B, 5*(3), 169–175.
52. Torchilin, V. P. (2001). Structure and design of polymeric surfactant-based drug delivery systems. *Journal of Controlled Release, 73*(2, 3), 137–172.
53. Jones, M. C., & Leroux, J. C. (1999). Polymeric micelles–a new generation of colloidal drug carriers. *European Journal of Pharmaceutics and Biopharmaceutics, 48*(2), 101–111.
54. Guo, Q., Guan, D., Dong, B., Nan, F., & Zhang, Y. (2015). Charge-conversional binary drug delivery polymeric micelles for combined chemotherapy of cervical cancer. *International Journal of Polymeric Materials and Polymeric Biomaterials, 64*(18), 978–987.
55. Alsuraifi, A., Curtis, A., Lamprou, D. A., & Hoskins, C. (2018). Stimuli responsive polymeric systems for cancer therapy. *Pharmaceutics, 10*(3), 136.

CHAPTER 8

Polymer Chemistry Towards Pandemic COVID-19

SONALEE DAS

Central Institute of Petrochemicals Engineering & Technology (CIPET)-IPT Lucknow, Amausi Indl. Area, Lucknow

ABSTRACT

COVID-19 pandemic has created a challenge globally in the healthcare sector regarding the availability of personal protective equipments (PPEs), medical devices, test kits and safety accessories. Polymers are playing a pivotal role in designing customized indigenous medical devices and products owing to its tunable properties and versatility. Further, to address the shortage researchers and manufacturers have utilized additive manufacturing (AM) technology for the development of PPEs, different medical parts and prototypes. The versatility of 3D printing technology has led to increased adoption worldwide for optimising the ongoing crisis and to combat the shortage in supply chain of PPEs. This book chapter would highlight the recent developments, polymeric materials used, technology adapted and the role of 3D printing for designing and producing different types of PPEs. The book chapter would help the readers gain deep insight regarding the viability, application of different polymers and 3D printing technology especially in healthcare sector for combating COVID-19 pandemic.

Polymer Applications in Medicine: Revolutionizing Treatment and Therapeutics.
Mohd. Imran Ahamed, Faheem Ahmad, and Ishaat M. Khan (Eds.)

DOI: 10.1201/9781779640871-8

8.1 INTRODUCTION

Currently, COVID-19 has created a pandemic situation affecting 154,228,070 people around the globe (dated on 4th may, 2021) [1]. In India, as on 4th May, 2021 the coronavirus cases have reached 20,282,833 along with death of around 222,408 [2]. COVID-19 being air-borne is usually transmitted via .human touch, air, or droplet inhalation and hence has high transmissibility [3]. The symptoms of COVID-19 includes body pain, dry cough, fatigue, respiratory distress, fever, stomach disorder and sore throat as shown in Figure 8.1 [4].

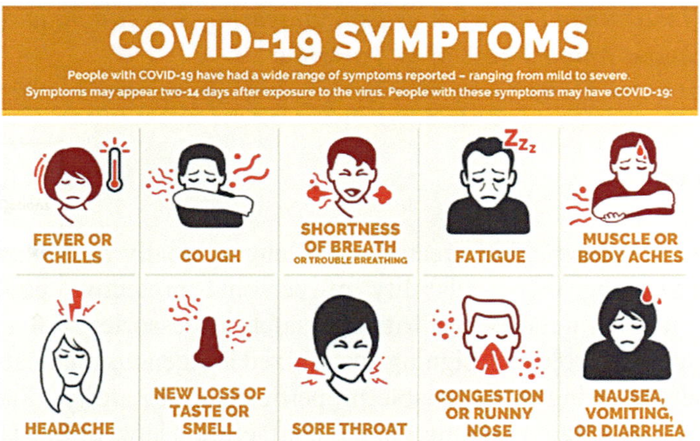

FIGURE 8.1 Common symptoms of COVID-19.

Image credit: Keuka College. https://www.keuka.edu/together-and-ready/what-are-most-common-covid-19-symptoms

Although vaccination for COVID-19 is now available for its treatment however, stringent monitoring is carried out to investigate its post effects. Hen ce, for curbing the effects of COVID-19 World Health Organization (WHO) has made it mandatory for taking various precautionary measures which includes hand hygiene, use of personal protective equipments, PPEs (i.e. mask, gloves, safety googles, face shields, gowns) and sterilized medical devices. Polymers owing to their versatility, sterile nature, cost effectiveness and ease of application have gained immense potential as the base material for developing personal protective equipments (PPE) as discussed below.

Further, with the rapid descent of COVID-19 there has been a huge demand for PPE kits resulting in acute shortage around the world. In the recent times it has also been observed that necessary medical equipments for treatment of infected patients were also in acute shortage [5]. Hence, to address the above issues there needs to be an alternative option for production of PPE kits and other essentials in large scales locally. In this context, additive manufacturing in the field of polymers has played a pivotal role in addressing the above issues owing to its accessibility and flexibility to fabricate complex geometries easily and quickly in almost minimal lead time [5-9].

Hence, this chapter will deal with the role of polymer chemistry (both synthetic and natural) and additive manufacturing for controlling and counteracting COVID-19.

8.2 APPLICATION OF DIFFERENT TYPES OF POLYMER IN COMBATING COVID-19 PANDEMIC

8.2.1 SYNTHETIC POLYMERS

8.2.1.1 POLYPROPYLENE

Xiong et al. [10] has recently reported about the development of surgical antimicrobial PP non-woven mask using conductive inorganic nanomaterial (boron nitride nanoparticles via. melt blown process and oxygen plasma treatment for activation. The author also used suspension of quaternary ammonium salt as an antibacterial agent. The incorporation of both quaternary ammonium salt as well as boron nitride can help in interacting with bacterial electrostatically for inactivating the penetration of bacteria into cell membrane as depicted in Figure 8.2 below.

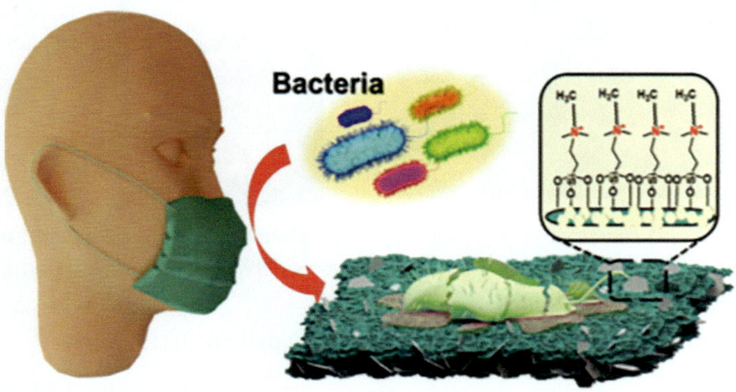

FIGURE 8.2 Antibacterial mechanism of QAC/h-BN/PP nanocomposite fibrous masks (2020).

Source: Reprinted with permission from Ref. [10]. Copyright 2021. American Chemical Society.

8.2.1.2 POLYSTYRENE

Recently, Li et al. [11] in a review reported about electret fibers face mask based on polystyrene/poly (vinylidene fluoride) hybrid via. electrospinning process. Being strong and weakly polar polymers PVDF and PS can be easily electrospun with high porosity and enhanced electret feature (Figure 8.3). The developed hybrid mask exhibited long shelf life, excellent filtration efficiency (99.752%) and low air resistance (72 Pa) etc. Similarly, Chen et al. [12] developed Lanthanum-doped nano-polystyrene antiviral mask *via*. mini-emulsion polymerization technique for rapid detection of anti-SARS-CoV-2 IgG antibodies.

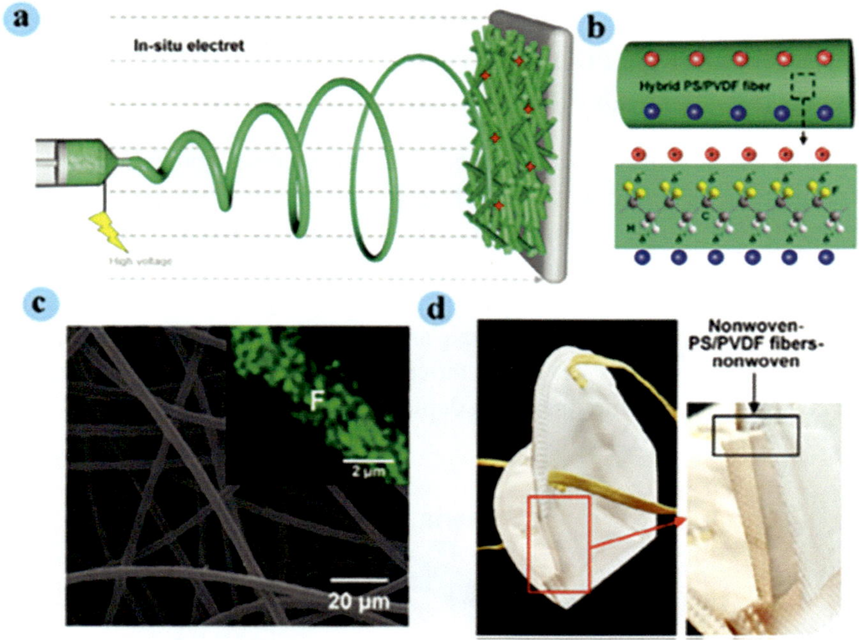

FIGURE 8.3 (a) Electrospinning process; (b) Overview of PVDF on electret effect; (c) Morphological image of electret PS/PVDF fibers (d) N95 respirator based on PS/PVDF fibers, 2020.

Source: Reprinted with permission from Ref. [11]. Copyright 2021. Elsevier.

8.2.1.3 POLYVINYL ALCOHOL

L. Yang et al. [13] developed face mask with super-absorbent features against sweat and moisture using poly (acrylic acid-co-acrylamide) produced via. wet-spinning process followed by preparation of composite layer using ethylene propylene and bamboo pulp fibers with high thermal resistance. Similarly, Mart et al. [14] developed face mask filter with a bio-functional coating of benzalkonium chloride for inactivation of SARS-CoV-2 rapidly. In another recent work Khanzada et al. [15] developed antimicrobial PVA-cross linked glutaraldehyde mask *via.* electrospinning process. From the results obtained it was concluded that the PVA based electrospun nanofiber mask indicated enhanced antimicrobial performance against the two strains i.e. Gram-positive (*Staphylococcus aureus*) as well as Gram-negative (*Escherichia coli*) bacteria.

8.2.1.4 POLYLACTIC ACID

Bulus et al. [16] face mask based on PLA/activated charcoal via. electrospinning process. The author observed that with the loading of 8% activated charcoal the composite face mask exhibited filtering efficiency ≥ 98%. Similarly, Vankova et al. [17] developed PLA based face mask using 3D-printing technique Fused Deposition Modelling (FDM)]. The developed mask exhibited compact structure with decontaminating efficiency against microorganism of 70 %. Similarly, Liu et al. [18] developed and designed adapter using 3-D printing technique by using PLA. The efficiency of the developed adapters was investigated using respiratory rate examination, as well as end-tidal CO_2 monitoring during and after 60 min. Westphal et al. [19] reported about flexible frames for producing face shields using 3D printing FDM and SLS technology using PLA and PETG filaments (1.75 mm diameter) biocompatible in nature suitable for biomedical use. The frames obtained via. FDM method was cheaper while those obtained from SLS method were expensive and smoother in nature.

8.2.2 NATURAL POLYMERS

8.2.2.1 COTTON AND CELLULOSE

Eissaand Zourob, et al. [20] developed cotton fiber based immune sensor electrochemical assays for sample collection as well as detection of COVID-1 within a low detection limit in an easy and cost effective way.

The authors used carbon electrodes for immobilizing Nucleocapsid antigen after functionalizing the surface. Similarly, Chauhan and Kumar et al. [21] developed protective clothes for frontline workers with antibacterial, antiviral, anti-stain, anti-pollution capability and anti-washable (durable) properties with excellent chemical, thermal stability and water repellency (164°water contact angle). Two strains were used i.e. *E. coli* and *A. nigerto* test the antifungal and antibacterial properties of the coating. Polysaccharides and anthraquinones present in Aloe vera induced antimicrobial, anti-viral and waterproof properties to the linen fabric. The authors used two anti-viral mechanisms i.e. Elimination of virus containing aerosol owing to its superhydrophobic property, and inhibition of protein synthesis owing to the presence of Aloe vera on the surface. On the other hand, Lee et al. [22] used natural and eco-friendly cellulose acetate polymer for the development of face shields. However, the major drawback of the polymer is its low hydrophobicity which was overcome by modifying with hexamethyldisilazane. The developed cellulose acetate based face shields exhibited huge transparency and super hydrophobicity.

8.2.2.2 CHITOSAN

Milewska et al. [23] recently developed N-(2-hydroxypropyl)-3-trimethylammonium chitosan chloride (HTCC) for the inhibition of COVID-19. The authors observed that the HTCC prevents virus penetration by interacting with the spike protein of the host cell. Further, it also inhibited the replication of COVID-19. Similarly, Alitongbieke et al. [24] developed a strategy for preventing and controlling COVID-19 using β-chitosan. The authors observed that the β-chitosan could provide significant therapeutic by destroying the angiotensin-converting enzyme II from attaching to human respiratory epithelial cells.

8.2.2.3 ALGINATE

Fabra et al. [25] reported about the use of bio-compatible, non-toxic Alginate as an anti-inflammatory, antioxidant, and anti-viral drug. Further, alginate can act as a therapeutic supplement for reducing inflammation related to COVID-19 and also enhance the immune system. Alginate can reduce inflammation by regulating release of cytokine storm and lymphopenia. El-Sekaily et al. [26] reported that alginate can improve the immunity by activating macrophages or by inactivating virus and producing specific antibody. In another work Sanmartín-Santos et al. [27] studied about the anti-viral activity of alginate nano-films imbibed with carbon fibers.

Additive manufacturing

ISO/ASTM 52900 defines additive manufacturing as a "process of joining materials usually layer upon layer to make parts from 3D model data" [28].

8.2.3 SUPPLY CHAIN OF ADDITIVE MANUFACTURING:

AM/3D printing has reduced the supply chain steps which involved mass segmentation, customization, variety, complexity, modularization and standardization [29] since demand on warehouse, transportation and IT systems gets reduced.

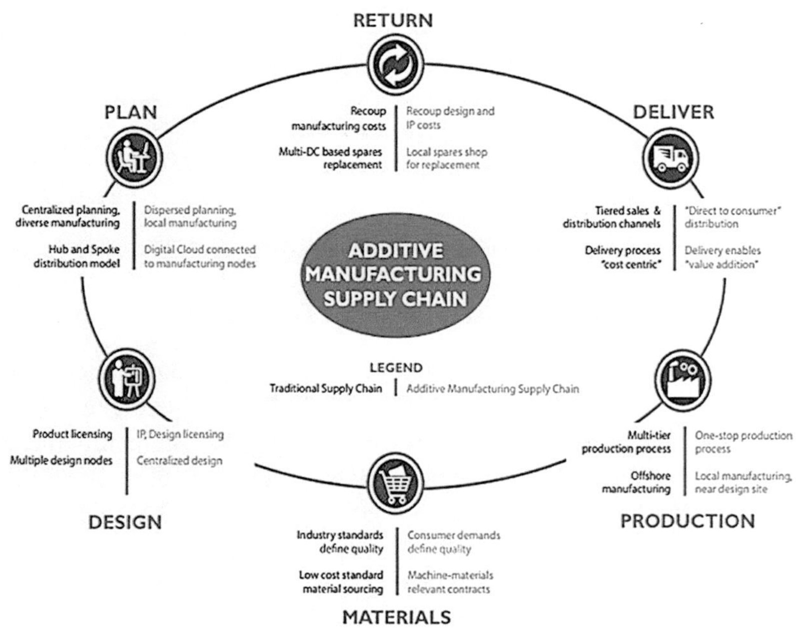

FIGURE 8.4 Supply chain of additive manufacturing [30].

Source: Reprinted from Ref. [30]. Reprinted from Croft Additive Manufacturing, 2021, Open Access: https://www.croftam.co.uk/the-role-of-additive-manufacturing-in-the-supply-chain

Salient features of AM supply chain is highlighted below [30-34],

- On-demand manufacturing process and design innovation are involved in AM process which significantly reduces requirement of ware-houses and transportation facility.
- Additive manufacturing has enabled the production of single part with multi-components by reducing the assembly costs and lead time thereby refining the supply chain. Further, part complexity also increases with improved function vis-a-vis the traditional conventional parts.
- Additive manufacturing has reduced the printing of inventory parts in aircraft industry thereby saving money by decreasing the holding cost of the inventory.
- Additive manufacturing has enabled to improve the creativity of the users in consumer goods industry without any constraint of time and money. This has fostered the development of local decentralized supply market chain.
- Additive manufacturing has reduced the material costs and waste generation by 90 % since it works by adding material layer by layer.

8.2.4 ADVANTAGES AND DISADVANTAGES OF ADDITIVE MANUFACTURING

8.2.4.1 THE MAJOR ADVANTAGES OF AM INCLUDE

8.2.4.1.1 Reduction in Waste, Cost and Lead time

As compared to the traditional manufacturing process material cost, lead time and waste generation is reduced by 90 % in additive manufacturing process. AM allows creation of parts near to manufacturing facility thereby eliminating the cost and time required for shipping parts globally. Further mass customization can be done at a relatively low cost [30, 35-37].

8.2.4.1.2 Energy saver

Additive manufacturing can help to reduce energy usage significantly as compared to traditional manufacturing processes, by reducing steps in production process as well as using less material. Further only 20-25 %

of energy would be required for re-manufacturing of replacement parts through additive manufacturing processes thereby facilitating on-demand manufacturing [38].

8.2.4.1.3 Decentralized manufacturing

Additive manufacturing can help in reducing the logistic need of designing since the later can be transferred digitally facilitating decentralized manufacturing and reducing logistical costs and environmental impacts [37].

8.2.4.1.4 Increasing creativity

Additive manufacturing allows design innovation by fostering creativity of the designer and enables engineers to go for more iteration with minimal cost [30].

8.2.4.1.5 Improvement in quality

Additive manufacturing helps in quality improvement of the prototype with intricate printing of small parts along with possible multiple iterations. Further, specific color and printers can also be used for making the part more attractive and informative. In addition, lightweight products with higher fuel efficiency for automotive and aerospace sectors can also be manufactured from polymers. Polymer matrix composites (PMCs) consist of organic or inorganic polymer as the matrix reinforced with short or continuous fiber. On application of load the fibers together transfer and uniformly distribute load within the matrix. Hence, PMC imparts high stiffness, high specific strength, fatigue, wear and corrosion resistance, high design flexibility and desirable thermal expansion characteristics [2, 4, 5]. In case of automotive components PMCs find application in door panel, bumper system, boot linen engine cover, refrigerated truck linens, connecting rod, dashboard, spoiler, seatback, pedal box system, wheel rim, fire engine, parcel shelves, chassis, and body stiffener.

AM also allows for designing complex geometries with fine finish and texture. AM helps in controlling the design by allowing in-house prototype production with high process visibility, control over design and timeline [30, 35-37].

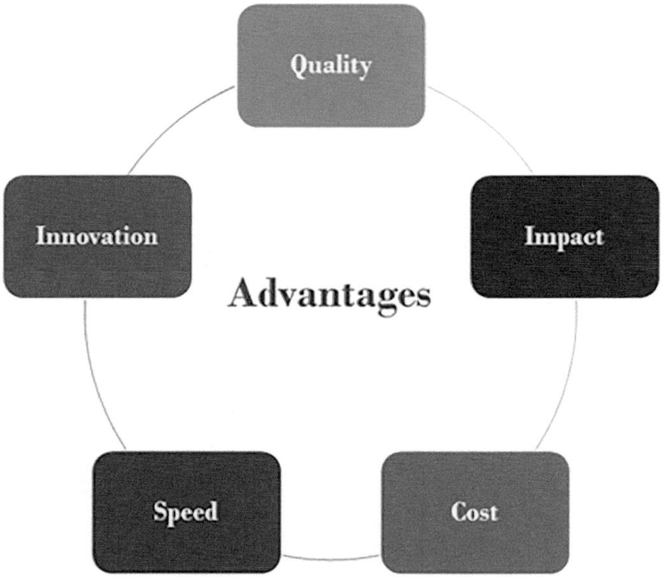

FIGURE 8.5 Advantages of additive manufacturing.

8.2.4.2 THE VARIOUS DISADVANTAGES OF ADDITIVE MANUFACTURING ARE DISCUSSED BELOW

8.2.4.2.1 Requirement of post-processing

Additive manufacturing requires post-processing to remove the support material and to impart surface finish and dimensional accuracy. The various methods involved in post processing include water jetting, sanding, chemical treatment etc. [41]. The various factors which influence the amount of post processing requirement include the product size, its application and 3D printing technology type. Although 3D printing promotes faster production, the manufacturing rate is lowered down by post processing which are of low quality as compared to other manufacturing techniques [36].

8.2.4.2.2 Reduced mechanical properties

Since additive manufacturing involves material build-up layer-by-layer with multiple interfaces which can undergo delamination under stress or certain orientations resulting in production of brittle products [39].

8.2.4.2.3 Material cost

The raw materials used for 3D printing are quite costly quite exhaustive. Further, the usage of raw materials is quite specific based on the applications i.e. food grade/medical grade etc. Further, the printable final products cannot be recycled. In addition, the 3D printed materials lack recyclability [35-36].

8.2.4.2.4 Flexibility in material selection

3D printing is only possible with the specified raw materials available. However, it lacks flexibil3D printing is only possible with the specified raw materials available. However, it lacks flexibility in selecting materials apart from the specific ones which creates hindrance for development of products with in-house developed fibers.

TABLE 8.1 Summary of Advantages Vis-à-Vis the Areas of Application of Additive Manufacturing [37]

Areas of Application	Advantages
Rapid Prototyping	Reduce time to market by accelerating prototyping
	Reduce the cost involved in product development
	Making companies more efficient and competitive in innovation
Production of spare parts	Reduce repair times
	Reduce labor cost
	Avoid costly warehousing
Small volume manufacturing	Small batches can be produced cost-efficiently
	Eliminate the investment in tooling
Customized unique items	Enable mass customization at low cost
	Quick production of exact and customized replacement parts on site
	Eliminate penalty for redesign
Very complex work pieces	Produce very complex work pieces at low cost
Machine tool manufacturing	Reduce labor cost
	Avoid costly warehousing
	Enables mass communication at low cost

TABLE 8.1 *(Continued)*

Areas of Application	Advantages
Rapid manufacturing	Directly manufacturing finished components
	Relatively inexpensive production of small number of parts
Component manufacturing	Enables mass customization at low cost
	Improves quality
	Shortens supply chain
	Reduce the cost involve in development'
	Help eliminate excess parts
On site and on-demand manufacturing of customized replacement parts	Eliminate storage and transportation costs
	Save money by preventing downtimes
	Reduce repair costs considerably
	Shorten supply chain
	The need for large inventory is reduced
	Allow product lifecycle leverage
Rapid repair	Significant reduction in repair time
	Opportunity to modify repaired components to the latest design

8.2.5 APPLICATION OF ADDITIVE MANUFACTURING USING POLYMERS

Additive manufacturing has emerged as a major driving technology in the field of healthcare during the pandemic period. The sudden surge of COVID-19 has led to the shortage in supply of PPE kits such as gloves, masks, test swabs and face shields etc. In this context additive manufacturing has emerged as one of the most desired fabrication process owing to its flexibility and easy accessibility to produce complex parts directly from CAD design file. The CAD design file can help in rapid manufacturing of prototypes that can significantly contribute towards addressing the shortage and combating COVID-19. Additive manufacturing has opened up flexible solution to foster up the creativity of individuals and for supply of various items locally thereby reducing the supply chain dependency. Further, as discussed in the earlier section additive manufacturing enables production of complex parts within a shorter lead time thereby providing an immediate response to the pandemic. Another important aspect of additive manufacturing is the availability of wide range of 3D-materials such as PEEK, PC (medical grade), ABS etc. that can find myriad of application in different areas of fabricating medical devices.

Additive manufacturing allows design feasibility for fabrication of different protective medical equipments such as hand sanitizer handles, door handles, face shields, face masks, ventilators, oxygen valves, adapters, test swabs etc. using different techniques such as fused deposition modelling (FDM), Stereolithography (SLA) and Selective laser sintering (SLS) to impart higher protection against the coronavirus [40].

TABLE 8.2 Different techniques used for fabrication of 3D printed items [40]

FDM

- **Hand sanitizer handles**
- **Door handle attachment**
- **Screw less hand-free door handle openers**
- **Visors/Face shields**
- **Face masks (e.g. surgical and N95 Respiratory)**
- **Non-invasive positive and expiratory pressure (PEEP) Masks**
- **3D printed quarantine booths**

SLA

- **Ventural type valves for respirators (needs regulatory approval first due to the materials used)**
- **COVID-19 test swabs**
- **3DP lung models for use in surgical planning**

8.3.3.1 SURGICAL MASK

As reported by the traditional surgical mask can be replaced with 3D printed adaptor valves coupled with full-face snorkelling masks and high-efficiency particulate air (HEPA) filter for combating COVID-19 effectively. Further, additive manufacturing is also utilized for fabricating mask parts and the open pump source for powered air-purifying respirators (PPE kit) [41-43]. However, Gierthmuehlen et al. [44], reported that the full-face snorkel mask provides only 85% filtering efficiency against particle size < 660 nm, which is much below the efficacy of N95 filters. Additive manufacturing also helps in the fabrication of mask and pump of powered air-purifying respirators (PAPR) (Class II devices, FDA) [45]. Half face mask using filter materials in an air inlet/outlet can be a substitute for surgical mask [46].

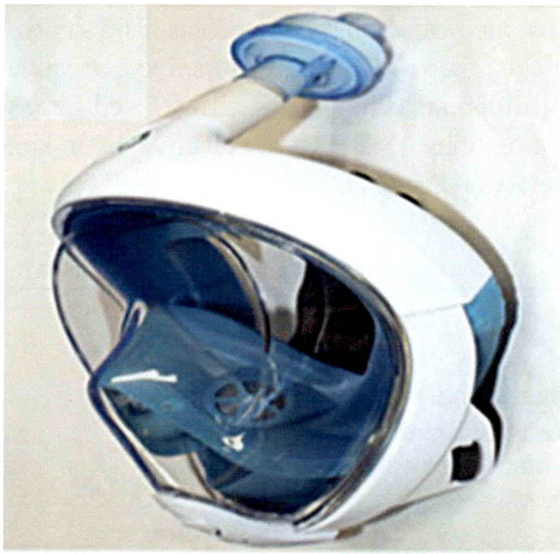

FIGURE 8.6 PPE snorkelling mask, adaptor and HEPA filter.

Source: Reprinted from Permission from Addi et.al. 2020. Open Access: https://www.jceionline.org/download/easybreath-decathlon-mask-an-efficient-personal-protective-equipment-ppe-against-covid-19-in-africa-7894.pdf [43]

8.3.3.2 VENTILATORS AND SPLITTERS

Additive manufacturing addressed the shortage of mechanical ventilators by fabrication of 3D printed splitters (FDA classified class II devices) [45] which allow the usage of single ventilator by two different patients [47]. Also, prototypes of splitters for multiplying the ventilator capacity have also been developed using 3D printing technology.

8.3.3.3 OXYGEN VALVES

French researchers have developed replacement valves for oxygen within a short period of few hours in collaboration with a local hospital [48]. Further, a hospital in Italy used 3D printing in association with a Brescia-based engineering firm, for fabrication of 100 oxygen respirator valves in 24 hours using SLS 3D printer as depicted in Figure 8.5 [49].

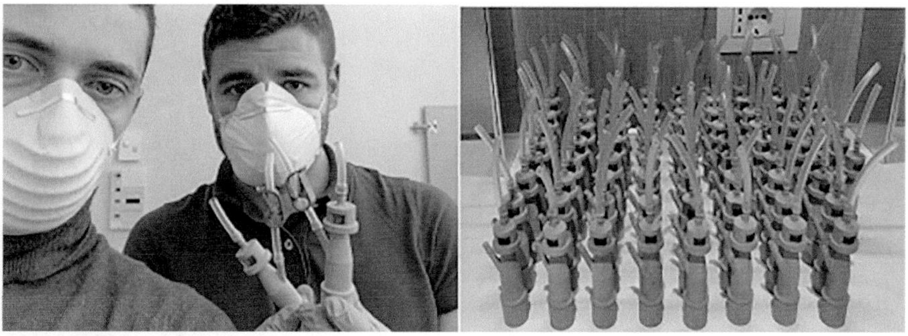

FIGURE 8.7 Oxygen valves.

Source: Reprinted from BBC News 2020. Open Access: https://www.bbc.com/news/technology-51911070 [49]

8.3.3.4 LUNG MODELS

During treatment of respiratory illness during the pandemic, specialist respirators were designed using 3D printing to take over the lung functionality during surgery. They were also simulated for their effectiveness for keeping human cells alive for a minimum period of 02 hrs [50].

8.3.3.5 HAND SANITIZER HOLDERS

Another important development was that of technique for mass production of hand sanitizer holders [51].

8.3.3.6 SUPPORT MATERIALS

Additive manufacturing/3D printing has also helped in designing parts to be used as a support material for surgical masks or N95 masks which are mandatory for healthcare professionals. The mask bands which create huge discomfort to the delicate skin behind the ears owing to prolonged use can be designed to enhance its wellness. In this context, NIH 3D Print Exchange repository have designed 3D printed ear savers/mask extenders as shown in the Figure 8.9 below to address the above issue [53]. In addition, Bellus3D have designed face mask fitter on 3D printed plastic frame to enhance the proper fitting of the masks by using face scan software [54].

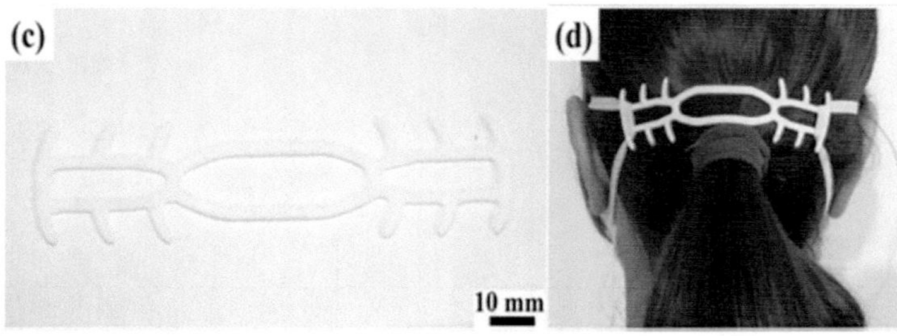

FIGURE 8.8 3D printed ear savers/mask extenders.

Source: Reprinted from NIH 3D Open Access: https://3d.nih.gov/entries/3dpx-013860 [53].

8.3.3.7 HANDS-FREE DOOR HANDLES

In order to reduce Coronavirus transmission through door handles, a commonly used medium, 3D printing was used to develop a lever for enabling the door to open using one's elbows. François et al. [55] used FFF technology to develop different hands-free tool kits.

8.3.3.8 FUNCTIONAL ANTIMICROBIAL POLYMERS USED IN ADDITIVE MANUFACTURING

In the recent decade, polymers have become one of the emerging materials to be used for bio-medical applications owing to their biocompatibility, elasticity and inertness. The polymeric materials can be tailor-made by additive manufacturing technology to foster its applicability in medical applications. Thermoplastic materials such as polycaprolactone, polyglycolic acid (PGA), PLA, polypropylene (PP), and polydioxanone (PDO) have been used for multiple applications such as knee implants and synthetic blood vessels [56-61].

Currently, PLA is the most common polymer used for additive manufacturing. For instance, PGL and PLA based materials being bio-resorbable as well as radiolucent can be used for the fabrication of melt-processed screws and pins for orthopaedic surgery [62-63]. Similarly, PCL owing to its biocompatible and biodegradable nature can be used for the fabrication of implantable devices. In this context, Elomaa and co-workers [62] have developed scaffolds based on photocrosslinkable PCL-based resin using SLA technique higher interconnectivity, porosity and negligible shrinkage as shown in Figure 8.9 below.

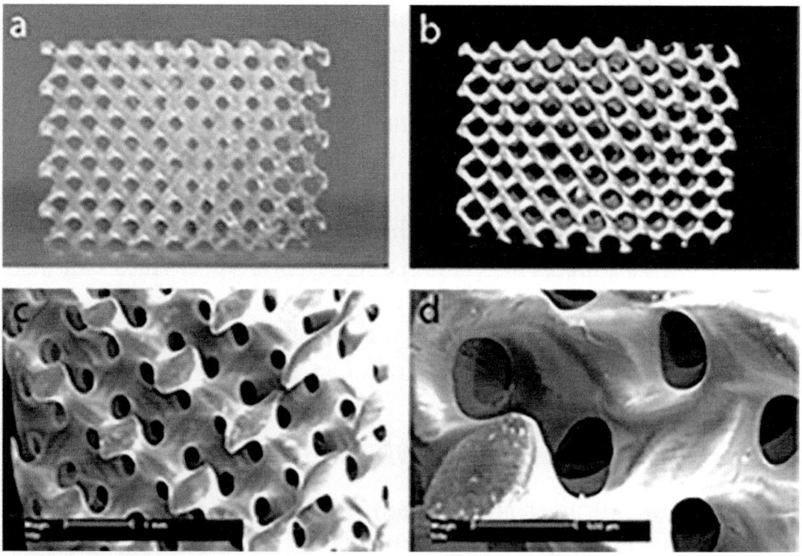

FIGURE 8.9 SEM images of scaffolds based on photocrosslinkable PCL-based resin.
Source: Reprinted with permission from Elomaa et.al. @ Elsevier, 2011 [62].

Peltola et al. [63] have designed novel antimicrobial composite based on PMMA and bio-active glass for the development of low cost craniofacial reconstructions. Ultra-high molecular weight polyethylene (UHMWPE), have been used for developing hip and knee join implants by additive manufacturing [64]. It can be also used for creating 3D printed structures using laser sintering process. Polyethersulfone (PES), polymethylmethacrylate (PMMA) or even PP membranes have been used for designing membranes for plasmapheresis which involves plasma transfusion from COVID recovered patients for treating infected patients [65]. The major drawback of AM related to higher stability of coronavirus on the surfaces of 3D printed masks, gloves and valves etc. can be addressed by using antimicrobial polymers and metals such as copper and silver [66-67]. Novel antimicrobial polymers have been attempted for 3D printing compatibility for development of medical devices to prevent microbial growth in various healthcare systems [68]. In this context, Borkow et al. [69] developed face mask reinforced with Cu (copper) and CuO (copper oxide) which reducing the risk against H1N1 and H9N2 contamination. The antibacterial mechanism of action is explained as follows Cu particles with nanoscale range of 10 nm increases the volume and total surface area for promoting its release in higher amounts [70]. Cu nanoparticles present on the polymer surface facilitate the adsorption of microorganisms (MOs) by initiating water diffusion through the matrix. The water with dissolved oxygen on reaching the polymer surface with reinforced Cu nanoparticles allows the activation of corrosion process by releasing Cu ions. As a consequence, the Cu ion along with hydroxyl radicals on reaching the surface of the composites damages the cell membrane, DNA, RNA of the MOs. Further, antimicrobial coatings on 3D printed devices can also be a suitable method for addressing the above limitation. Muro-Fraguas et al. [71] used plasma-polymerization technique for imparting antibacterial properties by coating acrylic acid (AcAc) on 3D printed PLA Petri dishes.

8.3.3.9 ISOLATION CHAMBERS AND WARDS

Additive manufacturing has also been used for the fabrication of isolation chambers and wards to inhibit the spread of coronavirus and reduce environmental contamination. For instance, the Chinese company Win Sun [72-73] have designed isolation wards for patient treatment and can also serve as a resting place for healthcare professionals. These 3D printed wards being lightweight can be re-located easily to different locations with easy power supply connections. 3D printing can be effectively used for creating isolation chambers or quarantine booth in large numbers within shorter time periods. They can also be sanitized resting wards for healthcare professionals. The building made can also be re-located to desired locations with easy accessibility to power connection [74-75]. One of the major benefits is that the construction waste can easily be used for printing new buildings.

8.3.3.10 NASOPHARYNGEAL SWABS

AM has also been used for the fabrication of nasopharyngeal swabs (FDA categorized Class I medical devices) [45] which are rod-shaped with synthetic filament coated head to collect nasal secretions. Various researchers such as Cox and Koepsell and Callahan et al. [76-77] have developed printable and sterilizable swabs with same efficiency as the commercial ones. Similarly, Arnold et al. [78] developed swabs by DLP process with an open lattice design. The swab was tested and the authors found 90% match vis-à-vis the commercial ones. Also, Ford et al. [79]

fabricated about 20 nasopharyngeal tips which displayed 94% match with the commercial synthetic ones. Similarly, Marianne et al., [80] have designed nasopharyngeal swabs by using SLS/PA12 technique. On the other hand, University of Southern Denmark have designed a robot for carrying out swab tests, thereby preventing the risk of infecting healthcare professionals [81].

8.3.3.11 FACE SHIELDS AND SAFETY GOOGLE

Other healthcare systems like face shields have also been prepared suing additive manufacturing technique while a Russian Company, 3D Bioprinting, used 3D printed tissues to predict toxicology and develop therapy for COVID-19 related or other disorders [82]. Farsoon, Huaxiang and LEHVOSS companies have used SLS, SLA or FFF technologies to design two different sizes of safety googles from acrylic material [83]. Major fields of application wherein 3D printing has benefitted medical and clinical fields are described below [84].

8.3.3.12 PERSONALIZED PRE-SURGICAL/TREATMENT AND PRE-OPERATIVE PLANNING

The technique also facilitates development of a 3D model of patient anatomy thereby helping the surgeon to plan the approach in an accurate manner and model customized prosthetics suitable for the desired patient [85-87]. The additive manufacturing technique using 3D printing allows to design prostheses components with increased accuracy, prior to implantation [88-90]. This would also result in decreasing the post-operative stays, reduced re-intervention rates, and lesser healthcare costs.

8.3.3.13 STUDY OF OSTEOPOROTIC CONDITIONS AND REPRODUCTION OF VASCULAR PATTERNS

The technique helps in understanding the bone condition accurately for a better treatment approach [91]. The efficiency of a cardiovascular system shall be studied prior-hand for treating coronary artery diseases [92]. 3D printing enables faster prototypes production conceptualized with innovative design concepts to existing ones.

8.3.3.14 IMPROVING MEDICAL AND PATIENT EDUCATION

Anatomical models developed using 3D printing would foster rapid learning and better understanding of the human body while improving the quality of medical education overall [93-94]. Additive manufacturing allows easy modelling of various physiological and pathological anatomy, while sharing the 3D models among institutions with fewer resources [95]. 3D printers having capabilities to print materials with varying densities and colours can further augment the anatomical details [96-97]. Furthermore, 3D printing can improvise communication in between doctor and patient by means of representing 3D anatomy. This would enhance the patient understanding vis-a-vis the 2D images obtained from magnetic resonance imaging (MRI) or computed tomography (CT) – Scan [98-99]. This technique can also facilitate storage of rare pathological conditions of patients through generation of a larger dataset and allow sophisticated training.

8.3.3.15 CUSTOMIZING ORGANS

3D printed organs can help to replace model of animal for investigating the drug toxicity [100]. Also, heart valves can be replicated to control the stiffness of valve's [101] while human ears can be replicated with moulds using bovine cartilage cells suspended in collagen [102]. 3D printing can also be utilized for personalized drug development with faster dissolution than normal pills, while facilitating drugs with patient-specific quantity [103].

8.4 FUTURE PROSPECTS

During this pandemic AM/3D printing has emerged as an essential technology with wide application in fabrication of various devices such as safety googles, face shields, face masks, swabs, valves and ventilators etc. Additive manufacturing has paved its way by opening new opportunities in terms of production, manufacturing possibilities and global supply chain. With the development of latest designs, techniques and software by users with their own experience care should be taken for building up of guidelines and centralized standards for proper validation of the parts. Further, exploitation of this unique technology needs to be carried out to explore its benefits and potential to revolutionize its applications in many facets of everyday life. Another limitation of this technology which remains a challenge for stakeholders is the high-volume manufacturing that can be addressed by collaborative ventures across different sectors and industries. Further limitations of additive manufacturing related to poor mechanical properties and post-processing requirement can be addressed in the coming times to gain high end output.

8.5 CONCLUSION

This book chapter discussed about the application of different polymers in combating COVID-19. Also, the application of additive manufacturing in the field of polymers its advantages and disadvantages, importance and application to restrict transmission of COVID-19. The demonstrated literature and studies indicated that there is ample opportunity in the field of polymers and additive manufacturing for developing sophisticated therapeutic supplements, masks, shields, anti-viral coatings to address the global concerns related to COVID-19. Further research is required for the replacement of synthetic polymeric materials with eco-friendly ones in order to address the growing issues related to global warming and plastic pollution. The advent of polymer additive manufacturing can be an effective solution for addressing the above issues with short lead times, improved accuracy, design reliability and higher productivity.

CONFLICT OF INTEREST

There is no conflict of interest.

KEYWORDS

- **polymers**
- **personal protective equipments**
- **additive manufacturing**
- **COVID-19**

REFERENCES

1. COVID-19 Coronavirus Pandemic, Worldometer
2. Coronavirus Cases, Worldometer
3. M. Tarfaoui, M. Nachtane, I. Goda, Y. Qureshi and H. Benyahia, Additive manufacturing in fighting against novel coronavirus COVID-19, *International Journal of Advanced Manufacturing Technology*, **2020**, 110, 2913–2927
4. https://www.keuka.edu/together-and-ready/what-are-most-common-covid-19-symptoms
5. Guo N and Leu MC, Additive manufacturing: technology, applications and research needs. *Frontiers of Mechanical Engineering*, **2013**, 8, 215–243
6. Wohlers T, Campbell I, Diegel O and Kowen J Wohlers, Report 2018—3D printing and additive manufacturing state of the industry—annual worldwide progress report. Wohlers Associates Inc., Fort Collins, ISBN 978-0-9913332-4-0
7. Franchetti M and Kress C, An economic analysis comparing the cost feasibility of replacing injection molding processes with emerging additive manufacturing techniques, *International Journal of Advanced Manufacturing Technology*, **2017**, 88, 2573–2579
8. Mueller T, Elkaseer A and Charles A et al, Eight weeks later—The unprecedented rise of 3D Printing during the COVID- 19 pandemic—a case study, lessons learned, and implications on the future of global decentralized manufacturing. *Applied Sciences*, **2020**, 10, 4135
9. Manero A, Smith P and Koontz A et al, Leveraging 3D printing capacity in times of crisis: recommendations for COVID-19 distributed manufacturing for medical equipment rapid response. *International Journal of Environmental Research and Public Health*, **2020**, 17, 1–17
10. Xiong SW, Fu P, Zou Q, Chen L, Jiang M, Zhang P, Wang Z, Cui L, Guo H and Gai JG, Heat conduction and antibacterial hexagonal boron nitride/polypropylene nanocomposite fibrous membranes for face masks with long-time wearing performance. *ACS Applied Material Interfaces*, **2021**, 13, 196–206
11. Li Y, Yin X, Si Y, Yu J and Ding B, All-polymer hybrid electret fibers for high efficiency and low-resistance filter media. *Chemical Engineering Journal*, **2020**, 398, 125626,
12. Chen Z, Zhang Z, Zhai X, Li Y, Lin L, Zhao H, Bian L, Li P, Yu L, Wu Y and Lin G, Rapid and sensitive detection of anti-SARS-CoV-2 IgG, using lanthanide-doped nanoparticles-based lateral flow immunoassay. *Analytical chemistry*, **2020**, 92, 7226–7231.
13. Yang L, Liu H, Ding S, Wu J, Zhang Y, Wang Z, Wei L, Tian M and Tao G, Superabsorbent fibers for comfortable disposable medical protective clothing. *Advanced Fiber Materials*, **2020**, 2, 140–149
14. Mart M, Tuñ A, Aachmann FL, Muramoto Y, Noda T, Takayama K and Serrano-aroca, Á, Protective face mask filter capable of inactivating SARS-CoV-2, and methicillinresistant Staphylococcus aureus and Staphylococcus epidermidis, *Polymer*, **2021**, 13, 207
15. Khanzada H., Salam A., Qadir,MB., Phan DN, Hassan T and Munir MU, Fabrication of promising antimicrobial aloe. *Materials*, **2020**, 13, 3884.

16. Buluş E, Buluş GS and Yakuphanoğlu F, Production of polylactic acid activated charcoal nanofiber membranes for COVID-19 pandemic by electrospinning technique and determination of filtration efficiency. *Journal of Materials Science: Materials in Electronics*, **2020**, 4, 21–26
17. Vaňková E, Kašparová P, Khun J, Machková A, Julák J, Sláma,M, Hodek J, Ulrychová L, Weber J, Obrová K, Kosulin K, Lion T and Scholtz V, Polylactic acid as a suitable material for 3D printing of protective masks in times of COVID-19 pandemic, *The Journal of Life & Environmental Sciences*, **2020**, 8, 1–20
18. Liu DCY, Koo TH, Wong JKK, Wong YH, Fung KSC, Chan Y and Lim HS, Adapting re-usable elastomeric respirators to utilise anaesthesia circuit filters using a 3D-printed adaptor - a potential alternative to address N95 shortages during the COVID-19 pandemic. *Anaesthesia*, **2020**, 75, 1022–1027
19. Westphal E, Mau R, Dreier T and Seitz H, 3D printing of frames for anti-coronavirus face shields using different processes and materials. *Transactions on Additive Manufacturing Meets Medicine*, **2020**, 2
20. Eissa S and Zourob M, Development of a low-cost cotton-tipped electrochemical Immunosensor for the detection of SARS-CoV-2, *Analytical chemistry*, **2021**, 93, 1826-1833
21. Chauhan P and Kumar A, Development of a microbial coating for cellulosic surface using aloe vera and silane. *Carbohydrate Polymer Technologies and Applications,* 2020, 1, 100015
22. Lee SE, Surface modifications of cellulose acetate film for the application of face shield. *Journal of Chemical Engineering and Materials Science*, **2020**, 8, 41-45
23. Milewska A, Chi Y, Szczepanski A, Barreto-Duran E, Dabrowska A, Botwina P, Obloza M, Liu K, Liu D, Guo X, Ge Y, Li J, Cui L, Ochman M, Urlik M, Rodziewicz-Motowidlo S, Zhu F, Szczubialka K, Nowakowska M and Pyrc K, HTCC as a polymeric inhibitor of SARS-CoV-2 and MERS-CoV. *Journal of Virology*, **2021**, 95
24. Alitongbieke G, Li XM, Wu QC, Lin ZC, Huang JF, Xue Y, Liu JN, Lin JM, Pan T, Chen YX, Su Y, Zhang GG, Leng B, Liu SW and Pan YT, Study on β-Chitosan Against the Binding of SARS-CoV-2S-RBD/ACE2. *bioRxiv*, **2020**
25. Fabra MJ, Falcó I, Randazzo W, Sánchez G and López-Rubio A, Antiviral and antioxidant properties of active alginate edible films containing phenolic extracts. *Food Hydrocolloids*, **2018**, 81, 96–103
26. El-Sekaily A, Helal M and Saad, A, Enhancement of immune tolerance of COVID-19 patients might be achieved with alginate supplemented therapy, *International Journal of Cancer and Biomedical Research*, **2020**, 4, 21-26
27. Sanmartín-Santos I, Gandía-Llop S and Serrano-Aroca Á, Low-cost alginate-based nanocomposite films showed high antiviral activity. *bioRxiv*, **2020**
28. ISO/ASTM International standard ISO/ASTM 52900 additive manufacturing—general principles—terminology. *International Organization for Standardization*, **2015**, 5, 1–26
29. Arora PK, Arora R, Haleem A and Kumar H, Application of additive manufacturing in challenges posed by COVID-19. *Materials Today: Proceedings*, **2020**, 38, 13-14
30. The Role of Additive Manufacturing in the Supply Chain, *Croft Additive Manufacturing*

31. Huang Samuel H, Peng L, Abhiram M, Liang Hou, Additive manufacturing and its societal impact: a literature review. *The International Journal of Advanced Manufacturing Technology*, **2013**, 67, 1191–1203
32. Liu Huang SH, Mokasdar A, Zhou H and Hou L, The impact of additive manufacturing in the aircraftspare parts supply chain: supply chain operation reference (scor) model based analysis, Production Planning and Control. **2013**, 25, 1169–1181,
33. Bogers M, Hadar R and Bilberg A, Additive manufacturing for consumer-centric business models:implications for supply chains in consumer goods manufacturing. *Technol. Forecast. Soc. Chang*, **2015**, 102, 225-239
34. Varsha Shree M, Dhinakaran V, Rajkumar V, Bupathi Ram PM, Vijayakumar MD and Sathish T, Effect of 3D printing on supply chain management. *Materials Today: Proceedings*, **2020**, 21, 958–963
35. Additive Manufacturing: Advantages and Disadvantages for PCB Prototyping, **2019**
36. WHAT ARE THE ADVANTAGES AND DISADVANTAGES OF 3D PRINTING?TWI
37. Mohsen Attaran, The rise of 3-D printing: The advantages of additive manufacturing over traditional manufacturing, *Business Horizons*, **2017**, 60, 677—688
38. Tofail Syed AM, Koumoulos Elias P, Bandyopadhyay A, Bose Susmita, Lisa O' Donoghue and Charitidis C, Additive manufacturing: scientific and technological challenges, market uptake and opportunities. *Materials Today*, **2018**, 21, 22-37
39. Zhang Y, Wu L, Guo X, Kane S, Deng Y, Jung Yeon-Gil, Lee Je-Hyun and Zhang J, Additive Manufacturing of Metallic Materials: A Review. *Journal of Materials Engineering and Performance*, **2018**, 27, 1–13
40. Larrañeta E, Dominguez-Robles J and Lamprou DA, Additive Manufacturing Can Assist in the Fight Against COVID-19 and Other Pandemics and Impact on the Global Supply Chain. *3D Printing and Additive Manufacturing*, **2020**, 7, 100-103,
41. Greig PR, Carvalho C, El-Boghdadly K, Ramessur S. Safety testing improvised COVID-19 personal protective equipment based on a modified full-face snorkel mask. *Anaesthesia*, **2020**, 75, 970-971
42. Kroo L, Kothari A and Hannebelle M et al, Pneumask:modified full-face snorkel masks as reusable personal protective equipment for hospital personnel. *medRxiv*, **2020**
43. Addi RA, Abdelhafid B and Mohamed C, Easybreath decathlon mask: an efficient personal protective equipment (PPE) against COVID-19 in Africa. *Journal of thoracic oncology*, **2020**, 11, 1–3
44. Gierthmuehlen M, Kuhlenkoetter B and Parpaley Y et al, Evaluation and discussion of handmade face-masks and commercial diving-equipment as personal protection in pandemic scenarios, PLOS ONE, **2020**, 15
45. Sinha MS, Bourgeois FT and Sorger PK, Personal protective equipment for COVID-19: distributed fabrication and additive manufacturing. *American Journal of Public Health*, **2020**, 110, 1162–1164
46. Longhitano G A, Nunes G B, Candido G and Lopes da Silva JV, The role of 3D printing during COVID-19 pandemic: a review. *Progress in Additive Manufacturing*, **2021**, 6, 19-37
47. Tino R, Moore R and Antoline S et al, COVID-19 and the role of 3D printing in medicine, *3D Printing in Medicine*, **2020**, 6, 1–8

48. 3D Printing for COVID-19, Part Two: Spare Valves for Oxygen Masks, 3D Print.com, The Voice of 3D Printing, **2020**
49. Researchers model COVID-19 infection in 3D human lung tissue, UAB Reporter, **2020**
50. 3D PRINTING COMMUNITY RESPONDS TO COVID-19 AND CORONAVIRUS RESOURCES, 3D Printing Industry, **2020**
51. Ear Savers for health workers, NIH 3D Print Exchange, **2020**
52. How to make Bellus3D's Face mask fitter|Bellus3D: High-quality 3D face scanning, **2020**
53. Materialise Acts: Our 3D Printing Response to COVID-19, **2020**
54. Carmen M. González-Henríquez, Mauricio A. Sarabia-Vallejos and Juan Rodriguez-Hernandez, Polymers for additive manufacturing and 4D-printing: Materials, methodologies, and biomedical applications. *Progress in Polymer Science*, **2019**, 94, 57-116
55. Teo AJT, Mishra A, Park I, Kim YJ, Park WT and Yoon YJ, Polymeric biomaterials for medical implants and devices. *ACS Biomaterials Science & Engineering*, **2016**, 2, 454–472
56. Ramot Y, Haim-Zada M, Domb AJ and Nyska A. Biocompatibility and safety of PLA and its copolymers. *Advanced Drug Delivery Reviews*, **2016**, 107, 153–162
57. Moore JEJ and Maitland DJ, Biomedical technology and devices, Second Edi Boca Raton: *CRC Press*, **2014**
58. Ntagiopoulos PG, Demey G, Tavernier T and Dejour D, Comparison of resorption and remodeling of bioabsorbable interference screws in anterior cruciate ligament reconstruction. *International Orthopaedics*, **2015**, 39, 697–706
59. Liu A, Xue G, Sun M, Shao H, Ma C and Gao Q, et al, 3D printing surgical implants at the clinic: a experimental study on anterior cruciate ligament reconstruction, *Scientific Reports*, **2016**, 6, 1–13
60. Narayanan G, Vernekar VN, Kuyinu EL and Laurencin CT, Poly (lactic acid)-based biomaterials for orthopaedic regenerative engineering, *Advanced Drug Delivery Reviews*, **2016**, 107, 247–276
61. Elomaa L, Teixeira S, Hakala R, Korhonen H, Grijpma DW and Seppälä JV, Preparation of poly(-caprolactone)-based tissue engineering scaffolds by stereolithography. *ActaBiomater*, **2011**, 7, 3850–3856
62. Peltola MJ, Vallittu PK, Vuorinen V, Aho AAJ, Puntala A and Aitasalo KMJ, Novel composite implant in craniofacial bone reconstruction. *European archives of oto-rhino-laryngology*, **2012**, 269, 623–628
63. Brach del Prever EM, Bistolfi A, Bracco P and Costa L, UHMWPE for arthroplasty: past or future? *Journal of Orthopaedics and Traumatology*, **2009**, 10, 1–8
64. Bohler, J., Donauer, K., Koster, W., Schollmayer, P., Wieland, H. and Horl, W, Biocompatibility of Four Plasmapheresis Membranes in Patients Treated for Hypercholesterolemia. *Journal of Nephrology*, **1991**, 11, 479-485
65. van Doremalen N, Bushmaker T and Morris DH et al, Aerosol and surface stability of SARS-CoV-2 as compared with SARSCoV-1, *The New England Journal of Medicine*, **2020**, 382, 1564–1567
66. Palza H, Antimicrobial polymers with metal nanoparticles. *International Journal of Molecular Science*, **2015,** 16, 2099–2116

67. Jorge M. Zuniga and Aaron Cortes, The role of additive manufacturing and antimicrobial polymers in the COVID-19 pandemic. *Expert Review of Medical Devices*, **2020**, 17, 477-481
68. Borkow G, Zhou SS, Page T and Gabbay J, A novel antiinfluenza copper oxide containing respiratory face mask. PLoSONE. **2010**
69. Gadhave R V, Vineeth S K, and Gadekar P T, Polymers and Polymeric Materials in COVID-19 Pandemic-A Review. *Open Journal of Polymer Chemistry*, **2020**, 10, 66-75
70. Muro-Fraguas I, Sainz-García A and López M et al, Antibiofilm coatings through atmospheric pressure plasma for 3D printed surgical instruments, *Surface Coatings Technology*, **2020**, 399
71. News-Yingchuang Building Technique (Shanghai) Co.Ltd. (WinSun), **2020**
72. Win Sun deploys 3D printed isolation wards for coronavirus medical staff - 3D Printing Media Network. **2020**
73. Choong Y Y C, Tan H W and Patel D C et al, The global rise of 3D printing during the COVID-19 pandemic. *Nature Reviews Materials*, **2020**, 5, 637-639
74. Advincula R C, Dizon J R C and Chen Q et al, Additive manufacturing for COVID-19: devices, materials, prospects and challenges. *MRS Communication*, **2020**, 10, 413-427,
75. Winsun 3D prints isolation wards to curb coronavirus outbreak. **2020**
76. Cox J L and Koepsell S A, 3D-printing to address COVID-19 Testing supply shortages. *Laboratory Medicine*, **2020**, 51, 45-46
77. Callahan CJ, Lee R and Zulauf KE et al, Open Development and clinical validation of multiple 3D-printed nasopharyngeal collection swabs: rapid resolution of a critical COVID-19 testing Bottleneck. *Journal of clinical microbiology*, **2020**, 58
78. Arnold F W, Grant G and Bressoud P F et al, A comparison efficacy study of commercial nasopharyngeal swabs versus a novel 3D printed swab for the detection of SARS-CoV-2, *UnivLouisv J Respir Infect*, **2020**, 4
79. Ford J, Goldstein T and Trahan S et al, A 3D-printed nasopharyngeal swab for COVID-19 diagnostic testing. *3d printing in medical*, **2020**, 6, 1–7.
80. 3D-Printed Test Swabs|NIH 3D Print Exchange, **2020**
81. Garrigou A, Critical review of the role of PPE in the prevention of risks related to agricultural pesticide use. *Safety Science*, **2020**, 123
82. P. He, J. Zhao and J. Zhang et al., Bioprinting of skin constructs for wound healing, *Burns & Trauma*, **2018**, 6
83. Safety goggles to protect against COVID-19—3D Printing Media Network, **2020**, 19
84. Ballard D H, Trace A P and Ali S. et al, Clinical applications of 3D printing. *Academic Radiology*, **2018**, 25, 52–65
85. Wong K C, 3D-printed patient-specific applications in orthopaedics. *Orthopedic Research and Reviews,* **2016**, 8, 57–66
86. Costello J P, Olivieri R J and Su L et.al., Incorporating three-dimensional printing into a simulation-based congenital heart-disease and critical care training curriculum for resident physicians. *Congenital Heart Disease*, **2015**, 10, 185–190
87. Frame M and Huntley J S, Rapid prototyping in orthopaedic surgery: a user's guide. *Scientific World Journal*, **2012**

88. Hosny A, Dilley J D, and Mathur M et al, Pre-procedural fit-testing of TAVR valves using parametric modeling and 3D printing. *Journal of Cardiovascular Computed Tomography*, **2018**, 18, 21-30
89. Vaishya R., Vijay V, Vaish A, and Agarwal A K, Computed tomography based 3D printed patient specific blocks for total knee replacement. *Journal of Clinical Orthopaedics and Trauma*, **2018**, 9, 254–259
90. Chen X., Possel J K, Wacongne C, Van Ham A F, Klink P C, and Roelfsema P R, 3D printing and modelling of customized implants and surgical guides for non-human primates. *Journal of Neuroscience Methods*, **2017**, 286, 38-55
91. Dodziuk H, Application of 3D printing in healthcare, *Kardiochirurgiai Torakochirurgia Polska*, **2016**, 13, 283–293
92. Stratasys, Case study, Printing Pathways to Medical Innovation. 3D Printing's Versatility Paves the Way for Medical Advancements by Cardiovascular Systems, Inc. **2022**.
93. Rosen K R, The history of medical simulation, *Journal of Critical Care*, **2008**, 23, 157–166
94. Garcia J, Yang Z, Mongrain R, Leask R L, and Lachapelle K, 3D printing materials and their use in medical education: a review of current technology and trends for the future. *BMJ Simulation and Technology Enhanced Learning*, **2017**, 4, 27–40
95. Walker V, Implementing a 3D printing service in a biomedical library. *Journal of the Medical Library Association*, **2017**, 105, 55–60
96. Wang K, Wu C, Qian Z, Zhang C, Wang B, and Vannan M A, Dual-material 3D printed metamaterials with tunable mechanical properties for patient-specific tissue-mimicking phantoms. *Additive Manufacturing*, **2016**, 12, 31-37
97. Lim K H A, Loo Z Y, Goldie S J, Adams J W, and McMenamin P G, Use of 3D printed models in medical education: a randomized control trial comparing 3D prints versus cadaveric materials for learning external cardiac anatomy. *Anatomical Sciences Education*, **2015**, 9, 213-221
98. Bernhard J C, Isotani S and Matsugasumi T et al, Personalized 3D printed model of kidney and tumor anatomy: A useful tool for patient education. *World Journal of Urology*, **2016**, 34, 337–345
99. Andolfi C, Plana A, Kania P, Banerjee,P P, and Small S, Usefulness of three-dimensional modeling in surgical planning, resident training, and patient education. *Journal of Laparoendoscopic & Advanced Surgical Techniques*, **2017**, 27, 512-515
100. Charbe N, McCarron P A, and Tambuwala M M, Three-dimensional bio-printing: a new frontier in oncology research. *World Journal of Clinical Oncology*, **2017**, 8, 21-36
101. Vukievic M, Mosadegh B, Little J K, and Little S H, Cardiac 3D printing and its future directions. *JACC: Cardiovascular Imaging*, 2017, 10, 171-184
102. Zhou G, Jiang H and Yin Z et al., In vitro regeneration of patient-specific ear-shaped cartilage and its first clinical application for auricular reconstruction, *EBioMedicine*, **2018**, 28, 287-302
103. COVID-19 Call to Action, 3D Systems, 2023

CHAPTER 9

Polymers in Tissue Engineering

K. KOWSUKI,[1] S. BRINDHA DEVI,[1] R. NAVAMATHAVAN,[1,*] and R. NIRMALA[2,*]

[1]*Division of Physics, School of Advanced Sciences, Vellore Institute of Technology (VIT), Chennai, Tamil Nadu, India*

[2]*Department of Biotechnology, Hindustan College of Arts and Science, affiliated to University of Madras, Padur, Chennai, Tamil Nadu, India*

*Corresponding author

ABSTRACT

The biomedical area has flourished during the last two decades due to a spike in demand for pharmaceutical items based on biomaterials and tissue engineering. For a variety of medicinal uses, a range of hybrid polymers, both synthesized and biological, are employed. Polymers appear in a variety of shapes and sizes, and they have the added benefit of being adjustable in terms of physical, chemical, and biological characteristics to meet the needs of specific applications. The study provides a brief history of the introduction and implementation of polymers in medicine in general, focusing on stability polymers initially, followed by polymers with degradation rates for the first biological process, and finally numerous additional multifunctional and responsive polymers. Biomedicinal polymers have been proven to include not just bulk materials, but also coatings and pharmaceutical nano-carriers for medicines. Following that, a review of the most often utilized polymer groups is given. The study's main part is then divided into sections regarding medical applications, with major application needs and currently employed polymer solutions highlighted.

Polymer Applications in Medicine: Revolutionizing Treatment and Therapeutics.
Mohd. Imran Ahamed, Faheem Ahmad, and Ishaat M. Khan (Eds.)

DOI: 10.1201/9781779640871-9

9.1 INTRODUCTION

Macromolecules in polymers are formed from several monomer subunits frequently. Polymer comes from the Greek word "poly," which means various, and "meros," which means parts. Polymers, therefore, signify a large number of components. Polymers make up the majority of large molecules, also referred to as macromolecules [1]. Small molecules termed monomers are the frequent units that act as the building blocks of a polymer. The delocalization of electrons in conducting polymers allows them to conduct electricity. These compounds can be either metallic conductors or semiconductors [2, 3]. Conducting polymers, in contrast to insulating polymers, are organic molecules. They have a high level of electrical conductivity, but their mechanical properties are inferior to those of other commercially available polymers. Foremost among the electrical characteristics, organic synthesis, and specialized scattering methods have been properties. Conducting polymers generated as nanoparticles are particularly interesting since their properties differ significantly from those of their bulk counterparts. The formation of conducting polymers at the nanoscale is now a foundation for a variety of innovative technological devices, including electrochromic displays, biosensors, and photovoltaic instruments, specifying too many characteristics of conducting polymers.

The method of a certain drug carrier system is also a crucial platform for development that mixes the principles of biomedical technology, nanotechnology, and pharmaceutical drug design. Over the last few decades, advances in material sciences have resulted in powerful advancements in this direction, particularly in drug delivery techniques. The most common medication delivery methods are said to be transdermal (TD), intramuscular (IM), subcutaneous (SC), and intravenous (IV). New materials such as polymeric hydrogels, lipids, carbohydrate polymers, inorganic carriers, and bio-macromolecular scaffolds, combined with a greater understanding of cancer biology, have made it possible to produce chemotherapeutic drugs targeted to specific locations through highly efficient therapeutic and drug delivery systems (DDS). In this context, in 1960, Freeman et al. used small iron particles to perform targeted drug delivery, a topic of study that has attracted interest [4]. Thus, according to World Health Organization (WHO) projections, the number of deaths from cancer-related causes, which are the most significant disorders, is expected to rise in the future. In the previous five years, the death rate has decreased due to an improved understanding of cancer biology and recent advances in analysis techniques and treatments [5, 6]. Chemotherapy (CT), as a standard cancer treatment, has many drawbacks, including low curative outcomes and severe side effects [7, 8]. Significant efforts have been made to optimize CT by combining it with other cancer treatment options, particularly photothermal therapy (PTT), which utilizes the heat effects of photothermal nano-agents produced by near-infrared (NIR) light to target tumor tissues (PTNAs) [9, 10]. The creation of PTNAs with significant photothermal properties and improved biocompatibility is the core issue in enhancing the efficacy of chemo-photothermal treatment in production [11]. On the other hand, the synthesis of SPNs requires high temperatures and organic solvents, which could result in higher industrial manufacturing costs and considerable safety risks. As a result, establishing an efficient, environmentally friendly technology for producing highly conductive polymer PTNAs is critical to making chemo-photothermal treatment a reality. Advanced PTNAs for chemo-photothermal treatment should have substantial distribution efficiency of anticancer drugs to tumor areas, in addition to improved photothermal performance and biodegradability [12]. The tumor microenvironment (TME) is distinguished from the normal physiological environment by redox potential, highly expressed H_2O_2, and acidic pH [13, 14]. Based on these discrepancies, the rational development of advanced nanomedicines with sensitive drug release capabilities in the TME could increase CT therapeutic potency while reducing the harmful effects of chemotherapeutics [15, 16]. Tissue engineering, a rapidly evolving area, has the potential to meet the growing need for tissue and organ transplantation while also significantly accelerating the identification of new therapies and drugs [17]. Many tissue engineering techniques have had gold standards in place for a long time. Fixing the neural gap using autologous superficial cutaneous nerves has been regarded as the gold standard for nerve regeneration and repair [18]. Tissue engineering has already been emphasized as a unique technique to interact with tissue and organ replacement owing to the intrinsic limits of autografts, such as side effects and complications, donor site access, and the formation of a secondary surgical field [19, 20]. Electrically conducting polymeric materials, defined as conductive polymers, are among the most promising materials for tissue engineering. Poly(3,4-ethylene dioxythiophene) (PEDOT), polystyrene sulfonate (PSS), polyaniline (PANI), polypyrrole (PPY), polythiophene, and polyphenylene sulfide are examples of intrinsically conducting polymers [21, 22]. They are used in many tissue engineering and biomedical applications due to their adjustable mechanical properties, simple fabrication techniques, and strong conductivity [23]. Since conductive materials are an important aspect of biomimicry, other important properties must be replicated to mimic the unique tissue architecture. Because of the complex structure of real tissues and organs, 3D bioprinting is a potential method for making biomimetic objects. 3D bioprinting is a technique that converts 3D digital models into functional tissue structures and organs using cell-laden bioinks [24]. 3D models are developed layer by layer, allowing excellent reproducibility and flexibility compared to traditional approaches [25]. Tissue engineering has emerged as a viable alternative to traditional transplantation procedures in recent years [26, 27]. The development of an artificial scaffold that can imitate the architecture of the natural extracellular matrix (ECM) is one of the main challenges in neural tissue engineering [28].

9.2 GENERAL PROPERTIES OF POLYMER

Polymers are used in a wide range of commercial products and technologies, including packaging, medical components, domestic items, and industrial parts. Polymers' fundamental advantage is the capability to be mixed in a large range of compositions, resulting in products with a wide range of physical and chemical properties [29, 30]. As a result, changing the physicochemical properties of a copolymer, the molecular weight, and polydispersity of the polymer, as well as the chemical characteristics and function of the monomer (aliphatic, aromatic, polar, nonpolar, or with unique functional groups) and its topologies (blocks, branching, or random) can adapt the properties for a specific application. Moreover, different suitable polymers can be blended to generate a variety of final qualities [31]. All of these characteristics are specified in this review, which focuses on polymers that commonly provide the most essential properties of polymers that were employed or enhanced to improve the effectiveness of analysis applications in the medical industry. Its first chapter includes an analysis of the structural, physical, and chemical properties of the most relevant polymers for this purpose [32]. To make conducting polymers, researchers used electrochemical polymerization, hydrothermal, electrospinning, chemical oxidation, vapor phase synthesis, solvothermal, self-assembly, solid-state methods, plasma polymerization, integration processes, and photochemical methods [33, 34]. Conducting polymers have low electrical conductivity and optical properties in their natural state; therefore, doping with the relevant components can increase these properties [35]. Polyacetylene has a conductivity of 10^5 S·cm^{-1}, but when the doping levels rise, its conductivity increases to 10^2 to 10^3 S·cm^{-1}, and its properties modify as well, based on the dopant element, providing it tunable qualities such as electrochemical or optical-mechanical functionality [36, 37]. These tables refer to the conducting polymers in five types, with advantages, disadvantages, and applications shown in Table 9.1. As seen in Figure 9.1, this is to determine the molecular structure of the conducting polymer.

TABLE 9.1 Types of Conducting Polymer

Conductive Polymer Type	Conductivity	Key Benefits	Main Drawbacks	Common Applications
Polypyrrole (PPy)	103~5×10^4 mS·cm^{-1}	High conductivity, excellent stability, enhanced biocompatibility, and improved mechanical strength	Brittle, prone to invisible oxidation, non-soluble in water	Antioxidants, tissue engineering, neural prosthetics, drug delivery, biosensors
Polyaniline (PANi)	10^2–10^8 mS·cm^{-1}	High conductivity, excellent stability, and water solubility	Poor flexibility, inadequate cell growth and adhesion, insufficient solubility	Food industry, tissue engineering, drug delivery, biosensors, antioxidants, actuators
Polythiophene (PT)	10^{-1}–10^{-4} mS·cm^{-1}	Good optical properties, biocompatibility, and versatile functionality	Poor stability, low solubility, reduced conductivity	Food industry, tissue engineering, biosensors
Poly (3,4-ethylene dioxythiophene) (PEDOT)	3×10^5–5×10^5 mS·cm^{-1}	Outstanding mechanical strength, biocompatibility, stability, and conductivity, water solubility (PSS-doped)	Lower mechanical strength compared to other polymers	Drug delivery, antioxidants, neural prosthetic electrodes
Poly (P-Phenylenevinylene) (PPV)	1–1×10^5 mS·cm^{-1}	Compatible with aqueous solutions, favorable optical properties, high stability	Slightly soluble in water, requires doping for increased conductivity	Photovoltaic devices, light-emitting diodes, biosensors

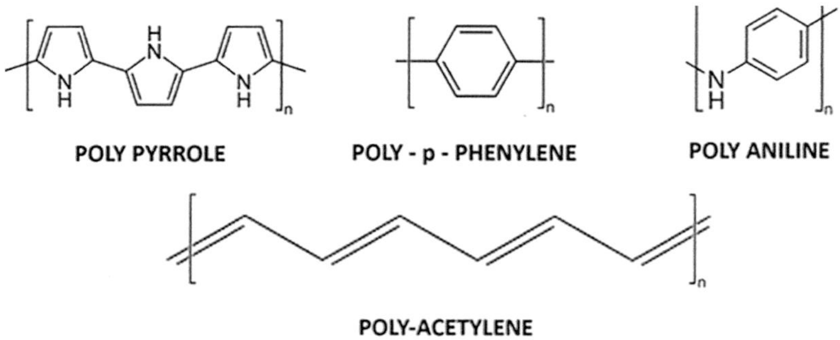

FIGURE 9.1 Molecular structure of conducting polymer.

Source: Adapted from Ref. [47]

9.3 APPLICATIONS

9.3.1 TARGETED DRUG DELIVERY

In the last several years, a substantial effort has been devoted to developing nanotechnology as a new basis for the delivery of drugs and specific targeting. Because it provides an appropriate method of delivering drugs of low molecular weight, as well as peptides, genes, or proteins, such large molecules can be delivered through either concentrated or targeted delivery to tissue. Activity polymers have been regarded as an effective method of drug delivery, and they have played a significant part in targeted drug administration, hence boosting therapeutic usage and decreasing negative effects to a system that focuses on pathological conditions in their initial stages, while also improving the status of the patient. In general, in cancer therapy, there is a residual reluctance to establish a controlled targeted drug delivery technique capable of treating cancer areas while preserving healthy cells [38, 39]. The biological functions of a medication can be realized at the targeted site through interactions between the drug and receptor; therefore, the maximal therapeutic effects and minimal side effects can only be detected when the drug is delivered to the active site at a certain pace and concentration. The result significantly improves the effectiveness of targeted medicine combinations. Targeted drug delivery, also referred to as "drug administration," is a potential method for achieving this goal and is a crucial technology for delivering pharmaceuticals to patients. This approach works by concentrating the medicine in the targeted spot rather than dispersing it throughout the body [40]. Drug carriers play an essential role in improving therapeutic delivery and are divided into three categories: nanoparticles (NPs), nanogels, and nanostructures. Examples of metal NPs include quantum dots [41, 42], dendrimers [43], fullerenes [44], polymers [45], and liposomes [46]. After intravenous injection, magnetic NPs primarily aggregate in the liver, lymph nodes, and spleen, as shown in Figure 9.1, but they could also travel to other parts of the body, including the brain and lungs, through blood circulation [47]. After injection into a tumor and exposure to a magnetic field, magnetic NPs will disperse in the tumor, as illustrated in the image as green patches of hypodermic needles [48]. Moreover, possibly as a result of NPs leaking from a tumor's circulation, a small number of NPs could be found in many other organs such as the brain, lungs, spleen, lymph nodes, and liver, as indicated by Figure 9.2 in green points [49]. Various systems to identify targeted drug delivery and to distinguish between passive and active targeting are illustrated [50]. Table 9.2 illustrates the benefits and drawbacks of targeted drug delivery methods when conducting polymers. In this graphical representation, Figure 9.3 depicts five generations of medication delivery systems.

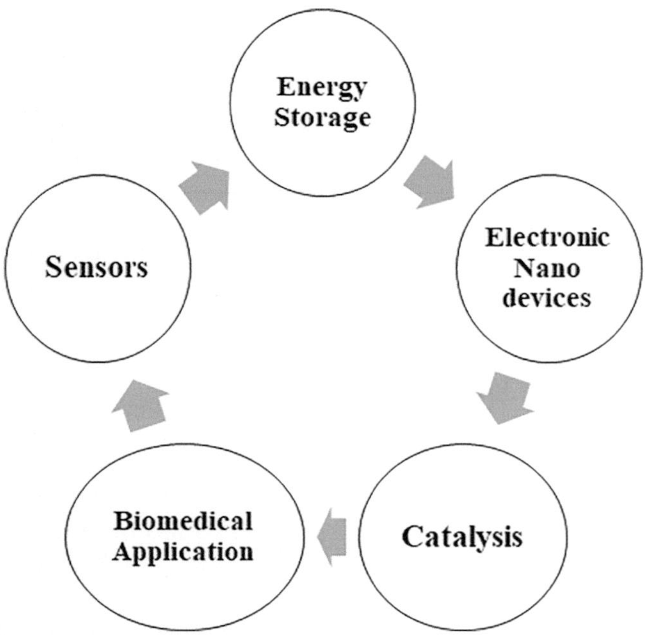

FIGURE 9.2 Conducting polymer properties.

Source: Adapted from Ref. [48]

TABLE 9.2 Advantages and Disadvantages

Advantages	Disadvantages
Reduced Dose of the Drug	**Immune Reactions Against Carrier Systems**
• Significantly lowers the amount of drug needed	• Immune system may recognize and react against the carrier
• Minimizes exposure to non-target tissues	• Potential for reduced efficacy and allergic reactions
Maximizes the Therapeutic Index	**Diffusion and Redistribution of Released Drug**
• Enhances therapeutic effect to adverse effect ratio	• Drug may diffuse away from the target site
• Allows higher doses without increased toxicity	• Decreased concentration at target site
Reduction of Drug Side Effects	**High Cost**
• Targets the drug specifically to the site of action	• Advanced delivery systems are expensive
• Decreases likelihood of off-target side effects	• Increased overall cost of treatment
Uniform Blood Level of Drug	**Rapid Clearance of Targeted Systems**
• Maintains consistent drug concentrations	• May be rapidly cleared from the body
• Prevents peaks and troughs in drug levels	• Results in shorter duration of action
	• May require more frequent dosing
Reduced Frequency of Drug Intake	**Insufficient Localization in Tumor Cells**
• Controlled and sustained release formulations	• May not localize effectively in tumor cells
• Improves patient compliance and convenience	• Leads to suboptimal drug delivery and therapeutic outcomes

9.3.2 CHEMOTHERAPY (CT)

CT is one of the most significant weapons in the treatment of cancers [51]. CT medications' anti-tumor impact is considerably enhanced by a variety of flexible carriers [52, 53]. MN@SRS has been used to deliver chemotherapeutic medications such as doxorubicin (Dox), dacarbazine, and others [54, 55]. Kim et al. described these biodegradable MN particles with an original water-soluble backer formed of porous silicon (p-Si). Dox and p-Si MNs were covalently bonded. This water-soluble backer was used to assist in the implantation of the MNs into the skin

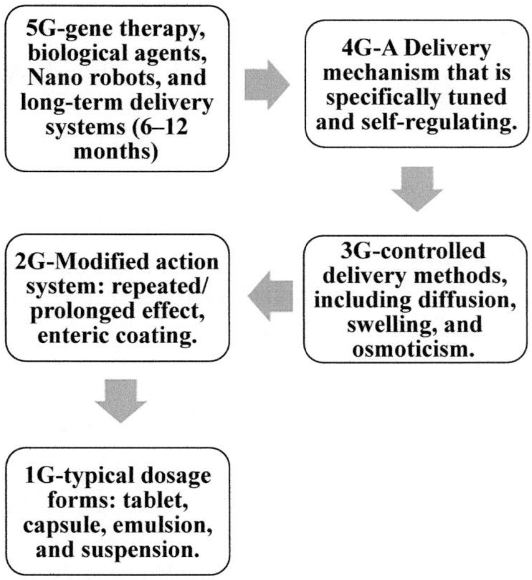

FIGURE 9.3 Generation of drug delivery.
Source: Adapted from Ref. [50]

for a short time before dissolving in one minute, allowing the MNs to circumvent the difficulty and irritation that standard flexible backing, such as PDMS backing, causes to patients. As a result, the p-Si MNs were implanted within tissues for several days, eventually hydrolyzing to biocompatible intermediates and releasing Dox at a steady pace. The study's findings revealed that MN@SRS had a higher anti-tumor activity with minimal skin lesions, which was ascribed to MN@SRS's extended-release feature, allowing for minimally invasive and long-lasting efficient drug delivery at the specific area [56]. MN@SRS was created by Luo et al. for continuous Dox delivery made of gelatin methacryloyl (GelMA), a novel biodegradable polymer. The cross-linking degree of GelMA can be used to modify therapeutic delivery rates and mechanical qualities. Specific GelMA MNs effectively infiltrated the skin, with a probable linkage between extended-release time and connection time, according to the results [57]. Until now, cancer treatment options include surgery, radiation, stem cell transplant, hormone therapy, chemotherapy, immunotherapy, and targeted therapy, with CT still being the most common [58]. Although efforts to develop ideal treatment solutions typically involve one or more treatments, practically every available option at the moment is essentially ineffective. The results are largely attributable to the cancer processes that are currently unexplained, such as the tumoral microenvironment's unique cellular and molecular complexity (poor lymphatic drainage, vascular endothelial pores, and heterogeneous architecture) [59, 60]. CT medicine (sometimes called antineoplastic substances or anticancer drugs) has long been used to slow or stop cancer cell proliferation [61]. The most often used chemotherapeutic medicines and their mechanisms of action are listed in CT regimens. Chemotherapeutic-based medicines are intrinsically related to significant and undesirable adverse reactions, despite their wide circulation (with reduced patient outcomes) [62, 63]. The low efficiency, low drug loading, and bioavailability of chemotherapeutic agents, as well as their poor pharmacokinetic and pharmacodynamic characteristics, lower service efficiency, nonspecific transmission of clarity (unintended off-target effects), concentration in usual tissues and organs (such as in the spleen and liver), and increased systemic toxicity due to immune stimulation, contribute to this problem [64, 65]. In addition to chemotherapeutics' inherent qualities, frequent exposure to tumor cells stimulates the development of resistance to the treatments through multidrug resistance (MDR) pathways, which act as a physiological barrier to regular chemotherapeutics [66]. The following are examples of prevalent cancer medication-resistant strains: (i) lipid changes in the cell membrane that limit cellular absorption, (ii) in these cellular membranes, the integrin export pump removes drug particles from the target cell, lowering the drug's intracellular levels (specifically, the appearance of the transmembrane P-glycoprotein in the cell membranes), (iii) mechanisms against apoptosis, and (iv) DNA impairment [67, 68]. As a result of the fluctuation in medication levels at tumor sites, multiple administrations are required, resulting in extreme pain, discomfort, and low patient acceptance through therapy rounds [69]. Dox is commonly used in CT, although it has been associated with severe toxicities and is impeded by MDR processes that involve P-glycoprotein [70]. Consequently, this CT is frequently employed as a "model drug" for different formulations to determine the efficacy and effectiveness of new methods, boosting Dox's therapeutic potential while minimizing the medication's daily dosage cardiotoxicity. Biopharmaceutical-based medications have emerged as viable CT replacements in recent years. Among the substances analyzed were proteins, nucleic acids, monoclonal antibodies (mAbs), cytokines, interferons, and other biological-based products, which are referred to as "biopharmaceuticals" [71, 72].

Table 9.3 refers to the characteristics of CT and its effects on the body, which are depicted in Figure 9.4.

TABLE 9.3 Properties of Chemotherapy (CT)

Types of Cancer	Types of Chemotherapy Regimen
Breast Cancer	• Doxorubicin: An anthracycline antibiotic that interferes with DNA replication. • Cyclophosphamide: An alkylating agent that prevents cell division. • 5-FU (5-Fluorouracil): A pyrimidine analog that inhibits DNA synthesis.
Lymphoma	• Vincristine: A vinca alkaloid that inhibits microtubule formation in the mitotic spindle. • Doxorubicin: An anthracycline antibiotic that interferes with DNA replication. • Cyclophosphamide: An alkylating agent that prevents cell division. • Allopurinol: Used to manage uric acid levels during treatment. • Gemcitabine: A nucleoside analog that inhibits DNA synthesis. • 5-FU (5-Fluorouracil): A pyrimidine analog that inhibits DNA synthesis.
Sarcoma	• Vincristine: A vinca alkaloid that inhibits microtubule formation in the mitotic spindle. • Doxorubicin: An anthracycline antibiotic that interferes with DNA replication. • Cyclophosphamide: An alkylating agent that prevents cell division. • Paclitaxel: A taxane that stabilizes microtubules and inhibits cell division. • Cisplatin: A platinum-based drug that causes DNA crosslinking and apoptosis. • Methotrexate: A folate antagonist that inhibits DNA synthesis.
Colo-Rectal Cancer	• Oxaliplatin: A platinum-based drug that causes DNA crosslinking and apoptosis. • Levoleucovorin: Enhances the effectiveness of 5-FU. • 5-FU (5-Fluorouracil): A pyrimidine analog that inhibits DNA synthesis.
Others	• Methotrexate: A folate antagonist that inhibits DNA synthesis. • Cisplatin: A platinum-based drug that causes DNA crosslinking and apoptosis. • Doxorubicin: An anthracycline antibiotic that interferes with DNA replication. • Paclitaxel: A taxane that stabilizes microtubules and inhibits cell division. • Gemcitabine: A nucleoside analog that inhibits DNA synthesis. • Levoleucovorin: Enhances the effectiveness of 5-FU. • Vincristine: A vinca alkaloid that inhibits microtubule formation in the mitotic spindle. • 5-FU (5-Fluorouracil): A pyrimidine analog that inhibits DNA synthesis. • Oxaliplatin: A platinum-based drug that causes DNA crosslinking and apoptosis. • Cyclophosphamide: An alkylating agent that prevents cell division.

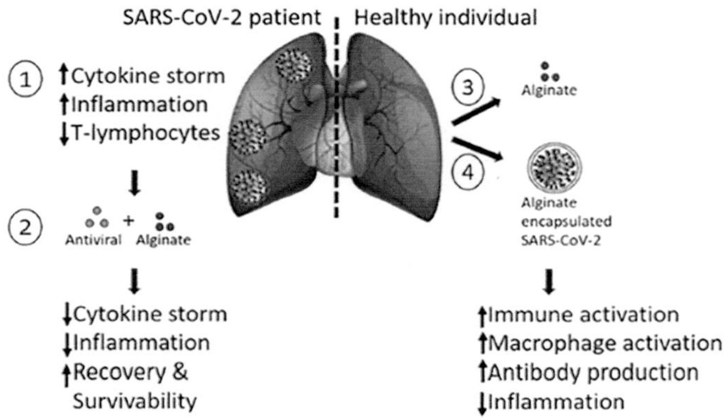

FIGURE 9.4 Effects on the body chemotherapy.

Source: Adapted from Ref. [75]

9.3.3 TISSUE ENGINEERING

Tissue engineering is a rapidly growing field in biomedicine that integrates biology as well as technology to enable tissue renewal, growth, and replacement [73]. The use of cell therapy and stem cells to restore blood tissue is particularly important in the tissue repair processes [74, 75]. Its performance in tissue regeneration is directly linked to the level of cell growth. Electrical activity has the capacity to stimulate and control cell development by engaging intrinsic signal transduction and modulating intracellular microenvironments [76]. Electrical impulses can regulate cellular responses and encourage migration, proliferation, cell orientation, and differentiation, all of which aid in tissue repair. Conversely, insufficient or excessive electrical impulses may have no effect or cause cell release independently [77]. To achieve the desired effects, both the intensity and duration of electrical stimulation must be properly regulated. Therefore, even identical electrical stimulation conditions can affect distinct cell responses. In particular, an electrical impulse intensity of less than 10 V/cm promotes cell orientation, while 0.1 V/cm to 12 V/cm promotes cell survival and phenotype for cell migration, and less than 2 V/cm promotes specific cell differentiation over an extended duration (over 7 days) [78]. When developing tissues and organs, magnetic, chemical, structural, mechanical, and electrical properties have all been taken into account. Electrical activity is an effective domain in the engineering of neural, cardiac, and musculoskeletal tissues because of all these features [79, 80].

Because conductive scaffolds contain conductive polymers, they may be suitable foundations for the development and expansion of heart, nerve, and muscle cells when exposed to the internal electric field [81, 82]. Conductive scaffolding, on the other hand, has gained attention due to its potential to electro-activate the cells of injured tissue using internal electric pulses instead of externally applied electric fields [83, 84]. As a result, the conductive nanosheets in this work might be employed as a variety of scaffolds for tissue engineering, particularly those with electrical signals. Tissue loss and organ loss generate various ailments or incidents that pose a severe threat to people's lives, especially as the population ages and their health deteriorates. Tissue engineering using scaffolds and seed cells is now being investigated as a way to heal or replace damaged tissues. Because of their superior biocompatibility, controlled invasive techniques, mechanical characteristics, and other qualities, injection hydrogels are generally employed in tissue engineering. Conductive polymer nanocomposites (CPNs), especially for electroactive tissues, can form an electroactive connection between hydrogels and damaged/healthy tissue, for example, neural, cardiac, and musculoskeletal muscle [85]. To achieve the necessary restoration effects, CPH conductivities must be similar to those of larger tissues, for example, skeletal muscle at 0.01 S/m, heart = 0.08 and 66 mN/mm, nerves = 0.0813 S/m. While injection CPHs have immense potential in tissue engineering as advanced conducting biomaterials, further research is needed into their biosafety and clinical translation. As a result, the study advances injection CPHs for skeletal muscle renewal, heart recovery, and neurological therapy, which will be described in this part. In tissue engineering, specialists and biologists attempt to generate whole organs or parts of organs to restore function in the lab to heal sick tissues, a process known as tissue engineering, which is part of the field of regenerative medicine. Producing three-dimensional tissues from two-dimensional layers of cells is a significant challenge that necessitates specialized skills and abilities. The proper cells are essential first and foremost. They can also be made as cell lines, but they must initially develop into the cells of the repaired tissues. Furthermore, when tissues are composed of a variety of cell types, multiple cell types are typically required. Solely 30% of the heart is made up of cardiomyocytes (contractile muscle cells), while the remainder consists of myofibroblasts, blood clot cells, and types of connective tissue cells found only in the heart. Secondly, these cells require scaffolds and structures to connect and develop to perform these specific roles, which include creating proteins found in cartilage and bones [86]. A three-dimensional tissue-engineered organ will ultimately require appropriate oxygen and cell nutrition, as well as the removal of cellular waste products. Furthermore, the three-dimensional substrate on which the cells grow for therapeutic transplantation must be "immunologically inert," meaning it must not trigger the immune system in the client's presence [87]. It could be advantageous for an implantable scaffold to be biologically degradable and slowly replaced over time, depending on the illness, so it can be subsequently completely replaced by the body's supporting tissue. When you examine some of these requirements, it's almost a miracle that this tissue engineering approach has worked at all. In rare situations, it has been possible not only to duplicate the intricate process of organic growth that occurs naturally within humans but also to successfully transfer organ pieces to patients [88]. Recent tissue-engineering success stories include patients with biomimetic vesicles for spina bifida and a tissue-engineered trachea (windpipe) for a young lady who was on the verge of dying from tuberculosis-related damage. On the other hand, imitating the typical tissue growth process in laboratories is still incredibly challenging for many tissues. Within an organism, intricate intercellular contacts and connections with the protein matrix, made up of proteins from the cells themselves, bring cells together in the correct format and keep them in the exact right location. The extracellular matrix is the name for this protein layer [89]. Cells release specific signaling molecules that bind to other cells and communicate information about where the cell must multiply, where they can migrate within a growing organ, and which routes must be characterized. Furthermore, a massive system of microscopic blood vessels throughout a whole organ design ensures proper oxygen, nutrition, and waste delivery. Given the vast disparities between tissues (such as the softness of skin or rigidity of bone versus gelatin), tissue-engineered organs and components necessitate a significant investment in science to become practically viable. The rapid advancement of stem cell research, on the other hand, has proven to be a potent new engine for tissue engineering research. The availability of adequate numbers of healthy specialized cells is required for successful lab manufacture of tissues and organs, and a stable stem cell source is a perfect solution. Bioreactors, like the massive devices that are used to make yeast or beer, should be designed to match the conditions for growth present in the body and also be suited for large-scale tissue engineering cell growth [90].

Figure 9.5 show the complete views of tissue engineering in conducting polymers and scaffold-based tissue engineering, respectively.

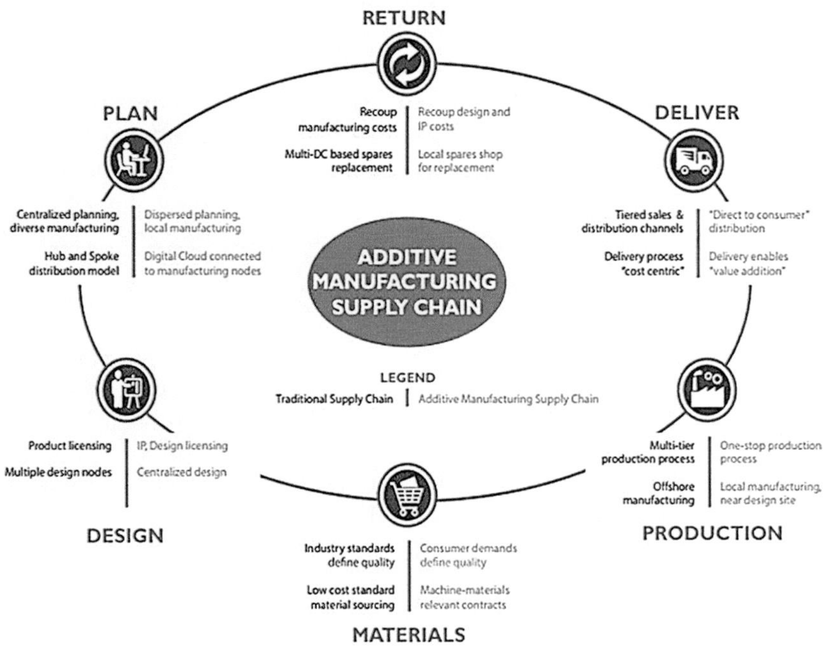

FIGURE 9.5 Structure of tissue engineering.

Source: Adapted from Ref. [87]

9.4 CONCLUSION

Conductive polymers' main advantage is their wide range of applications. The dopant is the key to this. The dopant used determines the polymer's characteristics and allows it to be functionalized for a specific application. Different types of polymers are now used in almost every sector of medicine. This wide range of applications is enabled by the numerous categories with customized formulas, such as cross-linking degrees, changed molecular weight, degree of crystallization in copolymer mixtures, and additional bioactive surface modifications. While engineering features such as flexibility, tensile rigidity, and elasticity were usually the much more essential considerations when choosing polymers, toxicity and biocompatibility must also be considered. Because these devices may disappear once they have served their purpose, biodegradation, as a more advanced attribute of particular polymers, finds application in an expanding variety of fields, from suture materials to orthopedic stabilizing materials to vascular stents. Controlled drug release applications are also largely due to the responsive degradation of polymers in response to specific triggers. These concepts are now the most active research sectors, and devices should be available on the market soon. These various degrees of easy modification allow conductive polymers a measure of control over their characteristics during production that no other material can equal. As a consequence, we predict many applications of this smart material in tissue engineering soon.

KEYWORDS

- **bio-medicinal polymers**
- **biomedicine**
- **chemotherapy**
- **conducting polymers**
- **conductive polymer nanocomposites**
- **conductive scaffolding**
- **nanoparticles**
- **targeted drug delivery**
- **tissue engineering**

REFERENCES

1. Yang, X., Dai, T., Zhu, Z., & Lu, Y. (2007). Electrochemical synthesis of functional polypyrene nanotubes via a self-assembly process. *Polymer, 48*, 4021–4027.
2. Raghavendra, S. C., Raibagkar, R. L., & Kulkarni, A. B. (2002). Conducting polymers. *Indian Journal of Pure & Applied Physics, 40*, 367.
3. Margolis, J. (1989). *Conductive Polymers and Plastics*. Chapman and Hall.
4. Prausnitz, M. R., Mitragotri, S., & Langer, R. (2004). Current status and future potential of transdermal drug delivery. *Nature Reviews Drug Discovery, 3*, 115–124.
5. Shih, H., & Lin, C. C. (2015). Photoclick hydrogels prepared from functionalized cyclodextrin and poly (ethylene glycol) for drug delivery and *in situ* cell encapsulation. *Biomacromolecules, 16*, 1915–1923.

6. Li, Y., Maciel, D., Rodrigues, J., Shi, X., & Tomas, H. (2015). Biodegradable polymer nanogels for drug/nucleic acid delivery. *Chemical Reviews, 115*, 8564–8608.
7. Mo, R., Jiang, T., & Gu, Z. (2014). Recent progress in multidrug delivery to cancer cells by liposomes. *Nanomedicine, 9*, 1117–1120.
8. Abdulrachman, D., Thongkred, P., Kocharin, K., Nakpathom, M., Somboon, B., Narumol, N., Champreda, V., Eurwilaichitr, L., Suwanto, A., & Nimchua, T. (2017). Heterologous expression of *Aspergillus aculeatus* endo-polygalacturonase in *Pichia pastoris* by high cell density fermentation and its application in textile scouring. *BMC Biotechnology, 17*, 15.
9. Soppimath, K. S., Aminabhavi, T. M., Kulkarni, A. R., & Rudzinski, W. E. (2001). Biodegradable polymeric nanoparticles as drug delivery devices. *Journal of Controlled Release, 70*, 1–20.
10. Shim, M. S., & Kwon, Y. J. (2012). Stimuli-responsive polymers and nanomaterials for gene delivery and imaging applications. *Advanced Drug Delivery Reviews, 64*, 1046–1059.
11. Gu, F. X., Karnik, R., Wang, A. Z., Alexis, F., Levy-Nissenbaum, E., Hong, S., Langer, R. S., & Farokhzad, O. C. (2007). Targeted nanoparticles for cancer therapy. *Nano Today, 2*, 14–21.
12. Sun, W., & Gu, Z. (2015). Engineering DNA scaffolds for delivery of anticancer therapeutics. *Biomaterials Science, 3*, 1018–1024.
13. Niazvand, F., Cheshmi, A., Zand, M., Nasr Azadani, R., Kumari, B., & Raza, A., et al. (2020). An overview of the development of composites containing Mg and Zn for drug delivery. *Journal of Composites and Compounds, 2*, 193–204.
14. Tartaj, P., del Puerto Morales, M., Veintemillas-Verdaguer, S., González-Carreño, T., & Serna, C. J. (2003). The preparation of magnetic nanoparticles for applications in biomedicine. *Journal of Physics D: Applied Physics, 36*, R182.
15. Senapati, S., Mahanta, A. K., Kumar, S., & Maiti, P. (2018). Controlled drug delivery vehicles for cancer treatment and their performance. *Signal Transduction and Targeted Therapy, 3*, 1–19.
16. Vajhadin, F., Ahadian, S., Travas-Sejdic, J., Lee, J., Mazloum-Ardakani, M., Salvador, J., Aninwene, G. E., Bandaru, P., Sun, W., & Khademhossieni, A. (2020). Electrochemical cytosensors for detection of breast cancer cells. *Biosensors and Bioelectronics, 151*, 111984.
17. Roy, A. M., Goel, A., Konda, M., & Verma, R. (2020). Cardiotoxicity and heart failure in patients receiving chemotherapy: A nationwide analysis. *Journal of Clinical Oncology, 38*, e19097.
18. Burstein, H. J. (2000). Side effects of chemotherapy. Case 1: Radiation recall dermatitis from gemcitabine. *Journal of Clinical Oncology, 18*, 693–694.
19. Gao, J., Wang, F., Wang, S., Liu, L., Ye, Y., Wang, Z., Wang, H., Chen, B., Jiang, J., Ou, J., Hest, J. C. M., Peng, F., & Tu, Y. (2020). Hyperthermia-triggered on-demand biomimetic nanocarriers for synergetic photothermal and chemotherapy. *Advanced Science, 7*, 1903642.
20. Wang, D., Yao, Y., He, J., Zhong, X., Li, B., Rao, S., Yu, H., He, S., Feng, X., Xu, T., Yang, B., Yong, T., Gan, L., Hu, J., & Yang, X. (2020). Engineered cell-derived microparticles Bi2Se3/DOX@MPs for imaging-guided synergistic photothermal/ low-dose chemotherapy of cancer. *Advanced Science, 7*, 1901293.

21. Cheng, L., Wang, C., Feng, L., Yang, K., & Liu, Z. (2014). Functional nanomaterials for phototherapies of cancer. *Chemical Reviews, 114*, 10869–10939.
22. Liu, T., Wang, C., Gu, X., Gong, H., Cheng, L., Shi, X., Feng, L., Sun, B., & Liu, Z. (2014). Drug delivery with PEGylated MoS2 nanosheets for combined photothermal and chemotherapy of cancer. *Advanced Materials, 26*, 3433–3440.
23. Ovais, M., Mukherjee, S., Pramanik, A., Das, D., Mukherjee, A., Raza, A., & Chen, C. (2020). Designing stimuli-responsive upconversion nanoparticles that exploit the tumor microenvironment. *Advanced Materials, 32*, 2000055.
24. Chen, B., Dai, W., He, B., Zhang, H., Wang, X., Wang, Y., & Zhang, Q. (2017). Current multistage drug delivery systems based on the tumor microenvironment. *Theragnostic, 7*, 538–558.
25. Karimi, M., Ghasemi, A., Sahandi Z. P., Rahighi, R., Moosavi, S. M. B., Mirshekari, H., Amiri, M., Pishabad, Z. S., Aslani, A., Bozorgomid, M., Ghosh, D., Beyzavi, A., Vaseghi, A., Aref, A. R., Haghani, L., Bahrami, S., & Hamblin, M. R. (2016). Smart micro/nanoparticles in stimulus-responsive drug/gene delivery systems. *Chemical Society Reviews, 45*, 1457–1501.
26. Ma, Z., Jia, X., Bai, J., Ruan, Y., Wang, C., Li, J., Zhang, M., & Jiang, X. (2016). MnO2 gatekeeper: An intelligent and O2-evolving shell for preventing premature release of high cargo payload core, overcoming tumor hypoxia, and acidic H_2O_2-sensitive MRI. *Advanced Functional Materials, 27*, 1604258.
27. Griffith, L. G., & Naughton, G. (2002). Tissue engineering—Current challenges and expanding opportunities. *Science, 295*, 1009–1014.
28. Zarrintaj, P., et al. (2020). Conductive biomaterials as nerve conduits: Recent advances and future challenges. *Applied Materials Today, 20*.
29. Vijayavenkataraman, S., et al. (2018). 3D bioprinting of tissues and organs for regenerative medicine. *Advanced Drug Delivery Reviews, 132*, 296–332.
30. Pal, R. K., et al. (2017). Mechanically robust, photopatternable conductive hydrogel composites. *Reactive and Functional Polymers, 120*, 66–73.
31. Heo, D. N., et al. (2019). Development of 3D printable conductive hydrogel with crystallized PEDOT: PSS for neural tissue engineering. *Materials Science and Engineering C, 99*, 582–590.
32. Hong Min, J., Patel, M., & Koh, W. G. (2018). Incorporation of conductive materials into hydrogels for tissue engineering applications. *Polymers, 10*, 1078.
33. Kim, B. S., Park, I. K., Hoshiba, T., Jiang, H. L., Choi, Y. J., Akaike, T., & Cho, C. S. (2011). Design of artificial extracellular matrices for tissue engineering. *Progress in Polymer Science, 36*, 238–268.
34. Cunha, C., Panseri, S., & Antonini, S. (2011). Emerging nanotechnology approaches in tissue engineering for peripheral nerve regeneration. *Nanomedicine, 7*, 50–59.
35. Ghosh, S., Maiyalagan, T., & Basu, R. N. (2016). Nanostructured conducting polymers for energy applications: Towards a sustainable platform. *Nanoscale, 8*, 6921–6947.
36. Shafiee, A., & Atala, A. (2017). Tissue engineering: Toward a new era of medicine. *Annual Review of Medicine, 68*, 29–40.
37. Billmeyer, F. W. (2007). *Textbook of Polymer Science*. Wiley India Pvt. Limited.
38. Odian, G., & Group, F. (2004). *Principles of Polymerization* (4th ed.). Wiley & Sons Ltd.

39. Pillay, V., Seedat, A., Choonara, Y. E., Toit, L. C., Kumar, P., & Ndesendo, V. M. K. (2013). A review of polymeric refabrication techniques to modify polymer properties for biomedical and drug delivery applications. *AAPS PharmSciTech, 14*, 692–711.
40. Li, D., Hu, D., Xu, H., Patra, H. K., Liu, X., Zhou, Z., et al. (2021). Progress and perspective of microneedle system for anti-cancer drug delivery. *Biomaterials, 264*, 120410.
41. Zeng, X., Luo, M., Liu, G., Wang, X., Tao, W., Lin, Y., et al. (2018). Polydopamine-modified black phosphorus nanocapsule with enhanced stability and photothermal performance for tumor multimodal treatments. *Advanced Science, 5*, 1800510.
42. Cheng, W., Zeng, X., Chen, H., Li, Z., Zeng, W., Mei, L., et al. (2019). Versatile polydopamine platforms: Synthesis and promising applications for surface modification and advanced nanomedicine. *ACS Nano, 13*, 8537–8565.
43. Lu, Y., Mantha, S. N., Crowder, D. C., Chinchilla, S., Shah, K. N., & Yun, Y. H. (2015). Micro stereolithography and characterization of poly(propylene fumarate)-based drug-loaded microneedle arrays. *Bio Fabrication, 7*, 045001.
44. Luo, Z., Sun, W., Fang, J., Lee, K., Li, S., & Gu, Z. (2019). Biodegradable gelatin methacryloyl microneedles for transdermal drug delivery. *Advanced Healthcare Materials, 8*, 1801054.
45. Kim, H., Lee, H. S., Jeon, Y., Park, W., Zhang, Y., Kim, B., et al. (2020). Bioresorbable, miniaturized porous silicon needles on a flexible water-soluble backing for unobtrusive, sustained delivery of chemotherapy. *ACS Nano, 14*, 7227–7236.
46. Di Silvio, L. (2007). 15—Bone tissue engineering and biomineralization. In A. R. Boccaccini & J. E. Gough (Eds.), *Tissue Engineering Using Ceramics and Polymers* (pp. 319–331). Woodhead Publishing.
47. Namsheer, K., & Rout, C. S. (2021). Conducting polymers: A comprehensive review on recent advances in synthesis, properties and applications. *RSC Advances, 11*, 5659–5697.
48. Knop, K., Hoogenboom, R., Fischer, D., & Schubert, U. S. (2010). Poly (ethylene glycol) in drug delivery: Pros and cons as well as potential alternatives. *Angewandte Chemie International Edition, 49*, 6288–6308.
49. Kumar, A., Zhou, L., Zhi, K., Raji, B., Pernell, S., Tadrous, E., Kodidela, S., Nookala, A., Kochat, H., & Kumar, S. (2021). Challenges in biomaterial-based drug delivery approach for the treatment of neurodegenerative diseases: Opportunities for extracellular vesicles. *International Journal of Molecular Sciences, 22*, 138.
50. Tewabe, A., Abate, A., Tamrie, M., Seyfu, A., & Siraj, E. A. (2021). Targeted drug delivery: From magic bullet to nanomedicine: Principles, challenges, and future perspectives. *Journal of Multidisciplinary Healthcare, 14*, 1711–1724.
51. Albulet, D., et al. (2017). Chapter 1—Nanotechnology for personalized medicine: Cancer research, diagnosis, and therapy. In A. Ficai & A. M. Grumezescu (Eds.), *Nanostructures for Cancer Therapy* (pp. 1–21). Elsevier.
52. McClellan, P., & Landis, W. J. (2016). Recent applications of coaxial and emulsion electrospinning methods in the field of tissue engineering. *BioResearch Open Access, 5*.
53. Chen, C., et al. (2019). Electrical stimulation as a novel tool for regulating cell behavior in tissue engineering. *Biomaterials Research, 23*.
54. Nuccitelli, R., et al. (2013). Nanosecond pulsed electric field stimulation of reactive oxygen species in human pancreatic cancer cells is Ca^{2+}-dependent. *Biochemical and Biophysical Research Communications, 435*, 580–585.

55. Li, Y., Li, X., Zhao, R., Wang, C. C., Qiu, F., Sun, B., Ji, H., Qiu, J., & Wang, C. C. (2017). Enhanced adhesion and proliferation of human umbilical vein endothelial cells on conductive PANI–PCL fiber scaffold by electrical stimulation. *Materials Science and Engineering C, 72*, 106–112.
56. Allahyari, Z., Haghighipour, N., Moztarzadeh, F., Ghazizadeh, L., Hamrang, M., Shokrgozar, M. A., & Gholizadeh, S. (2016). Optimization of electrical stimulation parameters for MG-63 cell proliferation on chitosan/functionalized multiwalled carbon nanotube films. *RSC Advances, 6*, 109902–109915.
57. Kai, D., Prabhakaran, M. P., Jin, G., & Ramakrishna, S. (2011). Polypyrrole-contained electrospun conductive nanofibrous membranes for cardiac tissue engineering. *Journal of Biomedical Materials Research Part A, 99*, 376–385.
58. Spearman, B. S., Hodge, A. J., Porter, J. L., Hardy, J. G., Davis, Z. D., Xu, T., Zhang, X., Schmidt, C. E., Hamilton, M. C., & Lipke, E. A. (2015). Conductive interpenetrating networks of polypyrrole and polycaprolactone encourage electrophysiological development of cardiac cells. *Acta Biomaterial, 28*, 109–120.
59. Zhao, Y. H., Niu, C. M., Shi, J. Q., Wang, Y. Y., Yang, Y. M., & Wang, H. B. (2018). Novel conductive polypyrrole/silk fibroin scaffold for neural tissue repair. *Neural Regeneration Research, 13*, 1455–1464.
60. Babapoor, G., Karimi, S. I., Golestaneh, M. A., & Mezjin, M. (2017). Coaxial electrospun PEG/PA6 composite fibers: Fabrication and characterization. *Applied Thermal Engineering, 118*, 398–407.
61. Kaur, G., Adhikari, R., Cass, P., Bown, M., & Gunatillake, P. (2015). Electrically conductive polymers and composites for biomedical applications. *RSC Advances, 5*, 37553–37567.
62. Kim, S., Jang, L. K., Jang, M., Lee, S., Hardy, J. G., & Lee, J. Y. (2018). Electrically conductive polydopamine-polypyrrole as high-performance biomaterials for cell stimulation *in vitro* and electrical signal recording *in vivo*. *ACS Applied Materials & Interfaces, 10*, 33032–33042.
63. Qazi, T. H., Rai, R., Dippold, D., Roether, J. E., Schubert, D. W., Rosellini, E., Barbani, N., & Boccaccini, A. R. (2014). Development and characterization of novel electrically conductive PANI–PGS composites for cardiac tissue engineering applications. *Acta Biomaterialia, 10*, 2434–2445.
64. Zarrintaj, P., Manouchehri, S., Ahmadi, Z., Saeb, M. R., Urbanska, A. M., Kaplan, D. L., & Mozafari, M. (2018). Agarose-based biomaterials for tissue engineering. *Carbohydrate Polymers, 187*, 66–84.
65. Guo, B., Qu, J., Zhao, X., & Zhang, M. (2019). Degradable conductive self-healing hydrogels based on dextran-graft-tetraaniline and N-carboxyethyl chitosan as injectable carriers for myoblast cell therapy and muscle regeneration. *Acta Biomaterialia, 84*, 180–193.
66. Wondimneh, B., Setty, S. A. D., Asfeha, G. G., Belay, E., Gebremeskel, G., & Baye, G. (2021). *Cancer Management and Research, 13*, 625–632.
67. Fengg, S. S. (2011). Chemotherapeutic engineering: Concept, feasibility, safety and prospect—A tribute to Shu Chien's 80th birthday. *Cellular and Molecular Bioengineering, 4*, 708–716.
68. Chambers, A. F., Groom, A. C., & MacDonald, I. C. (2002). Dissemination and growth of cancer cells in metastatic sites. *Nature Reviews Cancer, 2*, 563–572.

69. Redondo-Blanco, S., Fernández, J., Gutiérrez-del-Río, I., Villar, C. J., & Lombó, F. (2017). New insights toward colorectal cancer chemotherapy using natural bioactive compounds. *Frontiers in Pharmacology, 8*, 109.
70. Salvioni, L., Rizzuti, M. A., Bertolini, J. A., Pandolfi, L., Colombo, M., & Prosperi, D. (2019). Thirty years of cancer nanomedicine: Success, frustration, and hope. *Cancers, 11*, 1855.
71. Remesh, A. (2012). Toxicities of anticancer drugs and its management. *International Journal of Basic & Clinical Pharmacology, 1*, 2–12.
72. He, C., Tang, Z., Tian, H., & Chen, X. (2016). Co-delivery of chemotherapeutics and proteins for synergistic therapy. *Advanced Drug Delivery Reviews, 98*, 64–76.
73. Kartal-Yandim, M., Adan-Gokbulut, A., & Baran, Y. (2016). Molecular mechanisms of drug resistance and its reversal in cancer. *Critical Reviews in Biotechnology, 36*, 716–726.
74. Garcia-Mayea, Y., Mir, C., Masson, F., Paciucci, R., & Leonart, M. E. (2019). Insights into new mechanisms and models of cancer stem cell multidrug resistance. *Seminars in Cancer Biology, 60*, 166–180. https://doi.org/10.1016/j.semcancer.2019.07.022
75. Renu, K., GA, V., TP, B. P., & Arunachalam, S. (2018). Molecular mechanism of doxorubicin-induced cardiomyopathy: An update. *European Journal of Pharmacology, 818*, 241–253.
76. Naldini, L. (2015). Gene therapy returns to center stage. *Nature, 526*, 351–360.
77. Lohmueller, J., & Finn, O. J. (2017). Current modalities in cancer immunotherapy: Immunomodulatory antibodies, CARs, and vaccines. *Pharmacology & Therapeutics, 178*, 31–47.
78. Le, T. H., Kim, Y., & Yoon, H. (2017). Electrical and electrochemical properties of conducting polymers. *Polymers, 9*, 150.
79. Charles, M. (1995). Template synthesis of electronically conductive polymer nanostructures. *Accounts of Chemical Research, 28*, 61–68.
80. Bredas, J. L., & Street, G. B. (1985). Polarons, bipolarons, and solitons in conducting polymers. *Accounts of Chemical Research, 18*, 309–315.
81. Hakansson, E., Lin, T., Wang, H., & Kaynak, A. (2006). The effects of dye dopants on the conductivity and optical absorption properties of polypyrrole. *Synthetic Metals, 156*, 1194–1202.
82. Kim, D. H., Richardson-Burns, S. M., Hendricks, J. L., Sequera, C., & Martin, D. C. (2007). Effect of immobilized nerve growth factor on conductive polymers: Electrical properties and cellular response. *Advanced Functional Materials, 17*, 79–86.
83. Guimard, N. K., Gomez, N., & Schmidt, C. E. (2007). Conducting polymers in biomedical engineering. *Progress in Polymer Science, 32*, 876–921.
84. Muffly, T. M., Tizzano, A. P., & Walters, M. D. (2011). The history and evolution of sutures in pelvic surgery. *Journal of the Royal Society of Medicine, 104*, 107–112.
85. Lendlein, A. (2010). Polymers in biomedicine. *Macromolecular Bioscience, 10*, 993–997.
86. Törmälä, P. (1992). Biodegradable self-reinforced composite materials; manufacturing structure and mechanical properties. *Clinical Materials, 10*, 29–34.
87. Jiao, L., David, L., Kaplan, B., & Zreiqat, H. (2014). Scaffold-based regeneration of skeletal tissues to meet clinical challenges. *Journal of Materials Chemistry B, 2*, 7272.

88. Chandra, P. K., Soker, S., & Atala, A. (n.d.). Tissue engineering: Current status and future perspectives. In *Principles of Tissue Engineering* (pp. 1–35).
89. Gao, C. C., Yu, L., Liu, H. S., & Chen, L. (2012). Development of self-reinforced polymer composites. *Progress in Polymer Science, 37*, 767–780.
90. Lendlein, A., Behl, M., Hiebl, B., & Wischke, C. (2010). Shape-memory polymers as a technology platform for biomedical applications. *Expert Review of Medical Devices, 7*, 357–379.

CHAPTER 10

Role of Polymers in Cancer Therapy

NISAT ALAM,[1] HASINA NAJNIN,[1] MD. WAMIQUE HOSSAIN,[2] MAIDUL ISLAM,[3,*] SONAM SHAKYA,[3] ISHAAT M. KHAN,[3] and RANA ZAIDI[1]

[1]*Department of Biochemistry, School of Chemical and Life Sciences, Jamia Hamdard, New Delhi, India*

[2]*School of Biotechnology, Jawaharlal Nehru University, New Delhi, India*

[3]*Department of Chemistry, Faculty of Science, Aligarh Muslim University, Aligarh, Uttar Pradesh, India*

*Corresponding author

ABSTRACT

Cancer is one of the deadliest diseases, with a death rate of 13% worldwide, and it can affect any part of our body. The most important hindrance in cancer treatment is that the drugs used in chemotherapy (CT) cannot differentiate between healthy and cancerous cells. Therefore, the development of specific targeting processes and proper delivery of drugs to the target site is an urgent necessity in cancer therapy. To fulfill this purpose, polymers are engineered and employed in the biomedical field for specific binding with cancerous cells. The purpose of this chapter is to provide a brief overview of recent advances in the use of polymers in cancer treatment, with greater emphasis on polymer-drug conjugates (PDCs) for lung cancer.

Polymer Applications in Medicine: Revolutionizing Treatment and Therapeutics.
Mohd. Imran Ahamed, Faheem Ahmad, and Ishaat M. Khan (Eds.)

DOI: 10.1201/9781779640871-10

10.1 INTRODUCTION

Numbers of cancer patients have been increasing day by day, and it has become one of the most severe diseases in our era. Considering this critical situation, various research efforts are underway for the development of innovative drug delivery systems (DDS) that can precisely target cancer cells. Up to this point, the widely used and effective strategy is chemotherapy (CT), but it is not devoid of negative effects. A large proportion of drugs used in the therapy are not properly soluble in the medium, which induces rapid clearance through urine and reduces their bioavailability. Besides, these drugs often target healthy tissues and cause serious unwanted side effects. Another significant side effect is toxicity, as these compounds do not have uniform biodegradation limits and have to be administered repeatedly in higher doses to cancer patients. Sometimes, such treatment can develop multi-drug resistance.

Recently, concurrent administration of different drugs has shown improvement in cancer management [1]. The Polymeric Drug Delivery System (PDDS) offers a variety of options in developing carriers in the nanometer range, tissue engineering, and more. The polymeric drug delivery system has huge potential in theragnostics and nanotechnology, which offers incredible promises for carrying cancer drugs [2, 3]. Polymers and their composites in the nanometer range are utilized in different forms such as liposomes, micelles, and hydrogels. Polymers are renowned for their remarkable design capabilities, eco-friendly nature, and ease of production and cost-effectiveness [4]. Polymers, both natural and engineered, show great bio-adaptability. Nature-derived polymers have functional groups like '-OH' or '$-NH_2$,' thus effortlessly offering biocompatibility and biodegradability. On the other hand, lab-made polymers provide an opportunity to select building blocks from various substances and to develop a polymer useful for a particular application [5–7]. For example, lab-made biodegradable polymers possess special significance as they can be readily degraded in biological systems and create very little toxicity [8].

Dox (Doxorubicin/Adriamycin), 4-substituted 2,5-dimethoxyamphetamine, is an example of a commonly used chemotherapeutic agent that is used along with other drugs for certain therapies such as leukemia and lymphomas, various myelomas, and diseases of the bladder, stomach, chest, ovaries, lungs, and thyroid. However, small doses of DOX over several months increase the risk of dangerous side effects such as cardiomyopathy, myelosuppression, and acute intestinal infections [9]. Many research and review papers have been published, including co-delivery of chemotherapeutic drugs through the polymeric drug delivery system for the treatment of cancer [10–12]. However, therapeutic drugs are often administered independently, without using the appropriate polymeric delivery system to deliver both agents at the same time [13]. In this chapter, we discuss in detail the goals and therapeutic aspects of various polymer-based delivery systems for cancer treatment.

10.2 BIO-ABSORBABLE POLYMERS

Such polymers can undergo changes and are easily degraded inside biological systems due to phagocytosis and other cellular functions [14, 15]. Organic absorbent ingredients commonly used to treat cancer include polyesters, polyanhydrides, polyphosphoesters, polysaccharides, and proteins.

10.2.1 LAB-MADE POLYMERS

Polymers made from lactic acid monomer (PLA), a combination of lactic acid and glycolic acid monomers (PLGA), and ε-caprolactone monomer (PCL) are common examples of lab-made biodegradable polymers [14]. Lactic acid monomers of 'D-form,' 'L-form,' 'racemic' (both D and L form), and 'meso-form' are utilized for polycondensation or ring-opening polymerization (ROP) of lactide. Poly [D-lactic acid] (PDLA) and poly [L-lactic acid] (PLLA) produce a semi-crystalline structure, while poly [racemic lactic acid] (PDLLA) is formless. These polymers are eroded in biological systems by hydrolysis of the ester linkage, ultimately generating lactic acids [5, 16, 17]. Although PLLA and PDLLA have been thoroughly examined for biological applications, PDLA can be a more appropriate preparation for drug delivery as it represents a quicker deterioration time than other PLAs [5]. Co-polymerization techniques are utilized for PLGA polymer development with lactic and glycolic acids. The ROP procedure has been employed for the development of semi-crystalline PCL polymer [18]. PCL has a lower melting point of 59 to 64°C, thus it steadily degrades inside our body. Such polymers play an important role in certain tumor treatments that require a longer release profile. Different types of aliphatic and aromatic monomers are chosen for the development of polyanhydrides (PAHs). These types of polymers show superficial corrosive properties, and their degradation rate depends on the monomer's characteristics. Aliphatic PAHs decrease over the day, while aromatic PAHs decrease gradually over the years. Thus, researchers have the freedom to select the proper monomer from a broad dissociation range for a particular therapeutic approach. Various techniques like melted and interfacial polycondensation, along with ROP, have been employed for the synthesis of PAHs. However, monomers with high molecular weight can only be polymerized through melted polycondensation [19]. Because of their corrosive properties, the drug delivered through such polymers must be encapsulated, as drugs often contain nucleophilic groups [14]. Poly [(1,3-bis-carboxyfenoxipropen) -co- (sebaceous anhydride)] is one of the widely examined examples of co-polymers of PAHs. It is approved by the Food and Drug Administration (FDA) for brain cancer therapy, which is marketed as Gliadel Wafer [20]. Polyphosphoester (PPP) is another type of biodegradable polymer containing phosphorus, created in 1970 by Lapin and Penjek [21]. Because of their phosphorus bond, PPPs are well-suited for use in our body. After hydrolysis of PPPs, phosphate, alcohol, and dials are generated as the final products. The phosphorus group allows binding with different proteins and drugs; this characteristic provides an opportunity to develop biocompatible polymers suitable for specific drugs [6]. A drug named paclitaxel has been delivered to the body using PPP polymer [20].

10.2.2 NATURE DERIVED POLYMER

In nature, polymers are basically found in two chemical forms: proteins like gelatin and albumin, and polysaccharides such as dextran, cellulose, chitosan, and hyaluronic acid (HA). According to an underlying view, proteins are molecules of high atomic weight where the residues of α-amino acids are joined through peptide bonds and typically represent a 3D structure [22]. Albumin polymer-based DDS have the benefit that multicellular cancer cells absorb albumin readily for their nourishment, followed by lysosomal breakdown and immediate uptake by liquid-phase endocytosis. Due to lysosomal digestion, α-amino acids provide energy and nitrogen to the cancer cells [23]. Paclitaxel-albumin particles (commercially known as Abraxane®) are injected for breast cancer therapy [24]. After thermal degradation of the triple-helix collagen molecule, gelatin is synthesized inside animals. It is highly biodegradable and biocompatible, which makes it a potential choice for drug delivery [25].

Polysaccharides may have different sources; for example, carrageenan and alginate are derived from algae, guar gum and cellulose are derived from plants, while chitosan, heparin, chondroitin, and HA are procured from animal sources [26]. The effectiveness of polysaccharides can be altered via various chemical reactions like redox reactions, sulfation, ester formation, and amidation [27]. HA, chitosan, and dextran are widely investigated for cancer treatment. HA is a linear polysaccharide that belongs to the glycosaminoglycan family and is composed of an alternating disaccharide unit of β-1,3-N-acetyl-D-glucosamine and α-1,4-D-glucuronic acid by β (1 → 3) linkages. The use of HA provides various benefits such as high water solubility, biodegradability, biocompatibility, non-toxicity, non-immunogenicity, and simplicity of chemical changes [24]. Besides, a notable characteristic of HA is its binding capacity to CD144 and CD168; these are otherwise called receptors for hyaluronic acid-mediated motility (RHAMM). In the case of various cancers like leukemia, lymphoma, myeloma, glioma, and squamous cell carcinoma, cancerous cells express these receptors; thus, HA polymer-based drug delivery can be done specifically [28]. Chitosan has a cationic charge and is produced by desalination in an alkaline environment from chitin, an abundant natural polysaccharide. Chitosan has two units: D-glucosamine and N-acetyl glucosamine [26]. The biocompatibility and biodegradability of chitosan, in addition to its ability to adhere to mucosal surfaces, provide advantages in the field of drug delivery [29]. Besides these advantages, chitosan itself has anti-cancer properties, as tested in *in vitro* and *in vivo* conditions [30]. Dextran is another naturally occurring polymer that easily dissolves in water. Microscopic organisms produce dextran by utilizing sucrose via a catalytic reaction of dextransucrase. Enzymes like dextranase and glucosidase can degrade it inside the body. Moreover, it is also biocompatible and does not produce any toxic effects. It is mainly injected through the intravenous route [31, 32].

10.3 TYPES OF POLYMERS USED IN DDS FOR CANCER THERAPY

10.3.1 BLOCK CO-POLYMER CONJUGATES

Block Co-Polymer Conjugates refers to block co-polymers that contain at least one conjugate polymer fragment. They may be constructed using either an assemblage of different conjugated polymer fragments with various characteristics, or an assemblage of conjugated polymer fragments and non-conjugated polymer fragments. An amphipathic co-polymer framework is developed for the delivery of hydrophilic and hydrophobic drugs. The benefit of using this polymer is that it contains different blocks; each block is assigned for a particular usage. Poly[(1,3-bis-carboxyfenoxipropen)-co-(sebaceous anhydride)] is an excellent example of this type of polymer.

10.3.2 THERMO-SENSITIVE POLYMERS

Temperature-reactive polymers or thermo-sensitive polymers show a radical and uninterrupted difference in their actual characteristics with temperature [33]. These polymers have been developed based on the fact that there is a temperature difference between healthy and cancerous cells, as cancer cells are hyperthermic. Thus, the temperature-reactive polymers can aim at cancer cells or tumors and deliver potential drugs for therapy. Sometimes, a magnetic cargo is loaded in polymeric nanoparticles, which get activated with the magnetic field and overheat the cancer cell [34]. In medical applications, thermal sensitivity is the most popular stimulant property [35]. This type of polymer exhibits two phase distributions. One is the upper critical solution temperature (UCST) and the other is the lower critical solution temperature (LCST). UCST-type polymers are soluble in organic solvents through Van der Waals bonds, while LCST-type is soluble in aqueous solvents through hydrogen bonds along with hydrophobic and hydrophilic interactions.

10.3.2.1 PH-SENSITIVE POLYMERS

A pH-sensitive or pH-reacting polymer is a substance that reacts to the progress of the pH of an enclosed medium by shifting its direction. This property is due to the specific functional groups in the polymer chain. pH-sensitive substances can be either acidic or basic, reacting with one or the other acidic or basic pH values. Polymers such as primary amines can sense acidic pH (pH 5.0) and increase endosomal escape for therapeutic agents. This polymer can sense the pH difference between healthy and cancerous cells and precisely aim towards the cancerous cells for drug delivery, which causes fewer adverse effects. The usefulness of these polymers also increases because of the fact that there is a pH variation between different cells, tissues, organelles, and systemic fluids. To facilitate uncontrolled growth of cancerous cells, excessive energy production is required;

thus, a higher rate of aerobic respiration takes place inside these cells. Due to the rise in the glycolysis process, the external pH of cancerous tissue becomes acidic (pH 6.5 to 7.2). Furthermore, this type of polymer-made nanoparticles can specifically supply cargoes to cancer tissues, which can be delivered inside cells through the endo-lysosomal system [36].

10.3.3 OXIDATION/REDUCTION-SENSITIVE POLYMERS

In cancer cells, there is an imbalance between oxidizing compounds and antioxidants, which creates more oxidative stress and generates reactive oxygen species (ROS). Polymers that can be degraded by oxidation are used to sense cancerous cells. For example, arylboron (which gets converted to phenol and boric acid after oxidation) dependent on acid esters, or diallyl sulfide polymer (hydrophilicity increases after oxidation) are utilized in cancer treatment [37]. However, the main drawback of using such polymers is that complete oxidation of polymers cannot happen efficiently; thus, drugs cannot be supplied properly [38].

10.4 POLYMER-DRUG CONJUGATES (PDCS)

In PDC, otherwise known as polymeric pro-drugs, drugs are added to the preferred polymers for a selected purpose [39]. These convincing frameworks are remarkable and are made up of three units: soluble units, a target component, and a drug unit integrated with a support. The basic structure was first described by Helmut Ringsdorf in 1975 (Figure 10.1) [40].

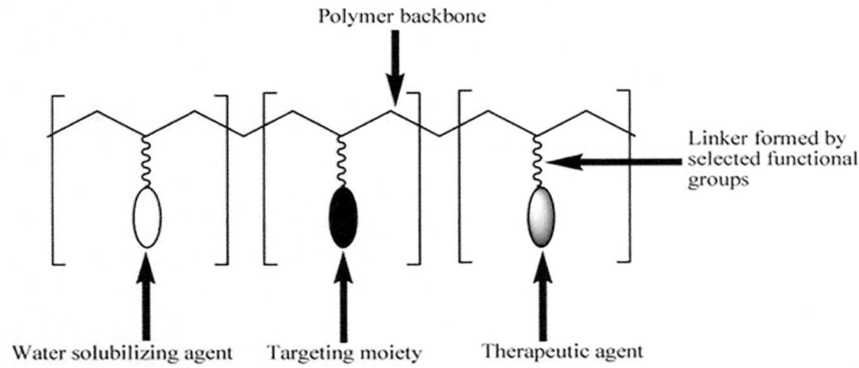

FIGURE 10.1 Diagram showing schematic representation of a polymer-drug conjugates.

The three units are designed to fulfill the main requirements of a polymer. The soluble unit facilitates proper mixing with the medium (water) [41], while the target component directs the transport of the conjugate towards specific cells/tissues. Vitamins like folic acid, sugars, antibodies, and peptides, and so forth, can act as target components and bind with their specific receptors [42]. The drug unit is attached to the support through a functional group linkage, which helps in loading, provides stability, and regulates the delivery of the conjugate drug to the specific site. Certain situations, such as changes in pH, expression of chemicals, or enzymes in infected organs/tissues, signal the drug release [43]. Disulfide, amide, azo, and hydrazine linkages have been utilized in such polymers. For example, HA and dihydro-artemisinin conjugates induce high cell death.

10.4.1 PDC IN LUNG CANCER THERAPY

There is a solid etiological relationship between tobacco smoke and cellular destruction with uncontrolled cell growth in the lungs. Lung cancer has become one of the most common cancers in males, while it is the fourth most common cancer in women, causing 1.3 million deaths each year worldwide. Past studies have shown that a cigarette contains a combination of several carcinogenic agents, including a tobacco-specific nitrosamine such as N'nitrosonornicotine, 4-(methylnitrosamino)-1-(3-pyridyl)-1-butanone (NNK), and polycyclic aromatic amines (PAHs) [44]. Although not all lung cancer patients (10–15%) are smokers [45, 46], other causative factors may include air pollutants, asbestos in the case of factory workers, passive cigarette inhalation, and/or genetic susceptibility. Chest radiography and computed tomography (CT) scans followed by biopsy can be used to diagnose lung cancer.

PDC is a beneficial approach to mitigate cancer cells, as direct administration of anti-carcinogenic drugs has various restrictions. PDC-mediated drug delivery provides greater solubility [47]. PDC can also be combined with two different drugs to increase the total activity synergistically [48]. For example, the carrier of PLA-b-P(α-BrCL) PDC exhibits synergistic effects and diminishes A549 cell proliferation. The PDC shows greater cytotoxicity and specific site binding than the drug administered alone [49, 50]. These qualities make PDC an important therapeutic initiative alongside traditional cancer drugs.

10.5 CONCLUSION

Different polymers have been studied, developed, and utilized as anti-cancer therapeutics. They show high functionality, target-specific binding, regulated release, bio-biodegradability, and less adversity inside the body, and can be a solution for MDR cancers. About 20 years ago, the first clinical trial of a PDC was started. Nowadays, several other trials are ongoing to generalize PDC usage in cancer therapies.

Cancer is a very fatal disease that destroys specific regions/tissues of our body and can spread to different parts through metastasis. There is a very low recovery rate in cancer, and chemotherapeutic drugs cause toxicity in the body. Frequent higher dose administration is required in cancer treatment, as the drugs have issues like low solubility, enzymatic decay, and short half-life. Sometimes the body becomes unresponsive to the drugs (MDR) as well. So, it is our primary necessity to develop a carrier that can deal with the above-mentioned problems.

Polymers are ideal candidates as they can encapsulate cancer drugs, and by specifically modifying them, we can regulate features like solubility, target binding, and sustained release profiles. Although vast research is needed for further clinical application and to understand their advantages and disadvantages.

KEYWORDS

- **cancer therapy**
- **chitosan**
- **drug delivery systems**
- **hyaluronic acid**
- **lung cancer**
- **polymer conjugates**
- **polymers**

REFERENCES

1. Rationalizing combination therapies. (2017). *Nature Medicine, 23*, 1113.
2. Qi, S. S., Sun, J. H., Yu, H. H., & Yu, S. Q. (2017). Co-delivery nanoparticles of anti-cancer drugs for improving chemotherapy efficacy. *Drug Delivery, 24*, 1909–1926.

3. Kumar, S., Singhal, A., Narang, U., Mishra, S., & Kumari, P. (2020). Recent progresses in organic-inorganic nanotechnological platforms for cancer therapeutics. *Current Medicinal Chemistry, 27*, 6015–6056.
4. Pan, J., Rostamizadeh, K., Filipczak, N., & Torchilin, V. P. (2019). Polymeric co-delivery systems in cancer treatment: An overview on component drugs' dosage ratio effect. *Molecules, 24*, 1035.
5. Ulery, B. D., Nair, L. S., & Laurencin, C. T. (2011). Biomedical applications of biodegradable polymers. *Journal of Polymer Science Part B: Polymer Physics, 49*, 832–864.
6. Nair, L. S., & Laurencin, C. T. (2007). Biodegradable polymers as biomaterials. *Progress in Polymer Science, 32*, 762–798.
7. Nair, L., & Laurencin, C. (2006). Polymers as biomaterials for tissue engineering and controlled drug delivery. In K. Lee & D. Kaplan (Eds.), *Tissue Engineering I. Advances in Biochemical Engineering/Biotechnology* (pp. 47–90). Springer Berlin Heidelberg.
8. Guo, X., Wang, L., Wei, X., & Zhou, S. (2016). Polymer-based drug delivery systems for cancer treatment. *Journal of Polymer Science Part A: Polymer Chemistry, 54*, 3525–3550.
9. Parveen, S., Arjmand, F., & Tabassum, S. (2019). Clinical developments of antitumor polymer therapeutics. *RSC Advances, 9*, 24699–24721.
10. Afsharzadeh, M., Hashemi, M., Mokhtarzadeh, A., Abnous, K., & Ramezani, M. (2018). Recent advances in co-delivery systems based on polymeric nanoparticle for cancer treatment. *Artificial Cells, Nanomedicine, and Biotechnology, 46*, 1095–1110.
11. Shen, S., Liu, M., Li, T., Lin, S., & Mo, R. (2017). Recent progress in nanomedicine-based combination cancer therapy using a site-specific co-delivery strategy. *Biomaterials Science, 5*, 1367–1381.
12. Eldar-Boock, A., Polyak, D., Scomparin, A., & Satchi-Fainaro, R. (2013). Nano-sized polymers and liposomes designed to deliver combination therapy for cancer. *Current Opinion in Biotechnology, 24*, 682–689.
13. Zhan, C., Wei, X., Qian, J., Feng, L., Zhu, J., & Lu, W. (2012). Co-delivery of TRAIL gene enhances the anti-glioblastoma effect of paclitaxel *in vitro* and *in vivo*. *Journal of Controlled Release, 160*, 630–636.
14. Ratner, B. D., Hoffman, A. S., Schoen, F. J., & Lemons, J. E. (2004). *Biomaterials Science: An Introduction to Materials in Medicine*. Elsevier Academic Press.
15. Vert, M., Li, S. M., Spenlehauer, G., & Guerin, P. (1992). Bioresorbable and biocompatibility of aliphatic polyesters. *Journal of Materials Science: Materials in Medicine, 3*, 432–446.
16. Maharana, T., Mohanty, B., & Negi, Y. S. (2009). Melt–solid polycondensation of lactic acid and its biodegradability. *Progress in Polymer Science, 34*, 99–124.
17. Södergård, A., & Stolt, M. (2002). Properties of lactic acid-based polymers and their correlation with composition. *Progress in Polymer Science, 27*, 1123–1163.
18. Limwanich, W., Meepowpan, P., Sriyai, M., Chaiwon, T., & Punyodom, W. (2021). Eco-friendly synthesis of biodegradable poly(ε-caprolactone) using L-lactic and glycolic acids as organic initiator. *Polymer Bulletin, 78*, 7089–7101.
19. Roskos, K., & Maskiewicz, R. (2002). Degradable controlled release systems useful for protein delivery. In L. Sanders & R. W. Hendren (Eds.), *Protein Delivery. Pharmaceutical Biotechnology* (pp. 45–92). Springer US.

20. Wolinsky, J. B., Colson, Y. L., & Grinstaff, M. W. (2012). Local drug delivery strategies for cancer treatment: Gels, nanoparticles, polymeric films, rods, and wafers. *Journal of Controlled Release, 159*, 14–26.
21. Lapienis, G., & Penczek, S. (1974). Kinetics and thermodynamics of the polymerization of the cyclic phosphate esters. II. Cationic polymerization of 2-methoxy-2-oxo-1,3,2-dioxaphosphorinane (1,3-propylene methyl phosphate). *Macromolecules, 7*, 166–174.
22. Fonseca, A. C., Ferreira, P., Cordeiro, R. A., Mendonça, P. V., Góis, J. R., Gil, M. H., & Coelho, J. F. (2013). Drug delivery systems for predictive medicine: Polymers as tools for advanced applications. In *New Strategies to Advance Pre/Diabetes Care: Integrative Approach by PPPM* (pp. 399–455). Springer, Dordrecht.
23. Chuang, T. G., Kragh-Hansen, U., & Otagiri, M. (2002). Pharmaceutical strategies utilizing recombinant human serum albumin. *Pharmaceutical Research, 19*, 569–577.
24. Kratz, F. (2008). Albumin as a drug carrier: Design of prodrugs, drug conjugates and nanoparticles. *Journal of Controlled Release, 132*, 171–183.
25. Elzoghby, A. O. (2013). Gelatin-based nanoparticles as drug and gene delivery systems: Reviewing three decades of research. *Journal of Controlled Release, 172*, 1075–1091.
26. Mizrahy, S., & Peer, D. (2012). Polysaccharides as building blocks for nanotherapeutics. *Chemical Society Reviews, 41*, 2623–2640.
27. Cumpstey, I. (2013). Chemical modification of polysaccharides. *ISRN Organic Chemistry, 2013*, 27.
28. Arpicco, S., Milla, P., Stella, B., & Dosio, F. (2014). Hyaluronic acid conjugates as vectors for the active targeting of drugs, genes and nanocomposites in cancer treatment. *Molecules, 19*, 3193.
29. Malafaya, P. B., Silva, G. A., & Reis, R. L. (2007). Natural–origin polymers as carriers and scaffolds for biomolecules and cell delivery in tissue engineering applications. *Advanced Drug Delivery Reviews, 59*, 207–233.
30. Dass, C. R., & Choong, P. F. M. (2008). The use of chitosan formulations in cancer therapy. *Journal of Microencapsulation, 25*, 275–279.
31. Baldwin, A. D., & Kiick, K. L. (2010). Polysaccharide-modified synthetic polymeric biomaterials. *Peptide Science, 94*, 128–140.
32. Koo, H., Yhee, J. Y., Kwon, I. C., Kim, K., & Subbiah, R. (2013). Polymeric nanoparticles in cancer therapy. In D. K. Yi & G. C. Papaefthymiou (Eds.), *Nano Biomaterials: Development and Applications*. CRC Press.
33. Sponchioni, M., Palmiero, U. C., & Moscatelli, D. (2019). Thermo-responsive polymers: Applications of smart materials in drug delivery and tissue engineering. *Materials Science and Engineering: C, 102*, 589–605.
34. Burkhart, A., & Ritter, H. (2014). Influence of cyclodextrin on the UCST- and LCST-behavior of poly(2-methacrylamido-caprolactam)-co-(N,N-dimethylacrylamide). *Beilstein Journal of Organic Chemistry, 10*, 1951–1958.
35. Mura, S., Nicolas, J., & Couvreur, P. (2013). Stimuli-responsive nanocarriers for drug delivery. *Nature Materials, 12*, 991–1003.
36. Dai, S., Ravi, P., & Tam, K. C. (2008). pH-responsive polymers: Synthesis, properties and applications. *Soft Matter, 4*, 435–449.

37. Huo, M., Yuan, J., Tao, L., & Wei, Y. (2014). Redox-responsive polymers for drug delivery: From molecular design to applications. *Polymer Chemistry, 5*, 519–528.
38. Broaders, K. E., Grandhe, S., & Fréchet, J. M. (2011). A biocompatible oxidation-triggered carrier polymer with potential in therapeutics. *Journal of the American Chemical Society, 133*, 756–758.
39. Pang, X., Yang, X., & Zhai, G. (2014). Polymer-drug conjugates: Recent progress on administration routes. *Expert Opinion on Drug Delivery, 11*, 1075–1086.
40. Elvira, C., Gallardo, A., Roman, J. S., & Cifuentes, A. (2005). Covalent polymer-drug conjugates. *Molecules, 10*, 114–125.
41. Larson, N., & Ghandehari, H. (2012). Polymeric conjugates for drug delivery. *Chemistry of Materials, 24*, 840–853.
42. Kumar, K. V. (2012). Targeted delivery of nanomedicines. *ISRN Pharmacology, 2012*, 1–9.
43. Patil, J. P., & Mahajan, H. S. (2015). A review on polymer drug conjugate—What, why and how? *International Journal of Pharmaceutical Sciences and Research, 6*, 4611–4621.
44. Alam, N., Najnin, H., Islam, M., Iqbal, S., & Zaidi, R. (2021). Development of a lung cancer model in Wistar rat and *in silico* screening of its biomarkers. *Current Computer-Aided Drug Design, 17*, 458–468.
45. Thun, M. J., Hanan, L. M., Adams-Campbell, A. L., Boffetta, P., Buring, J. E., Feskanich, D., Flanders, W. D., Jee, S. H., Katanoda, K., Kolonel, L. N., et al. (2008). Lung cancer occurrence in never-smokers: An analysis of 13 cohorts and 22 cancer registry studies. *PLoS Medicine, 5*, 1357–137.
46. Kumar, E., Singh, M., Meena, J., Singhvi, P., Thiyagarajan, D., Saneja, A., & Panda, A. K. (2019). Hyaluronic acid-dihydroartemisinic conjugate: Synthesis, characterization and *in vitro* evaluation in lung cancer cells. *International Journal of Biological Macromolecules, 133*, 495–502.
47. Chen, Y., Peng, F., Song, X., Wu, J., Yao, W., & Gao, X. (2018). Conjugation of paclitaxel to C-6 hexanediamide-modified hyaluronic acid for targeted drug delivery to enhance antitumor efficacy. *Carbohydrate Polymers, 181*, 150–158.
48. Wang, W., Zhao, B., Meng, X., She, P., Zhang, P., Cao, Y., & Zhang, X. (2018). Preparation of dual-drug conjugated polymeric micelles with synergistic anti-cancer efficacy *in vitro*. *Journal of Drug Delivery Science and Technology, 43*, 388–396.
49. Lou, T., Magnusson, J., Preat, V., Frederick, R., Alexander, C., Bosquillon, C., & Vanbever, R. (2016). Synthesis and *in vitro* evaluation of polyethylene glycol-paclitaxel conjugates for lung cancer therapy. *Pharmaceutical Research, 33*, 1671–1681.
50. Yang, S., Wang, Y., Ren, Z., Chen, M., Chen, W., & Zhang, X. (2018). Stepwise pH/reduction-responsive polymeric conjugates for enhanced drug delivery to tumor. *Materials Science and Engineering: C, 82*, 234–243.

CHAPTER 11

Role of Polymers in Medicine/Disease: A Special Focus on Oral Vaccination

SHABNAM,[1] MD. WAMIQUE HOSSAIN,[1] HASINA NAJNIN,[2] NISAT ALAM,[2] HABIBA SULTANA,[3] and MAIDUL ISLAM[4,*]

[1]*School of Biotechnology, Jawaharlal Nehru University, New Delhi, India*

[2]*Department of Biochemistry, School of Chemical and Life Sciences, Jamia Hamdard, New Delhi, India*

[3]*Department of Chemistry, Vidyasagar University, Midnapore, West Bengal, India*

[4]*Department of Chemistry, Faculty of Science, Aligarh Muslim University, Aligarh, Uttar Pradesh, India*

*Corresponding author

ABSTRACT

Polymers can be attractive substances for delivering drugs and immunization in recent years. Polymers, particularly degradable ones, show unique and exceptional qualities such as compatibility, degradability, and lower toxic effects in biological systems. The main concern of oral medication and vaccination is bioavailability, as they are less soluble and broken down by gastrointestinal enzymes and/or the acidic environment of the stomach. Oral vaccination systems in polymeric carriers have the potential to provide targeted immunological responses for extended periods of time without the requirement for booster doses, reducing the need for repeated injections and experienced staff, which are necessary in parenteral vaccination. Polymer structures build shields around drugs or antigens to prevent them

Polymer Applications in Medicine: Revolutionizing Treatment and Therapeutics.
Mohd. Imran Ahamed, Faheem Ahmad, and Ishaat M. Khan (Eds.)

DOI: 10.1201/9781779640871-11

from proteolytic degradation and acidic decay. In this book chapter, we discuss polymers, different types of polymers, and how they are useful for medication and vaccination; we especially focus on oral vaccination.

11.1 INTRODUCTION

The genesis of vaccinology was in 1796 when Edward Jenner investigated the cowpox virus [1, 2]. Vaccination protects against various infectious and non-infectious diseases and has saved many lives over the past two centuries [3].

Vaccines are biological preparations that allow for the active induction of immunity against rare diseases. Various vaccination processes have been developed and are currently in use. Live attenuated vaccinations, inactivated vaccinations, toxoid vaccinations, protein-based subunit vaccinations, DNA vaccinations, and vector vaccination processes are often employed to build strong immunity in our bodies [4–7]. Traditional vaccines are prone to degradation and have a limited half-life, with side effects such as inflammatory reactions that can cause discomfort at the time of vaccination at the injection site. Oral vaccination, as opposed to the standard vaccination approach, minimizes the discomfort of immunization and lowers the risk of wound inflammation at the injection site. Furthermore, because powerful and comprehensive immune responses may be produced using oral vaccination, the cost is significantly lower compared to traditional methods. Some illnesses caused by intracellular microorganisms are not preventable or treatable with vaccinations. These diseases require vaccine formulations that stimulate both cellular and humoral immune responses [8]. Due to the strong intestinal immunity and the greater benefit of vaccination through the oral route, a variety of cells providing immunity are found within the small and large intestines. The Peyer's patches in the small intestine and lymphoid follicles in the large intestine, for example, are crucial for antigen presentation and proper immune system functioning in order to verify and combat infection. Several measures have been implemented to improve the vaccine's immunological response and produce sustained release and mucosal immunity: employing an effective adjuvant, adopting a systemic shipment procedure, and utilizing suitably functional antigen displaying sites [9–12].

Polymers are generally biocompatible and biodegradable in nature; some polymers can protect vaccinogens from acidic pH and enzymatic degradation.

To be specific, PLG, PLGA, PEG, and PELA are the common polymer-based nanoparticles for vaccine delivery. Denaturation of these polymers by various physiological enzymes may decrease their potential. Water-soluble chitosan and HA (hyaluronic acid) are other novel natural biodegradable polymers under this system. Hence, polymer-based nanoparticle transportation of viral antigens for convenient oral delivery would show a good way of oral vaccine delivery strategy. There are many benefits to choosing oral vaccination, but the main drawback is that the antigen may be degraded by acidic conditions or enzymatic reactions in the intestinal tract, cannot express due to mucosal layers, and/or must keep up with microorganisms [13, 14]. Mucosal immune systems targeting oral vaccines are coated in specific materials that provide the appropriate immunological response for a longer duration, escaping the requirement for booster doses and reducing the need for repeated injections and experienced staff, as in parenteral vaccination. These polymer-based delivery methods can also protect medications from the acidic environment of the gut.

Biodegradable polymers such as chitosan, alginate, poly(lactic acid-co-glycolic acid), and others have been examined in this chapter in terms of their role, uses, and prospects.

11.2 WHAT ARE POLYMERS?

The polymerization of monomeric units of any substance results in polymer formation. Polymer is derived from the Greek phrase "many parts." Each of the components is referred to as a monomer (which means "one portion" in Greek). A polymer is a chain, with each of its links being a monomer. Those monomers can be simple—consisting of just one or two atoms—or complex structures including a dozen or more atoms. These materials, many of them artificial, are built from repeating chains of smaller chemical units. Polymers are large molecules made by bonding (chemically linking) a series of building blocks.

11.2.1 TYPES OF POLYMER

11.2.1.1 NON-BIODEGRADABLE POLYMER

Non-biodegradable polymers can be defined as those polymers that are resistant to environmental degradation and hence end up in the form of waste. Polystyrene, polyethylene, and other non-biodegradable polymers are examples. They are mainly used as hardware substances. They also contribute to solid waste and harm the environment. There is less use of non-biodegradable polymers in drug delivery and oral vaccination processes.

11.2.1.2 BIODEGRADABLE POLYMER

Biodegradable substances can be derived from nature or manufactured in labs, and they disintegrate both in and out of cells. In the event of *in vivo* degradation, which can be enzymatic, non-enzymatic, or both, biocompatible, non-toxic, and harmless by-products are produced, which are then removed by various metabolic pathways inside the human body. Biodegradable polymers are sometimes known as "biopolymers" because they are generated mostly from natural sources. While it's vital to remember that biodegradability is a feature of polymers that isn't affected by other factors of their origin, it may be changed by altering the sequencing at the molecular level. Over the last several years, the number of such compounds utilized as adjuvants in the supervised administration of drugs has expanded considerably. The bio-substances used in drug administration can be categorized into the following:

a. Synthetic biodegradable polymers are created through a synthetic chemical process that includes relatively hydrophobic materials like-hydroxy acids, polyanhydrides, and others, as well as
b. Naturally occurring polymers like complex sugars (hyaluronan, chitosan) and inorganics (hydroxyapatite) [15–17] exhibit a wide diversity of materials used in drug delivery, resulting from the numerous illnesses, dose ranges, and unique requirements that may be encountered. Biocompatibility is significant, but it's vital to remember that it's not an inherent quality of a material; it's dependent on the biological environment and the tolerability of specific drug-polymer-tissue interactions.

11.2.1.3 NATURE-DERIVED DERIVED AND MAN-MADE POLYMERS

Polymers derived from nature, including chitosan, cellulose, dextran, and so forth have all been investigated for use in vaccine production. Chitosan is widely used in vaccines due to its biodegradability, biocompatibility, nontoxicity, and ease of shape and size modification [18–20]. Derivatives of chitosan, such as poly-lactic and glycolic acid unit (PLGA), poly-caprolactone (PCL), poly-lactic acid (PLA), poly-ethylene glycol (PEG), and others, are examples of synthetic polymers. In our various studies, chitosan derivatives such as O-2'-hydroxypropyl tri-methyl ammonium chloride chitosan (O-2'-HACC) and N-2-hydroxy-propyl di-methyl-ethyl ammonium chloride chitosan (N-2-HFCC) are also synthesized and used for vaccination [21–23]. These chitosan derivatives have better water solubility than chitosan due to the addition of epoxypropyl dimethyl ethyl ammonium chloride (EEA) to the amide group. These types of polymers are widely used for antigen delivery in mucosal layers, as they are highly biocompatible, biodegradable, less toxic, and possess a sustained release pattern [24–26].

11.2.1.4 PHYSIOCHEMICAL PROPERTIES OF POLYMERS

Chitosan readily combines with DNA to create a polyelectrolyte complex, making DNA very resistant to nuclease destruction. The numerous hydroxyl and amino groups in the chitosan backbone make it simple to chemically alter and boost its targeting ability [27, 28]. PLGA is a very well-known polymer for use in vaccines [29]. PEG has been known for coating PLA nanoparticles, and it typically increases nanoparticle solubility, reducing aggregation and protein interaction, which creates firmness on the gene carrier's exterior and improves transfer efficiency [30]. To increase surface quality and material removal, it's crucial to understand the mechanical properties of polymer-based nanomaterials and how they interact with different types of surfaces [31].

11.2.1.5 PROTEINS ENCAPSULATED INTO POLYMERS

Because the gastrointestinal tract epithelial barrier limits oral bioavailability, protein delivery alone poses a significant problem. Because digestive enzymes have a limited half-life in the body, they are prone to gastrointestinal degradation, and most of them are unable to pass through specific biological barriers [32]. Proteins can be embedded in a polymer matrix to assist their function and integrity in the body, preventing hydrolysis and enzymatic destruction. It can sometimes guide therapeutic proteins to a specific target region, increasing their bioavailability [29]. Diverse proteins and peptides are encapsulated in chitosan nanomaterial for medication delivery [33]. Encapsulation into nanoparticles has become common in pharmaceutics, improving peptidyl drug delivery and bioavailability, such as desmopressin [34, 35].

11.2.1.6 NUCLEIC ACIDS ENCAPSULATED INTO POLYMERS

Nucleic acids are weak, fragile, and bear a negative charge, which brings undesirable consequences to delivery processes. So, positively charged polymers can be used to embed nucleic acids in a polymer matrix [36]. Chitosan can encapsulate and concentrate plasmid DNA for creating nanoparticle complexes that can stick to the epithelial cells of the intestine, travel across mucosal borders through microfold cells, and blot with epithelial cells along with immune cells in gut-associated lymphoid tissue (GALT) [37, 38]. High levels of cytokines such as interleukins and interferons are expressed here, demonstrating that this type of polymer can be used as an effective delivery method for DNA. Thus, it can also be utilized as adjuvants in vaccination processes for triggering humoral and cell-based immunity [39].

11.3 ROLE OF POLYMERS

11.3.1 NATURAL POLYMER

11.3.1.1 CHITOSAN

Chitosan is chemically α-(1-4)2-amino 2-deoxy β-D-glucan. Chitosan is most important for nasal delivery [40] (Figure 11.1). The mucoadhesive characteristics of chitosan-derived nanoparticles restrict quick nasal clearance, extending antigen retention duration in the nasal mucosa. Due to a loss in mucociliary clearance, this may prolong the contact duration between nose-associated lymphoid tissue and the formulation. Due to the utilization of adherent adhesive chitosan particles, the standard nasal residence period for dosing solutions may be enhanced by a factor of four [41]. Vaccines based on chitosan nanoparticles have been widely employed in the creation of vaccines against Newcastle disease, Neospora, hepatitis B virus, and *Clostridium botulinum* type A neurotoxins, to name a few. The chitosan-DNA nanoparticles were efficient against *T. pyogenes* infection illnesses and provided options for the creation of new chitosan nanoparticle-encapsulated vaccines [43]. Intranasally administered chitosan-DNA nanospheres enhance IgA and IgG, Tc cells, and interferon-gamma levels [44].

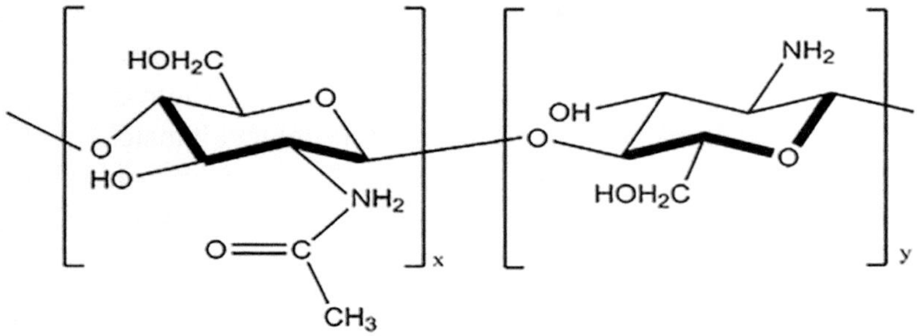

FIGURE 11.1 Chemical structure of chitosan.

11.3.1.2 HYALURONIC ACID (HA)

Hyaluronic acid (HA), commonly known as hyaluronan, is a bioadhesive polymer that occurs naturally in the body. HA is a polymer that is a linear polysaccharide in nature. The intercellular space of higher animals, such as the vitreous humor of the eye, contains HA, a mucopolysaccharide primarily composed of D-glucuronic acid and N-acetyl-D-glucosamine [44]. Following the intranasal vaccine injection made up of bio-adhesive HA, there is significant immunological activity induced against the antigens of the LKT63 influenza virus [45]. Many HA-drug conjugates, polyelectrolyte microcapsules, and hydrogel delivery methods have been developed using HA [46, 47]. Bioconjugation of HA with medicinal compounds can increase drug solubility and provide a longer-lasting release and better drug targeting [48]. HA combined with tri-methyl chitosan can generate a firm nanostructure for IgG binding [49].

11.3.1.3 ALGINATE

Alginates are a form of polysaccharide that is found in nature, such as in brown seaweed. Chemically, they are composed of 1–4 covalently linked, linearly ordered L-guluronic acid and D-mannuronic acid chains (*see* Figure 11.2). Alginate-coated medicine is used for greater bioavailability.

Alginate, recognized for its mucoadhesive qualities, allows it to alternately adhere to mucosal membranes due to its anionic composition, which is advantageous for transmucosal drug delivery systems (DDS). Furthermore, studies reveal that alginate-based compounds are pH-sensitive and that controlling the release mechanisms that encapsulate biomolecules from alginate drug-carrying vehicles "mechanically" might be advantageous [50].

Though alginate is not immunogenic by nature, protein additions are common since it is derived from natural sources. Chitosan particles, which adsorb antigens, are encapsulated with sodium alginate. According to studies, these nanoparticles suppress ovalbumin release in lab-made stomach acid. Furthermore, this type of polymer shows no cellular mortality in *in vitro* studies [51].

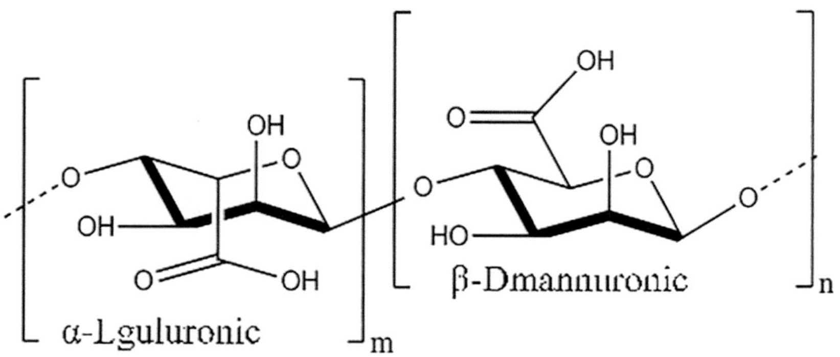

FIGURE 11.2 Chemical structure of alginate.

11.3.1.4 PULLULAN

Pullulan is a natural non-ionic water-soluble linear polysaccharide made up of a strange combination of glycosidic linkages and linked maltotriose residues. Nanostructures based on pullulan offer important research significance in constructing superior vaccine transmission systems because they have particular qualities such as non-toxicity and non-carcinogenicity [52].

11.3.1.5 INULIN

This is a plant-derived, low-cost dietary fiber that is hydrophilic and a linear polysaccharide, connected by a fructose unit chain and glycosidic linkages [53, 54]. When combined with antigens, inulin has a more effective adjuvant property as it boosts both cellular and humoral immune responses [55]. High molecular weight inulin nanoparticles have been proven in studies to be useful as innovative drug delivery methods or other compounds of interest [56, 57].

11.3.1.6 DEXTRAN

Dextrans are branched polysaccharides made up of D-glucopyranosyl straight chain units that are 1,6 connected and branch at 1,3 connections. Dextran is a neutral bacterial exo-polysaccharide with a repeating glucose component that is largely biocompatible and biodegradable. It's perfect for nanomedicine, nanomedicine carriers, cell imaging systems, and biosensors because of its simple and unique biopolymer characteristics. Most notably, it is water-soluble and does not cause cytotoxicity following medication administration [58].

11.3.1.6 GELATIN

Gelatin is a naturally occurring polymer and protein that is mostly found in connective tissues. Collagen is denatured in a controlled manner to produce it. Because of its non-toxic nature and biodegradability, this water-soluble polymer has a variety of uses in the medical field [59]. Hydrophobic medications have been released in a controlled/sustained manner using gelatin-based delivery devices [60]. Hydrophobic medicines and macromolecules like proteins have exhibited controlled/sustained release using gelatin-based delivery methods [61, 62]. However, these systems have several drawbacks, such as low mechanical strength. The use of crosslinking chemicals such as glutaraldehyde, on the other hand, improves the stability and shape of gelatin-based compositions. The degree of crosslinking can affect the variable release profiles of the encapsulated medicines [63, 64].

11.3.2 POLYMER-BASED SYNTHETIC NANOPARTICLES

11.3.2.1 PLGA

The different proportions of lactic acid and glycolic acid employed in the polymer development process produce different types of PLGA. The molar ratio of their copolymer determines whether PLGA is accessible in amorphous or crystalline form. Another important attribute of PLGA is its glass transition temperature, which ranges from 40 to 60°C. PLGA-PEG nanoparticles were used to encapsulate amphotericin B to increase the solubility of PLGA-PEG and also to target macrophages in visceral leishmaniasis-infected tissues. The nanoparticles were more effective than free amphotericin B [65]. The regulated release of tetanus toxoid (TT) from TT-PLGA microspheres has been widely explored [66]. Antigens encapsulated in PLGA/PLA-based nanoparticles can be delivered to antigen-presenting cells in a regulated and sustained manner [67, 68]. PEG increases PLA nanostructures' stability in GI fluid and promotes nanoparticle transmission to the lymphatic system, according to studies [69]. Extensive and thorough analyses of pharmacokinetics, biodistribution, and toxicity can be used to overcome the limitations of PLGA nanoparticles [70].

11.3.2.2 POLYPEPTIDES

Polypeptides include polyaspartamide P [Asp (DET)], poly(γ-glutamic acids) (γ-PGA), and poly-L-lysine (PLL). PLL peridium polystyrene nanoparticles were used to concentrate plasmids encoding chicken ovalbumin. The complexes extend the lifespan of mice carrying CT26 by encoding DNA for tumor antigens and cytokines, and by blocking tumor development along with metastasis. Intraperitoneally, colon carcinoma is a kind of cancer that affects [71].

11.3.2.3 PCL

PCL is a hydrophobic, slowly degradable polymer having a semi-crystalline structure. For this reason, PCL nanoparticles have been utilized for vaccination in mucosal areas [72]. In comparison to previous antigenic preparations, chitosan-coated PCL stimulates significant humoral and cellular immune responses [73]. Antigens of varying doses are adsorbed onto nanoparticles in constant proportions. The nasal secretions of mice produced the same humoral and mucosal antibodies [74]. An ecotropic diblock copolymer comprising methyl polyethylene glycol (PEG) and polycaprolactone is used to distribute hydrophobic medicines [75].

11.3.2.4 Polyanhydride (PAH)

Carboxylic acids with anhydride linkages form the monomers for the development of such a type of polymer. Water instability, biodegradability, and safety are all advantages of polyanhydride (PAH) [76, 77]. Various PAHs comprising 1,6-bis(p-carboxyphenoxy)hexane (CPH), sebacic anhydride, and 1,8-bis(p-carboxyphenoxy)-3,6-dioxaoctane (CPTEG) have also been reported. Antigen-presenting cells that imitate pathogens can be excited by amphiphilic PAH nanoparticles [78]. The particles are correctly phagocytosed and identified in phagosomes by antigen-presenting cells.

11.3.2.5 DENDRIMERS

Dendrimers are comparable to dendrites in that they are highly branching, symmetrical, and radial macromolecules. Dendrimers have a lot of branch points that are spherical with uniform size in nanometers. Dendrimers have a 3D structure that allows them to penetrate through cell membranes, making them superior nano delivery materials to traditional polymers [79]. Cationic dendrimers have been widely employed for medication and gene delivery due to their unique characteristics [80–82].

11.4 ORAL VACCINATIONS

11.4.1 VACCINATION THROUGH ORAL ROUTES

Oral vaccination of animals and humans is mostly ineffectual in providing effective mucosal and/or systemic immunity. This is due to the minimal amount of antigen that persists in the gut after being degraded during the intestinal wall crossing. Oral delivery of a variety of proteins is beneficial in activating mucosal and systemic immune responses. Specific binding to the epithelial membrane of the gastrointestinal tract (GIT) is required for the uptake of these molecules by the GIT epithelium. The identification of these molecules, as well as their potential use as 'carriers' for co-transporting tiny peptides known as haptens, proteins, and nanoparticles through the GIT epithelium, are explored.

11.4.2 CONCEPTS OF ORAL VACCINATION

The idea of medication or antigen encapsulation is nearly comparable in antigen delivery for oral vaccination. When tiny molecules/immunogens such as proteins or entire cellular organisms are administered, the main goal is to send them to the right place without changing their inherent properties, resulting in the therapeutic and immunological responses that are intended. In most circumstances, the oral route is unquestionably the best option for therapy, but the main issue is the chemical stability of the supplied drugs until they reach the desired location. Degradation of pharmacological compounds in the acidic pH (pH 1.5 to 3.5) in the stomach, and/or degradation by enzymes produced by the intestine and liver are the main challenges. Hydrolysis, dealkylation, desulfuration, and oxidation are all significant metabolic events in pre-systemic metabolism. Finally, the bioavailability of medicinal molecules and vaccination through the oral route is harmed, as there is a possibility that antigens might not reach the right place to sensitize our immunological cells for the required immune response [83].

11.4.3 ORAL VACCINATION DELIVERY APPROACH

Poor bioavailability of orally taken medications, as defined by the biopharmaceutical categorization system or BCS, is generally related to solubility and permeability difficulties. In such a setting, biodegradable polymers have gotten a lot of interest as a way to solve the bioavailability issues. The following measures can be used to address the drawbacks of oral medication administration.

Application of complexing agents to polymers: Enteric coating with polymeric polymers assists in overcoming medication hydrolytic instability at low gastric pH. However, utilizing polymer compounds to shield medications from metabolism which is pre-systemic in the gut lumen is rather difficult. However, in the presence of complexing agents such as EDTA and diethyl netriaminepenta acetic acid (DTPA), several polymers have shown promise inhibitory efficacy against intestinal enzymes by chelating with enzyme cofactors such as. Ca^{2+}, Zn^{2+} and so forth [84, 85].

11.4.4 IMMUNOLOGICAL RESPONSES AND MUCOSAL IMMUNITY

In order to administer vaccines orally, it is necessary to have a thorough understanding of the processes that activate the mucosal immune system.

In many ways, mucosal immunization is preferable to systemic vaccination. The mucosal immune network is deliberately situated to provide protection against external infections and antigens at the sites where these foreign substances enter the circulatory system. Mucosa-associated lymphoid tissue (MALT) and gut-associated lymphoid tissue (GALT) make up the majority of the mucosal immune system. The lungs, urinary system, and sexual organs are all protected by MALT, whereas the intestinal area is protected by GALT. GALT is made up of Peyer's patch-like lymphoid follicles, solitary lymphoid tissues, and non-associated cells found in the lamina propria and intra-epithelial portions of the gut wall [86, 87].

11.4.4.1 PEYER'S PATCH (PP)

The principal acquisition location for infections or antigens contacting the intestinal wall is PP. PP is a collection of lymphoid follicles that line the small intestine's mucosa and submucosa layers. M cells (specialized epithelial cells), macrophages, dendritic cells, as well as B-lymphocytes and T-lymphocytes, are all present. The PP application site produces initial immunological responses mediated by secretory IgA (S-IgA).

11.4.4.2 DENDRITIC CELLS (DCS)

Dendritic cells are common types of antigen-presenting cells (APCs) discovered in Peyer's patch's sub-epithelial zone. Immature DCs collect antigens that enter Peyer's patch from the intestinal lumen and travel to lymph nodes, where they trigger T cells and B cells to start the immunological response. DCs mature phenotypically and functionally when cytokines (IL-1, TNF) mediate inflammatory stimuli produced against viral/bacterial elements like lipopolysaccharide/viral RNA.

11.4.4.3 MACROPHAGES

The phagocyte system is mostly made up of macrophages, which are a type of differentiated cell. Monocytes, promonocytes, and monoblasts are the sources of macrophages (Figure 11.3). They induce and regulate immunological responses. They are the primary cells of the innate immune system, with several functions, including collecting and destroying foreign particles, presenting and processing antigens, and eliminating apoptotic bodies (mostly by macrophages of the M2 subtype). The diagram below illustrates the phagocytic activity of macrophages [88].

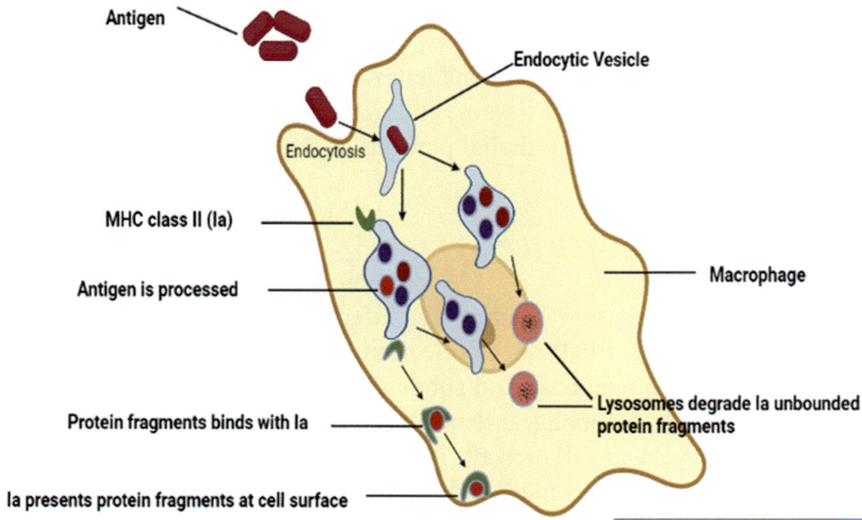

FIGURE 11.3 Endocytosis and following processing of antigens by macrophage.
Source: Drawn using biorender.

11.4.4.4 M CELLS

The antigen must first assault GALT in order to break through the epithelial barrier and produce an effective mucosal and systemic immune response. M cells play a critical part in this process because they control the migration of microbes and antigens into GALT regions capable of producing defensive responses. M cells have tiny cytoplasmic vesicles, some lysosomes, and short microvilli that let antigens [89, 90], innocuous substances [91], and microbes [92] enter the GALT faster. Normally, M cells carry immunogenic compounds from the lumen surface to Peyer's patch pocket areas without modifying them chemically. M cells in PP have been regarded as an interesting target for vaccine delivery because they can efficiently absorb and transfer a range of antigenic compounds to APCs [93, 94]. Qi et al. suggested the notion of a dome trap to highlight the process of blockading supplied by M cells. Approaches created with foreign particle collecting mechanisms in mind by M cells enhance immunity, and it's also easier to avoid the dome trap while delivering medications into the circulation of the systemic via the mucosal route [95]. However, only a few receptors and their glands are found on M cells at this time, but the majority of them are located in adjacent intestinal cells. As a result, vaccination by M cell receptors remains a difficult undertaking [96]. Toll-like receptor-4 (TLR-4), 51 integrins, and platelet-activating factor receptor (PAFR) are some of the most essential pathogen recognition receptors (PRRs) found on the human and mouse M cell surface for antigen recognition. Specific molecular patterns seen in bacteria, such as peptidoglycans and lipopolysaccharides, can be recognized by these receptors. This sort of affinity is necessary for microbe internalization; therefore, targeting such PRRs might be a good way to boost the absorption of oral vaccination formulations [97, 98].

11.4.4.5 B CELLS

B cells are triggered after detecting foreign antigenic compounds with surface-bound antibodies or immunoglobulins. B cells become antibody-secreting plasma cells after activation, allowing them to effectively eliminate pathogens at the intestinal lumen. Pathogens engage with the mucosal immune system, triggering an immune response [99].

11.5 APPLICATIONS OF POLYMERS IN ORAL VACCINATION

Various medicinal compounds, antigens such as proteins, and microorganisms are administered through the oral route utilizing biodegradable polymers, as detailed in the preceding sections. Polymers are utilized not only to keep therapeutic molecules chemically stable but also to transport them to a specific location to induce the desired therapeutic or immunological response.

a. Chitosan is a biodegradable polymer that is inert, biocompatible, and non-toxic. It is widely employed in biomedical applications. Numerous reports on its usage in drug delivery and oral vaccination are known. For example, Bordetella bronchiseptica dermonecrotoxin (BBD) was encapsulated in microspheres of chitosan, according to Jiang et al. In this study, BBD-inserted chitosan spheres (CMs) were delivered to the intestinal macrophages to examine if BBD may help with atrophic rhinitis [100].

b. Chitosan is also used to treat stomach ulcers caused by the *Helicobacter pylori* bacteria. Tetracycline-coated chitosan microspheres have been demonstrated to be far more efficient than tetracycline given orally in the treatment of ulcers caused by *H. pylori* [101].
c. Biodegradable polymeric nanoparticles are being investigated as potential vaccination adjuvants [102]. Chitosan has been found to promote T-helper 1 cell activation after immunization through the mucosal route as a vaccine adjuvant [103].

11.6 CONCLUSION AND FUTURE PERSPECTIVE

Biodegradable polymers have been widely employed in the field of targeted drug administration and immunization for the past two decades, primarily to achieve desired therapeutic efficacy while minimizing toxicity concerns. Oral medication and vaccine administration in polymeric micro/nanoparticulate systems have several advantages over standard formulations. The delivery mechanism for oral distribution should transport medications and antigens in stable forms and prevent them from degrading in the harsh environment of the stomach and intestinal lumen. Natural and synthetic biodegradable polymer-based methods emerge as viable options for medicine and vaccine administration in this area. Polymers used to make nanoparticles have a lot of promise as adjuvants for vaccinations and delivery systems [104]. The fundamental objective of developing polymer-based DDS in recent years has been to increase therapeutic efficacy while limiting the development of drug resistance [105]. The main concern that prevents such vaccines from being used in clinical trials is localized toxic effects. However, polymers with unique properties such as innate immune modulation, biocompatibility, mucosal adherence, and low toxicity have made it easier to create safe and effective carrier systems. The vital obstructions to be overcome in the future are to maintain critical and uniform properties in the polymer as well as understand the effects of these polymers in a biological system. With technological developments and a greater understanding of the physicochemical features of polymer-based particle systems, much more efficient medication and vaccine delivery methods can be devised, such as size, shape, and charge, as well as the processes that stimulate the immune system or produce a therapeutic response. Adjuvants or delivery vehicles should ideally be able to activate both humoral and cellular immune systems. We can add new appealing vaccination systems in the future by incorporating some other attractive properties such as prolonged release, targeted and alternative delivery techniques, and polymer-based delivery routes [106, 107].

KEYWORDS

- **antigen-presenting cells**
- **B cells**
- **biodegradable polymers**
- ***Bordetella bronchiseptica* dermonecrotoxin**
- **chitosan**
- **dendrimers**
- **dextrans**
- **hyaluronic acid**
- **oral vaccination**

REFERENCES

1. Chung, E. H. (2014). Clinical experimental vaccine: Vaccine allergies. *Clinical & Experimental Allergy, 50*, 50–57.
2. Silin, D. S., Lyubomska, O. V., Jirathitikal, V., & Bourinbaiar, A. S. (2007). Oral vaccination: Where are we? *Expert Opinion on Drug Delivery, 4*(4), 323–340.
3. Mitragotri, S., & Lahann, J. (2009). Physical approaches to biomaterial design. *Nature Materials, 8*, 15–23.
4. Govindarajan, D., Meschino, S., Guan, L., Clements, D. E., Meulen, J. T., Casimiro, D. R., Coller, B., & Bett, A. J. (2015). Preclinical development of a dengue tetravalent recombinant subunit vaccine: Immunogenicity and protective efficacy in nonhuman primates. *Vaccine, 33*, 4105–4116.
5. Li, J., Yu, J., Xu, S., Shi, J., Xu, S., Wu, X., Fu, F., Peng, Z., Zhang, L., & Zheng, S. (2016). Immunogenicity of porcine circovirus type 2 nucleic acid vaccine containing CpG motif for mice. *Virology Journal, 13*, 1–7.

6. Sergeyev, O., & Barinsky, I. (2016). Synthetic peptide vaccines. *Voprosy Virusologii, 61*, 5–8.
7. Ptepte, S. H., Stephenson, R. J., Simerska, P., Groves, P., Aljohani, S., Eskandari, S., Toth, I., & Doolan, D. L. (2016). Systematic evaluation of self-adjuvating lipopeptide nano-vaccine platforms for the induction of potent CD8+ T cell responses. *Nanomedicine, 11*, 137–152.
8. Vijaya, B. J., Sean, M. G., & Aliasger, K. S. (2013). Biodegradable particles as vaccine antigen delivery systems for stimulating cellular immune responses. *Human Vaccines & Immunotherapy, 9*, 2584–2590.
9. Di, G. S., Quattrocchi, V., & Zamorano, P. (2015). Use of adjuvants to enhance the immune response induced by a DNA vaccine against bovine herpesvirus-1. *Viral Immunology, 28*, 343–346.
10. Liu, F., Sun, X. J., Fairman, J., Lewis, D. B., Katz, J. M., Levine, M., Tumpey, T. M., & Lu, X. H. (2016). A cationic liposome-DNA complexes adjuvant (JVRS-100) enhances the immunogenicity and cross-protective efficacy of pre-pandemic influenza A (H5N1) vaccine in ferrets. *Virology, 492*, 197–205.
11. Manoj, S., & Babiuk, L. A. (2004). Approaches to enhance the efficacy of DNA vaccines. *Critical Reviews in Clinical Laboratory Sciences, 41*, 1–39.
12. Xu, J. H., Dai, W. J., Wang, Z. M., Chen, B., Li, Z. M., & Fan, X. Y. (2011). Intranasal vaccination with chitosan-DNA nanoparticles expressing pneumococcal surface antigen A protects mice against nasopharyngeal colonization by *Streptococcus pneumoniae*. *Clinical and Vaccine Immunology, 18*, 75–81.
13. Zhu, Q., Talton, J., Zhang, G., et al. (2012). Large intestine-targeted, nanoparticle releasing oral vaccine to control genitorectal viral infection. *Nature Medicine, 18*, 1291–1296.
14. Belyakov, I. M., Hel, Z., Kelsall, B., et al. (2001). Mucosal AIDS vaccine reduces disease and viral load in gut reservoir and blood after mucosal infection of macaques. *Nature Medicine, 7*, 1320–1326.
15. Uhrich, K. E., Cannizzaro, S. M., Langer, R. S., & Shakesheff, K. M. (1999). Polymeric systems for controlled drug release. *Chemical Reviews, 99*, 3181–3198.
16. Nair, L. S., & Laurencin, C. T. (2007). Biodegradable polymers as biomaterials. *Progress in Polymer Science, 32*, 762–798.
17. Anderson, J. M., & Shive, M. S. (1997). Biodegradation and biocompatibility of PLA and PLGA microspheres. *Advanced Drug Delivery Reviews, 28*, 5–24.
18. Chattopadhyay, S., Chen, J. Y., Chen, H. W., & Hu, C. M. J. (2017). Nanoparticle vaccines adopting virus-like features for enhanced immune potentiation. *Nano Theragnostic, 1*, 244–260.
19. Andeira, A. C., de Oliveira Matos, A., Evangelista, B. S., da Silva, S. M., Nagib, P. R. A., de Moraes Crespo, A., & Amaral, A. C. (2019). Is it possible to track intracellular chitosan nanoparticles using magnetic nanoparticles as contrast agent? *Bioorganic & Medicinal Chemistry, 27*, 2637–2643.
20. Hu, Q., Bae, M., Fleming, E., Lee, J., & Luo, Y. (2019). Biocompatible polymeric nanoparticles with exceptional gastrointestinal stability as oral delivery vehicles for lipophilic bioactive. *Food Hydrocolloids, 89*, 386–395.
21. Jin, Z., Li, W., Cao, H. W., Zhang, X., Chen, G., Wu, H., Guo, C., Zhang, Y., Kang, H., Wang, Y. F., & Zhao, K. (2013). Antimicrobial activity and cytotoxicity of

N-2-HACC and characterization of nanoparticles with N-2-HACC and CMC as a vaccine carrier. *Chemical Engineering Journal, 221*, 331–341.
22. Jin, Z., Li, D., Dai, C. X., Cheng, G. G., Wang, X. H., & Zhao, K. (2017). Response of live Newcastle disease virus encapsulated in N-2-hydroxypropyl dimethyl ethyl ammonium chloride chitosan nanoparticles. *Carbohydrate Polymers, 171*, 267–280.
23. Dai, C. X., Kang, H., Yang, W. Q., Sun, J. Y., Liu, C. L., Cheng, G. G., Rong, G. Y., Wang, X. H., Wang, X., Jin, Z., & Zhao, K. (2015). O-2′-Hydroxypropyl trimethyl ammonium chloride chitosan nanoparticles for the delivery of live Newcastle disease vaccine. *Carbohydrate Polymers, 130*, 280–289.
24. Wickline, S. A., Neubauer, A. M., Winter, P. M., Caruthers, S. D., & Lanza, G. M. (2007). Molecular imaging and therapy of atherosclerosis with targeted nanoparticles. *Journal of Magnetic Resonance Imaging, 25*, 667–680.
25. Akagi, T., & Akashi, M. (2006). Development of polymeric nanoparticles-based vaccine. *Nihon Rinsho, 64*, 279–285.
26. Mundargi, R. C., Babu, V. R., Rangaswamy, V., Patel, P., & Aminabhavi, T. M. (2008). Nano/microtechnologies for delivering macromolecular therapeutics using poly(D,L-lactide-co-glycolide) and its derivatives. *Journal of Controlled Release, 125*, 193–209.
27. Zhao, X., Yin, L. C., Ding, J. Y., Tang, C., Gu, S. H., Yin, C. H., & Mao, Y. M. (2010). Thiolate trimethyl chitosan nanocomplexes as gene carriers with high *in vitro* and *in vivo* transfection efficiency. *Journal of Controlled Release, 144*, 46–54.
28. Li, X., Deng, X., Yuan, M., Xiong, C., Huang, Z., Zhang, Y., & Jia, W. (2000). *In vitro* degradation and release profiles of poly-DL-lactide-poly (ethylene glycol) microspheres with entrapped proteins. *Journal of Applied Polymer Science, 78*, 140–148.
29. Danhier, F., Ansorena, E., Silva, J. M., Coco, R., Le Breton, A., & Préat, V. (2012). PLGA-based nanoparticles: An overview of biomedical applications. *Journal of Controlled Release, 161*, 505–522.
30. Namvar, A., Bolhassani, A., Khairkhah, N., & Motevalli, F. (2015). Physic-chemical properties of polymers: An important system to overcome the cell barriers in gene transfection. *Biopolymers, 103*, 363–375.
31. Ibrahim, K., Khalid, S., & Idrees, K. (2017). Nanoparticles: Properties, applications and toxicities. *Arabian Journal of Chemistry, 5*, 1878–5352.
32. Talmadge, J. E. (1993). The pharmaceutics and delivery of therapeutic polypeptides and proteins. *Advanced Drug Delivery Reviews, 10*, 247–299.
33. George, D. M., Alexandru, M. G., Cornelia, B., & Ludovic, E. B. (2016). Polymeric protective agents for nanoparticles in drug delivery and targeting. *International Journal of Pharmaceutics, 510*, 419–429.
34. Daniel, P., Nazende, G. T., & Marc, S. (2017). Influence of different stabilizers on the encapsulation of desmopressin acetate into PLGA nanoparticles. *European Journal of Pharmaceutics and Biopharmaceutics, 118*, 48–55.
35. Ribeiro, S., Hussain, N., & Florence, A. T. (2005). Release of DNA from dendriplexes encapsulated in PLGA nanoparticles. *International Journal of Pharmaceutics, 298*, 354–360.
36. Kim, I. S., Lee, S. K., Park, Y. M., Lee, Y. B., Shin, S. C., Lee, K. C., & Oh, I. J. (2005). Physicochemical characterization of poly(L-lactic acid) and

poly(D,L-lactide-co-glycolide) nanoparticles with polyethyleneimine as gene delivery carrier. *International Journal of Pharmaceutics, 298*, 255–262.
37. Ishii, T., Okahata, Y., & Sato, T. (2001). Mechanism of cell transfection with plasmid/ chitosan complexes. *Biochemical et Biophysical Acta, 1514*, 51–64.
38. Mao, S., Sun, W., & Kissel, T. (2010). Chitosan-based formulations for delivery of DNA and siRNA. *Advanced Drug Delivery Reviews, 62*, 12–27.
39. Zhao, K., Han, J. Y., Zhang, Y., Wei, L., Yu, S., Wang, X. H., Jin, Z., & Wang, Y. F. (2018). Enhancing mucosal immune response of Newcastle disease virus DNA vaccine using N-2-hydroxypropyl trimethyl ammonium chloride chitosan and N,O-carboxymethyl chitosan nanoparticles as a delivery carrier. *Molecular Pharmaceutics, 15*, 226–237.
40. Yu, S., Xu, X., Feng, J., Liu, M., & Hu, K. (2019). Chitosan and chitosan coating nanoparticles for the treatment of brain disease. *International Journal of Pharmaceutics, 560*, 282–293.
41. Bertocchi, B., Carpentier, R., & Betbeder, D. (2017). Nasal nano vaccines. *International Journal of Pharmaceutics, 530*, 128–138.
42. Huang, T., Song, X. H., Jing, J., Zhao, K. L., Shen, Y. M., Zhang, X. Y., & Yue, B. (2018). Chitosan-DNA nanoparticles enhanced the immunogenicity of multivalent DNA vaccination on mice against *Trueperella pyogenes* infection. *Journal of Nanobiotechnology, 16*, 1477–3155.
43. Kumar, M., Behera, A. K., Lockey, R. F., Zhang, J., Bhullar, G., de la Cruz, C. P., Chen, L. C., Leong, K. W., Huang, S. K., & Mohapatra, S. S. (2002). Intranasal gene transfer by chitosan-DNA nanospheres protects BALB/c mice against acute respiratory syncytial virus infection. *Human Gene Therapy, 13*, 1415–1425.
44. Kici, S., Ilgin, P., Butun, S., & Sahiner, N. (2011). Hyaluronic acid hydrogel particles with tunable charges as potential drug delivery devices. *Carbohydrate Polymers, 84*, 1306–1313.
45. Singh, M., Briones, M., & O'Hagan, D. T. (2001). A novel bio adhesive intranasal delivery system for inactivated influenza vaccines. *Journal of Controlled Release, 70*, 267–276.
46. Kamaly, N., Yameen, B., Wu, J., & Farokhzad, O. C. (2016). Degradable controlled-release polymers and polymeric nanoparticles: Mechanisms of controlling drug release. *Chemical Reviews, 116*, 2602–2663.
47. Kupper, S., Kłosowska-Chomiczewska, I., & Szumała, P. (2017). Collagen and hyaluronic acid hydrogel in water-in-oil microemulsion delivery systems. *Carbohydrate Polymers, 175*, 347–354.
48. Oh, E. J., Park, K., Kim, K. S., Kim, J., Yang, J. A., Kong, J. H., et al. (2010). Target-specific and long-acting delivery of protein, peptide, and nucleotide therapeutics using hyaluronic acid derivatives. *Journal of Controlled Release, 141*, 2–12.
49. Verheul, R. J., Slütter, B., Bal, S. M., Bouwstra, J. A., Jiskoot, W., & Hennink, W. E. (2011). Covalently stabilized trimethyl chitosan–hyaluronic acid nanoparticles for nasal and intradermal vaccination. *Journal of Controlled Release, 156*, 46–52.
50. Mohamed, E., Jie, H., & Mohan, E. (2015). Bioinspired preparation of alginate nanoparticles using microbubble bursting. *Materials Science and Engineering: C, 46*, 132–139.

51. Borges, O., Silva, M., de Sousa, A., Borchard, G., Junginger, H. E., & Cordeiro-da-Silva, A. (2008). Alginate-coated chitosan nanoparticles are an effective subcutaneous adjuvant for hepatitis B surface antigen. *International Immunology, 8*, 1773–1780.
52. Kawada, J., Wada, H., Isobe, M., Gnjatic, S., Nishikawa, H., Jungbluth, A. A., et al. (2012). Heteroclitic serological response in esophageal and prostate cancer patients after NY-ESO-1 protein vaccination. *International Journal of Cancer, 130*, 584–592.
53. Zhang, L., Li, G., Gao, M., Liu, X., Ji, B., Hua, R., Zhou, Y., & Yang, Y. (2016). RGD-peptide conjugated inulin-ibuprofen nanoparticles for targeted delivery of epirubicin. *Colloids and Surfaces B: Bio Interfaces, 144*, 81–89.
54. Gupta, N., Jangid, A. K., & Pooja, D., & Kulhari, H. (2019). Inulin: A novel and stretchy polysaccharide tool for biomedical and nutritional applications. *International Journal of Biological Macromolecules, 132*, 852–863.
55. Petrovsky, N., & Cooper, P. D. (2011). Carbohydrate-based immune adjuvants. *Expert Review of Vaccines, 10*, 523–537.
56. Jiménez-Sánchez, M., Pérez-Morales, R., Goycoolea, F. M., Praznik, M. M. W., Loeppert, R., Bermúdez-Morales, V., Guadalupe, Z. P., Ayala, M., & Olvera, C. (2019). Self-assembled high molecular weight inulin nanoparticles: Enzymatic synthesis, physicochemical and biological properties. *Carbohydrate Polymers, 215*, 160–169.
57. Zhang, L., Li, Y., Wang, C., Li, G., Zhao, Y., & Yang, Y. (2014). Synthesis of methylprednisolone loaded ibuprofen modified inulin-based nanoparticles and their application for drug delivery. *Materials Science and Engineering: C, 42*, 111–115.
58. Banerjee, A., & Bandopadhyay, R. (2016). Use of dextran nanoparticle: A paradigm shift in bacterial exopolysaccharide-based biomedical applications. *International Journal of Biological Macromolecules, 87*, 295–301.
59. Jain, J. P., Ayen, W. Y., Domb, A. J., & Kumar, N. (2011). Biodegradable polymers in drug delivery. *Biodegradable Polymers in Clinical Use and Clinical Development, 4*, 1–58.
60. George, A., Shah, P. A., & Shrivastav, P. S. (2019). Natural biodegradable polymers-based nano-formulations for drug delivery: A review. *International Journal of Pharmaceutics, 561*, 244–264.
61. Laha, A., Sharma, C. S., & Majumdar, S. J. (2017). Sustained drug release from multilayered sequentially cross-linked electro spun gelatin nanofiber mesh. *Materials Science and Engineering: C, 76*, 782–786.
62. Wang, P., Li, Y., Zhang, C., Feng, F., & Zhang, H. (2020). Sequential electrospinning of multilayer ethyl cellulose/gelatin/ethyl cellulose nanofibrous film for sustained release of curcumin. *Food Chemistry, 308*, 125599.
63. Bajpai, A., & Choubey, J. (2006). *In vitro* release dynamics of an anticancer drug from swellable gelatin nanoparticles. *Journal of Applied Polymer Science, 101*, 2320–2332.
64. Treesuppharat, W., Rojanapanthu, P., Siangsanoh, C., Manuspiya, H., & Ummartyotin, S. (2017). Synthesis and characterization of bacterial cellulose and gelatin-based hydrogel composites for drug-delivery systems. *Biotechnology Reports, 15*, 84–91.
65. Kumar, R., Sahoo, G. C., Pandey, K., Das, V., & Das, P. (2015). Study the effects of PLGA-PEG encapsulated amphotericin B nanoparticle drug delivery system against *Leishmania donovani*. *Drug Delivery, 22*, 383–388.

66. Maria, M., Naveed, A., & Asimur, R. (2017). Recent applications of PLGA-based nanostructures in drug delivery. *Colloids and Surfaces B: Bio Interfaces, 159*, 217–231.
67. Gupta, R. K., Singh, M., & O'Hagan, D. T. (1998). Poly(lactide-co-glycoside) microparticles for the development of single-dose controlled-release vaccines. *Advanced Drug Delivery Reviews, 32*, 225–246.
68. Jaganathan, K. S., & Vyas, S. P. (2006). Strong systemic and mucosal immune responses to surface-modified PLGA microspheres containing recombinant hepatitis B antigen administered intranasally. *Vaccine, 24*, 4201–4211.
69. Vila, A., Sánchez, A., Tobío, M., Calvo, P., & Alonso, M. J. (2002). Design of biodegradable particles for protein delivery. *Journal of Controlled Release, 78*, 15–24.
70. Shweta, S., Ankush, P., Shiv Poojan, K., & Rajat, S. (2016). PLGA-based nanoparticles: A new paradigm in biomedical applications. *Trends in Analytical Chemistry, 80*, 30–40.
71. Zhang, M. M., Hong, Y. H., Chen, W. J., & Wang, C. (2017). Polymers for DNA vaccine delivery. *ACS Biomaterials Science & Engineering, 3*, 108–125.
72. Haas, J., Kumar, M. N. R., Borchard, G., Bakowsky, U., & Lehr, C. M. (2005). Preparation and characterization of chitosan and trimethyl chitosan-modified poly(ε-caprolactone) nanoparticles as DNA carriers. *AAPS PharmSciTech, 6*, E22–E30.
73. Gupta, N. K., Tomar, P., Sharma, V., & Dixit, V. K. (2011). Development and characterization of chitosan-coated poly-ε-caprolactone nanoparticulate system for effective immunization against influenza. *Vaccine, 29*, 9026–9037.
74. Jesus, S., Soares, E., Costa, J., Borchard, G., & Borges, O. (2016). Immune response elicited by an intranasally delivered HBsAg low-dose adsorbed to poly-epsilon-caprolactone-based nanoparticles. *International Journal of Pharmaceutics, 504*, 59–69.
75. Farhadi, M., Haniloo, A., Rostamizadeh, K., & Faghihzadeh, S. (2018). Efficiency of flubendazole-loaded mPEG-PCL nanoparticles: A promising formulation against the protoscoleces and cysts of *Echinococcus granulosus*. *Acta Tropica, 187*, 190–200.
76. Li, M., Rouaud, O., & Poncelet, D. (2008). Microencapsulation by solvent evaporation: State of the art for process engineering approaches. *International Journal of Pharmaceutics, 363*, 26–39.
77. Sharma, R., Agrawal, U., Mody, N., & Vyas, S. P. (2015). Polymer nanotechnology-based approaches in mucosal vaccine delivery: Challenges and opportunities. *Biotechnology Advances, 33*, 64–79.
78. Petersen, L. K., Ramer-Tait, A. E., Broderick, S. R., Kong, C. S., Ulery, B. D., Rajan, K., Wannemuehler, M. J., & Narasimhan, B. (2011). Activation of innate immune responses in a pathogen-mimicking manner by amphiphilic polyanhydride nanoparticle adjuvants. *Biomaterials, 32*, 6815–6822.
79. Huang, D., & Wu, D. C. (2018). Biodegradable dendrimers for drug delivery. *Materials Science and Engineering: C, 90*, 713–727.
80. Li, J., Liang, H. M., Liu, J., & Wang, Z. Y. (2018). Poly(amidoamine) (PAMAM) dendrimer-mediated delivery of drug and pDNA/siRNA for cancer therapy. *International Journal of Pharmaceutics, 546*, 215–225.

81. Alemzadeh, E., Dehshahri, A., Izadpanah, K., & Ahmadi, F. (2018). Plant virus nanoparticles: Novel and robust nanocarriers for drug delivery and imaging. *Colloids and Surfaces B: Bio Interfaces, 167*, 20–27.
82. Lancelot, A., Gonzalez-Pastor, R., Claveria-Gimeno, R., Romero, P., Abian, O., & Martin-Duque, P. (2018). Cationic poly(ester amide) dendrimers: Alluring materials for biomedical applications. *Journal of Materials Chemistry B, 6*, 3956–3968.
83. de Sousa, I. P., & Bernkop-Schnürch, A. (2014). Pre-systemic metabolism of orally administered drugs and strategies to overcome it. *Journal of Controlled Release, 192*, 301–309.
84. Bernkop-Schnürch, A., & Krajicek, M. E. (1998). Mucoadhesive polymers as platforms for peroral peptide delivery and absorption: Synthesis and evaluation of different chitosan–EDTA conjugates. *Journal of Controlled Release, 50*, 215–223.
85. Suchaoin, W., & Bernkop-Schnürch, A. J. (2017). Nanocarriers protecting toward an intestinal pre-uptake metabolism. *Nanomedicine, 12*, 255–269.
86. Kagnoff, M. (1993). Immunology of the intestinal tract. *Gastroenterology, 105*, 1275.
87. Langkamp-Henken, B., Glezer, J. A., & Kudsk, K. A. (1992). Immunologic structure and function of the gastrointestinal tract. *Nutrition in Clinical Practice, 7*, 100–108.
88. Unanue, E. R., & Allen, P. M. (1987). The basis for the immunoregulatory role of macrophages and other accessory cells. *Journal of Immunology, 236*, 551–557.
89. Owen, R. L. (1977). Sequential uptake of horseradish peroxidase by lymphoid follicle epithelium of Peyer's patches in the normal unobstructed mouse intestine: An ultrastructural study. *Gastroenterology, 72*, 440.
90. Wolf, J. L., & Bye, W. A. (1984). The membranous epithelial (M) cell and the mucosal immune system. *Annual Review of Medicine, 35*, 95–112.
91. O'Hagan, D. T. (1994). Microparticles as oral vaccines. In D. T. O'Hagan (Ed.), *Novel Delivery System for Oral Vaccines* (pp. 175–205). Boca Raton, FL: CRC Press.
92. Russel, G. J., & Walker, W. A. (1990). Role of intestinal barriers and antigen uptake. In S. R. Targan & F. Shanahan (Eds.), *Immunology and Immunopathology of the Liver and Gastrointestinal Tract* (pp. 15–31). New York: Igaku-Shoin.
93. Neutra, M. R., Frey, A., & Kraehenbuhl, J. P. (1996). Epithelial M cells: Gateways for mucosal infection and immunization. *Cell, 86*, 345–348.
94. Holmgren, J., & Czerkinsky, C. (2005). Mucosal immunity and vaccines. *Nature Medicine, 11*(Suppl.), S45–S53.
95. Brayden, D. J., Jepson, M. A., & Baird, A. W. (2005). Keynote review: Intestinal Peyer's patch M cells and oral vaccine targeting. *Drug Discovery Today, 10*, 1145–1157.
96. Qi, J., Zhuang, J., Lv, Y., Lu, Y., & Wu, W. (2018). Exploiting or overcoming the dome trap for enhanced oral immunization and drug delivery. *Journal of Controlled Release, 275*, 92–106.
97. Azizi, A., Kumar, A., Diaz-Mitoma, F., & Mestecky, J. (2010). Enhancing oral vaccine potency by targeting intestinal M cells. *PLoS Pathogens, 6*, e1001147.
98. Devriendt, B., De Geest, B. G., Goddeeris, B. M., & Cox, E. (2012). Crossing the barrier: Targeting epithelial receptors for enhanced oral vaccine delivery. *Journal of Controlled Release, 160*, 431–439.

99. Macpherson, A. J., Geuking, M. B., & McCoy, K. D. (2005). Immune responses that adapt the intestinal mucosa to commensal intestinal bacteria. *Immunology, 115*, 153–162.
100. Jiang, H. L., Park, I. K., Shin, N. R., Yoo, H. S., Akaike, T., & Cho, C. S. (2004). Controlled release of *Bordetella bronchiseptica* dermonecrotoxin (BBD) vaccine from BBD-loaded chitosan microspheres *in vitro*. *Archives of Pharmacal Research, 27*, 346–350.
101. Hejazi, R., & Amiji, M. (2002). Stomach-specific anti-*H. pylori* therapy. I: Preparation and characterization of tetracycline-loaded chitosan microspheres. *International Journal of Pharmaceutics, 235*, 87–94.
102. Jin, Z., Gao, S., Cui, X., Sun, D., & Zhao, K. (2019). Adjuvants and delivery systems based on polymeric nanoparticles for mucosal vaccines. *International Journal of Pharmaceutics, 572*, 118731.
103. Moran, H. B., Turley, J. L., Andersson, M., & Lavelle, E. C. (2018). Immunomodulatory properties of chitosan polymers. *Biomaterials, 184*, 1–9.
104. Kumar, V., Dandapat, S., Kumar, A., & Kumar, N. (2014). Preparation and characterization of chitosan nanoparticles "alternatively, carrying potential" for cellular and humoral immune responses. *Advances in Animal and Veterinary Sciences, 2*, 414–417.
105. Gao, W. W., Chen, Y. J., Zhang, Y., Zhang, Q. Z., & Zhang, L. F. (2018). Nanoparticle-based local antimicrobial drug delivery. *Advanced Drug Delivery Reviews, 127*, 46–57.
106. Gutjahr, A., Philip, C., Coolen, A. L., Monge, C., Boisgard, A. S., Paul, S., & Verrier, B. (2016). Biodegradable polymeric nanoparticles-based vaccine adjuvants for lymph nodes targeting. *Vaccine, 4*, 1–16.
107. Zhao, L., Seth, A., Wibowo, N., Zhao, C. X., Mitter, N., Yu, C. Z., & Middelberg, A. P. J. (2014). Nanoparticle vaccines. *Vaccine, 32*, 327–337.

Index

S

T

U

V